**BOOKCELLAR
FREEBIE**

Evidence-Based Medicine
and the Search for a
Science of Clinical Care

Evidence-Based Medicine and the Search for a Science of Clinical Care

Jeanne Daly

University of California Press
BERKELEY / LOS ANGELES / LONDON

Milbank Memorial Fund
NEW YORK

University of California Press
Berkeley and Los Angeles, California

University of California Press, Ltd.
London, England

© 2005 by The Regents of the University of California

Library of Congress Cataloging-in-Publication Data

Daly, Jeanne.
 Evidence-based medicine and the search for a science of clinical care / Jeanne Daly.
   p. ; cm. — (California/Milbank books on health and the public ; 12)
   Includes bibliographical references and index.
   ISBN 0-520-24316-1 (cloth : alk. paper)
   1. Evidence-based medicine.
[DNLM: 1. Evidence-Based Medicine. 2. Biomedical Research. WB 102 D153e 2005] I. Title. II. Series.
R723.7.D356   2005
616 — dc22   2004019930

Manufactured in the United States of America

13 12 11 10 09 08 07 06 05
10 9 8 7 6 5 4 3 2 1

The paper used in this publication meets the minimum requirements of ANSI/NISO Z39.48–1992 (R 1997) (*Permanence of Paper*).

Contents

Foreword

The Milbank Memorial Fund is an endowed operating foundation that engages in nonpartisan analysis, study, research, and communication of significant issues in health policy. Since 1905 the Fund has worked to improve and maintain health by encouraging persons who make and implement health policy to use the best available evidence. The Fund makes available the results of its work in meetings with decision makers and publishes reports, books, and the *Milbank Quarterly,* a multidisciplinary journal of population health and health policy.

Evidence-Based Medicine and the Search for a Science of Clinical Care is the twelfth of the California/Milbank Books on Health and the Public. The publishing partnership between the Fund and the press seeks to encourage the synthesis and communication of findings from research that could contribute to more effective health policy.

Jeanne Daly has written the first comprehensive history of research on the effectiveness of health care interventions in populations that has in recent years become associated with the phrase "evidence-based medicine." Those who conduct this research, and the increasing number of health professionals who apply its findings to clinical practice, use a particular, and sometimes controversial, definition of evidence.

Evidence is, for them, the antonym of authority derived from experience and opinion. Proponents of evidence-based medicine insist that clinicians should integrate the best available evidence with their experience and their understanding of patients' values. Most of them also want to persuade clinicians, policy makers, and patients to accord the highest value to evidence from interventions that is derived from statistical inferences about data collected and assessed in ways that maximize the elimination of bias. Daly's history makes plain why this definition of evidence has enthusiasts as well as detractors among researchers, clinicians, managers, and policy makers.

Daly conducted exhaustive research in several countries. She derives compelling insights, and many good stories, from her interviews with central figures in the research associated with evidence-based medicine. Wherever possible, she supports what she learned in these interviews with evidence from archival sources and wide reading in the pertinent scientific literature.

Daniel M. Fox
President

Samuel L. Milbank
Chairman

By Way of Background

This book has gone through an extensive reviewing process set in place by Daniel Fox, president of the Milbank Memorial Fund, and Lynne Withey, director of the University of California Press. This process gave me extensive guidance from excellent reviewers, with particularly useful comments coming from those working in areas outside my own disciplinary scope. Some of the reviewers expressed interest in why a sociologist should dedicate years to analyzing evidence-based medicine and its precursors. What were my qualifications for writing the book? This prologue provides a brief, if circuitous, explanation.

I was born on a farm in South Africa that bordered on the Limpopo River. I grew up with few of the technological tools for life that I now take for granted: electricity, a flush toilet, medical care. When I went to university, my aim was to devote myself to science and technology: I enrolled to study nuclear physics as the most direct route to the dream of "power too cheap to meter." But this was South Africa in the 1960s. The University of Natal, where I studied, was in the grip of political unrest, and reluctantly I was drawn into an understanding that the political reality of the lives of black South Africans was far more important than my own lack of modern conveniences. I loved the science laboratory, but real life was outside in the community.

Disillusioned with the apparently entrenched power of the Nationalist government, I emigrated to Australia. By now my aims were political. When I enrolled to study for a master's degree in environmental science,

I wanted to analyze the occupational risk of exposure to ionizing radiation in the uranium mines in Namibia. To my surprise I found that my hard-won analytical skills were of little use. In the debates of the International Commission on Radiological Protection, the science of radiation was far less relevant than how the commission reached agreement about what counts as an acceptable hazard — by interpreting the science in terms of value judgments about the risks and benefits involved. I needed sociology for this analysis.

After retraining in sociology, I conducted a study of the patient's experience of diagnostic technology. It became clear that patients were unconcerned about risk or benefits and more concerned about the process of testing. Analyzing that problem required that I go through another painful mutation, that of becoming a qualitative researcher. While I was developing the methods for this qualitative study, some of the cardiologists with whom I was working dismissed my method: they saw it as impressionistic and intuitive. I was surprised. Given my experience of the laboratory, their own processes of decision making in clinical practice seemed a far cry from rigorous science.

In the 1980s, when I discovered the work that McMaster University was doing, I was immediately enchanted. This was the answer to the problem that increasingly concerned me: did the tangible benefits gained by patients from the diagnostic process really balance out the potential harm done by raising uncertainty about the normality of their hearts? It was at this stage that I decided to start interviewing people engaged in the new discipline of clinical epidemiology to chronicle its development.

The people I interviewed showed remarkable generosity in giving time to what was initially an exploratory study. Only a proportion of the interviews are reported here, but all the interviews contributed to my understanding of the topic. I was, and remain, most grateful for the insights these individuals shared with me; my admiration for their work is undimmed. However, as a critical sociologist, I cannot resist analyzing both the positive and the negative aspects of any enterprise, with the aim of possibly changing it for the better. I hope those I interviewed will forgive any suggestions that turn out to be based on inappropriate analysis or a lack of understanding.

I carried out the first round of interviews with funding from the Public Health Research and Development Committee of the Australian National Health and Medical Research Council. These interviews were conducted jointly with Dr. Ian McDonald, a cardiologist from Saint Vincent's Hospital, Melbourne. He had a parallel interest in technology assessment and in developing a secure foundation for the skills involved in the art of medicine, and he provided invaluable insight into how clinical processes interlock to produce good patient management. Without his encouragement, I might well have turned to more accessible research topics; but finally, any misinterpretations of which I am guilty are my own.

My first manuscript on the subject concentrated on clinical epidemiology and did not capture the attention of the publishers to whom I submitted it. The manuscript would have died a quiet death were it not for the intervention of Daniel Fox. He saw the need for a book analyzing the new phenomenon of evidence-based medicine. Extending my manuscript to address this topic seemed a simple task. It was not. After the Milbank Memorial Fund provided funds for another round of interviews, a painstaking task of editing commenced. There have been times when Dan's exacting demands seemed impossible to meet, but he has always been right about the directions he recommended. In the area of policy analysis, I am sure I could have done better, but this is an academic area about which I am singularly ignorant. While Dan's unequivocal support and incisive criticism have produced a much improved manuscript, I am solely responsible for its failings.

Note on Method

This book is largely based on personal interviews with people selected as key informants on the development of evidence-based medicine. I chose my interviewees after noting repeated references to their work in the published literature and after discussion with study participants as the study progressed. I also interviewed authors of the major textbooks on clinical epidemiology and related initiatives. In addition, as the need arose to address specific aspects of the area, I selected participants to fill these gaps, such as in the section addressing key criticisms of evidence-based medicine.

Inevitably there are omissions. There will be people whose contributions I have overlooked or failed to appreciate. In some cases, I found that important contributors had died and, unlike in the case of Archie Cochrane, there was insufficient archival or published material for me to construct an account of their contributions. Furthermore, I have selectively focused on contributors from the United States, Canada, and Europe, with the one exception being contributors from South Africa. I have omitted a number of other interviews that focused on information not immediately relevant to this focus.

My interviews were unstructured, and they started with open-ended questions: "What drew you to this field? What can you tell me about the development of this area? What was your role?" Interviews lasted anywhere from one hour to several hours spread across a number of days. I extracted from the interviews those passages that epitomized the views of each participant. All participants were offered the opportunity to review the sections of the manuscript that dealt with their contributions and to correct the account — to comment on the interpretation and indicate what they saw as their most important publications in the field.

I conducted the first interview in 1989. I followed with a round of interviews in 1991, a smaller round in 1997, and the last round in 2000, with a few interviews conducted more recently. Some participants were interviewed several times. All participants were invited to update their accounts when the manuscript was complete to indicate if they still held the views reported. In very few cases have views changed markedly over time. Where views have undergone an important shift, I refer to "early" and "late" views and give the dates of the interviews.

The Problem with Interviews

The use of qualitative methods has clear advantages: the methods are adaptable and can be used in innovative ways to address specific problems (see Daly et al. 1997, chap. 11). In this case, the challenge was to analyze the views of people too well known to be anonymous. There are also clear disadvantages to qualitative methods, especially in this case, where I rely primarily on interview data. Some of the material raised difficult issues of interpretation. With some leading participants, there was marked similarity among various interviews, even those conducted by other researchers. In some cases the same anecdotes were repeated almost word for word. This raises the question of whether what was recorded is a formulated and sanitized version of what happened. This is especially true in the tendency to promote a Great Man theory of the changes that occurred. My view is that the stories I recorded represent the way that the people interviewed want to see themselves portrayed, especially in describing the roles they played in the development of this field. I have quoted the interviews in sufficient detail for readers to be able to make their own judgments about the stories told, the great people who told them, and how Great the Man actually was. My own views are recorded at the start of chapter 4.

This brings me to claims made by participants about key events and factual details of their own work. I made every attempt to corroborate these statements from other sources, but where I was unable to do so, I reported the event as the view of one particular participant. In some cases, I found contradictory accounts of the same event. Where I was unable to resolve these contradictions, I did not report the event.

Finally, however, the disadvantages in relying on interviews are balanced by what was, for me, a primary consideration: almost all the study participants are extremely well published, and the text gives references to major works that supplement the interview accounts. Why then did I not rely on peer-reviewed publications as the primary source for my account? Certainly this would have been possible, but the material is often technical and inaccessible to the average reader. In contrast, the personal accounts supply vivid personal details that bring the work to life. Above all, the personal interviews offer a unique account of participants' personal commitment to the field, of what drew them to commit themselves to a field less promising than a career in a clinical specialty or the biomedical laboratory.

Other Sources

The publications of each participant served as my second resource for the book. These publications amplified points raised in interviews, as well as corroborated the biographies. In rare cases where the published literature appeared to contradict what was said in the interview, I asked participants to explain the differences.

My third resource was archival material, which was particularly useful in the case of Archie Cochrane, who had died before interviews started. Many of the interview participants have been interviewed by other researchers, and these interviews were available in archives for the purposes of comparison. I should note here that archival material in this field is scarce, still under embargo because of time rules, or not yet catalogued. This would be a good time to collect available material as a resource for future researchers.

Lastly, there is a large and intimidating literature from the various disciplines involved in analyzing the history and politics of medicine. My aim has been to make sufficient references to these sources so that an interested reader can make initial contact with this literature. A more detailed account runs the risk of making parts of this text inaccessible to readers not accustomed to the careful detail and meticulous cross-referencing provided by these disciplines.

CHAPTER I

Introduction

Evidence, Science, and Certainty

In the 1970s, attention focused on the central clinical task of medical care: patient management. At this time, there was no generally accepted formal way of ensuring a consciously scientific, critical approach to clinical decision making. Biomedical knowledge underpinned medical practice, but biomedicine did not address the application of this knowledge in actual clinical practice. Questions were being asked about the validity of using traditional clinical authority as the basis for clinical decision making, and there were no grounds for appeal except by reference to the very authority that was being questioned. One response was to make clinical care more scientific by developing a new clinical science, additional to the science of biomedicine. This would provide clinicians with a secure foundation for their clinical task.

Evidence-based medicine produced scientific evidence of a critically important aspect of patient care, its interventions. It generated scientific studies of what worked and what did not work in clinical practice itself. It equipped clinicians with scientific methods for critically assessing the literature to determine the extent to which published studies, and reviews of similar studies in a field, applied to a specific patient. Instead of having to face the dishearteningly subjective task of basing their decisions on "intuitions we could not explain" (Sackett et al. 1991, p. ix), clinicians had available to them a science that generated objective knowledge of effective interventions based, where possible, on the results of unbiased experiments. Clinicians could make decisions on the basis of the best available evidence or at least be aware of the strength of the evidence for a particular decision.

Evidence-based medicine emphasizes scientific evidence, rather than the views held by eminent practitioners, as the basis for clinical practice. It provides clinicians with greater certainty in choosing between competing interventions when deciding how to care for a patient. While evidence-based medicine would seem to be a self-evident good, it has been the subject of fierce criticism. It has been accused of being authoritarian, of privileging a narrow definition of evidence, and of having serious limitations in its capacity to answer clinical questions (Feinstein and Horwitz 1997). It stands accused of, among other things, denigrating clinical experience (Benech et al. 1996) and aligning itself with managed care, a party to coercion, control, and covert rationing (Hunter 1996; Frankford 1994).

Given these criticisms, it is worth balancing admiration for the achievements of evidence-based medicine with a more critical stance. My first aim in this book is to demonstrate that evidence-based medicine has increased knowledge of which clinical interventions actually work. Evidence-based medicine has provided improved tools for clinical decision making. This contribution is, however, constrained by a primary focus on the technical aspects of clinical care, its interventions.

What evidence-based medicine does not resolve are those problems that fall outside the scope of either biomedicine or evidence-based medicine. The greater conceptual hurdle is to generate a science appropriate for the whole of clinical practice, in all its complexity, including the social and political contexts of patients and the health care system. A secondary aim of this book is, therefore, to evaluate the performance of evidence-based medicine against this broader agenda, identify limitations, and suggest future developments.

The remainder of this chapter charts the two major formats of evidence-based medicine. I then turn to the central problem that precipitated these changes — uncertainty about decision making in clinical care — and to issues of science that underlie the directions taken. The following chapters deal with evidence-based medicine through the eyes of key participants in its development. My discussion begins with Canada and the United States and the intellectual traditions that helped to shape clinical epidemiology as an activity for clinician-researchers (chapter 2) and then moves on to a detailed analysis of the major center for practice of evidence-based medicine at McMaster University in Hamilton, Canada. This is where evidence-based medicine was first formally conceptualized (chapters

3 and 4). I conclude this theme with the criticisms that colleagues have directed at this Canadian version of evidence-based medicine (chapter 5). I then turn to a different format for evidence-based medicine, that of the Cochrane Collaboration, a network for identifying and synthesizing evidence for decision making. In the United Kingdom the intellectual inspiration that underpinned evidence-based medicine was influenced by the commitment of researchers to the National Health Service (chapter 6). This intellectual heritage disseminated to other centers, including centers in Canada and the United States, and led, in time, to the international Cochrane Collaboration (chapter 7). An interesting contrast with Britain, Canada, and the United States is the center committed to evidence-based medicine in South Africa (chapter 8). The chapter addresses the contribution of evidence-based medicine to a less industrialized country, one with a seriously compromised health system, where issues of political governance are evident and immediate. Chapter 9 returns to critical comment on evidence-based medicine from the perspective of this global initiative, recognizing achievements and limitations. The conclusion returns to the issues raised in the following sections.

Assembling the Evidence

Evidence-based medicine is a coherent scientific approach to clinical decision making. Considerable intellectual effort was involved in generating the new approach. It would be all too easy to ascribe the rise of evidence-based medicine to the persuasive power of a small number of insightful and articulate people who contributed to the rise of evidence-based medicine from the 1970s onward. There seemed to be the need for a practical science of clinical care to help clinicians make more scientific decisions about patient care. These people rose to the challenge, and they helped shape the institutions that emerged.

This book outlines and analyzes the activities of the leaders in the field of evidence-based medicine; there are important stories of individual initiative to be acknowledged. Most of the people who set the changes in motion are still alive. I identified contributors to this initiative through their published work, including the early textbooks. What interested me was learning what drew them to this new field and how they saw its development and their own contributions. I identified other participants through recommendations made during interviews, and I continued to interview contributors from Canada, the United States, Europe, and

South Africa. Interviews were supplemented by archival research, and this was especially important when key figures had died. By means of a close reading of published primary sources, particularly the relevant research literature, I corroborated and contextualized individual accounts (see the Note on Method for more details).

But circumstances can amplify the effect of individual actions. A web of circumstance links the participants with each other, with medical care in general, with the bodies that fund medical care, and with the medical past. The various chapters of the book aim to locate these personal histories within a larger context that identifies the flow of ideas across time, across disciplines, and across countries. As a result, no pure heroes emerge in the piece.

Two major initiatives stood out as providing a secure foundation for the new approach. One was the development of clinical epidemiology in Canada and the United States. Evidence-based medicine was the form in which clinical epidemiology promoted its findings to practicing clinicians, who were its primary target. The other development was the formation of the Cochrane Collaboration. Started in the United Kingdom, the Cochrane Collaboration is an international network that synthesizes evidence of what works and what does not work in health care. Its target audience includes not only clinicians but also consumers and health policy makers. Both initiatives drew on earlier contributions to the analysis of health care and, in particular, drew on the methods developed at earlier times. The two strands of development intertwined in the 1990s, brought together by a shared commitment to the synthesizing of scientific studies of clinical care. This synthesis provided not only the basis for a more critical scientific approach to care but also a foundation for funding decisions made by health policy makers. Despite the similarities in the two main approaches, there are important differences.

Two Approaches to Evidence-Based Medicine

Clinical epidemiology made its appearance in medical schools especially in Canada and the United States in the late 1960s. Focused on the application of quantitative methods to the empirical study of clinical practice, clinical epidemiology represented a new way of thinking about clinical care that its proponents described as representing a paradigm shift (Feinstein 1983). The aim of clinical epidemiology was not to displace biomedicine or clinical skill in patient care but to develop an additional, explicit, and comprehensive science of the way in which biomedical knowledge is implemented at the bedside. It took as its starting point the actual clinical setting, dealing with live patients rather than their biochemistry. It was a two-pronged approach.

In order to focus on the clinical setting, clinical epidemiology drew on the methods of epidemiology and biostatistics to develop systematic ways of ensuring that the best clinical data are collected and accurately interpreted, leading to well-justified treatment or management plans. So, for example, Sackett and colleagues (1985) showed that management decisions do not follow in an uncomplicated way from diagnostic data. Few diagnostic tests identify the presence of disease directly. What clinicians need to identify is the cutoff point above which patients are seen as likely to have the disease and below which patients are seen as unlikely to be diseased. This cutoff point determines the capacity of the test to detect disease when the disease is present (its sensitivity) or to identify correctly the absence of disease (its specificity). If an illness is serious and highly treatable at low cost, then it is reasonable to set a cutoff point to include 99.5 percent of patients who could have the disease, even if some of them are false positive diagnoses. On the other hand, if a disease is serious, with little in the way of treatment, we might want to set a cutoff point that excludes more patients who could have the disease, so that only those with a higher likelihood are diagnosed and treated. Explicit analysis of the assumptions that underlie particular cutoff points allows the clinician to interpret test data accurately when faced with a particular patient. How common the disease is in the population to which a patient belongs (its prevalence) is a further consideration. For example, the probable accuracy of a positive diagnosis of heart disease is higher in an old than a young patient. Such considerations are central in avoiding the pitfalls of preconceptions in clinical practice.

Applying these critical attitudes makes the tasks of clinical practice a more rigorous and self-conscious activity. But if the methods of epidemiology and biostatistics were useful in establishing better procedures for clinical practice, argued researchers at McMaster University, then the rules of evidence derived from these methods would also be useful in critically appraising the medical literature. Evaluating the results of published studies for scientific rigor establishes which studies should influence clinical practice. The same considerations of rigor apply when conducting primary research in clinical care. The research method seen as best able to generate firm scientific evidence of interventions in clinical practice was the randomized controlled trial. In its simplest form, patients are randomly assigned to a group receiving the treatment under investigation and to a control group receiving standard treatment, a placebo or no treatment at all. If the two groups are initially the same, and then are treated in exactly the same way in all other respects, any difference in outcome must be attributable to the treatment.

The next requirement for success was institutionalization of these initiatives. Clinical epidemiology first became a distinct clinical discipline at McMaster University, under David Sackett. The success of clinical epidemiology derives from the twin promises that it would both place clinical care on a firm footing and provide a basis for policy making. The randomized controlled trial was used to study some of the more complex issues related to the administration of health care. Nurse practitioners, for example, were shown to be an effective substitute for primary care physicians in terms of clinical effectiveness and safety, a result even more striking when the lower costs were taken into account (Spitzer et al. 1974). In alliance with health economists, the researchers addressed thorny issues like the high cost of neonatal intensive care for infants with very low birth weights (Boyle et al. 1983). The McMaster University clinical epidemiologists saw these controversial results as useful for health policy. Health economists who joined the Department of Clinical Epidemiology and Biostatistics provided expertise in the assessment of costs involved. The expectation in the department was that health policy makers and governments could draw on these studies to decide how best to spend the health care dollar.

By the early 1990s, randomized controlled trials were providing a solid basis of scientific evidence for clinicians committed to practicing evidence-based medicine, an appealing notion defined by McMaster University's Gordon Guyatt as "the application of scientific method in determining the optimal management of the individual patient" (1991, p. A-16). Evidence-based medicine provided a neat encapsulation of the activities presented as a new paradigm of clinical care (Evidence-Based Medicine Working Group 1992).

Another, parallel initiative of the department was to make evidence-based medicine a practical reality for any clinician. The problem facing clinicians was that trials are usually too complex for the individual clinician to conduct, especially in light of the large sample sizes required. The proliferation of randomized controlled trials in the medical literature created a problem in even keeping up-to-date with the literature in an area. McMaster University simplified the enterprise considerably by collecting evidence from trials conducted from across the world and making them available in a simplified form. In 1991, the American College of Physicians established the *ACP Journal Club* to collect and publish evaluations of new medical evidence soon after it was published in medical journals. In 1995, the journal *Evidence-Based Medicine* was started with the same procedures as the *ACP Journal Club,* but the accumulated evidence was made available on CD-ROM.

Evidence from the growing number of trials in every clinical area could be collected and presented in simplified form, but the bigger challenge was to generate an overview of this evidence, especially when different trials in the same area produced contradictory results. Formerly, the synthesis of evidence from various studies conducted in an area took the form of a narrative review, which could be selective as well as biased by the reviewer's views and affiliation. What was needed next was to collect all the studies done in an area, to exclude any that did not meet quality criteria for excluding bias, and then to conduct a meta-analysis, a statistical method for combining the results of the studies to produce an overall estimate of effectiveness or some other form of systematic review of the evidence. The methods of meta-analysis, developed by social scientists, were already being applied to clinical interventions (Hunt 1999). The Cochrane Collaboration provided an important coordinating role in the systematic review of evidence for clinical interventions.

Iain Chalmers of the United Kingdom met Murray Enkin of Canada at a conference in New York in 1978. Both had trained as obstetricians, and they decided to collaborate in setting up a database for storing the large mass of accumulated obstetric evidence from trials. The aim of their collection was to provide information on effective care in pregnancy and childbirth (Chalmers et al. 1986). Enkin was from Hamilton and was associated with McMaster University but not, at that stage, with the Department of Clinical Epidemiology and Biostatistics. He and Chalmers saw the potential of their data set for a new joint initiative involving not only the McMaster University researchers but also other researchers across the globe. Indeed, if such a database were to be properly comprehensive, it would require a large voluntary workforce collecting evidence of trials, both those published and those still being conducted, which could then be synthesized into a single database with easy electronic access. What they generated was the *Oxford Database of Perinatal Trials.*

From this initiative came the Cochrane Collaboration, an international network of researchers and consumers engaged in the vast task of collating and synthesizing studies (mainly randomized controlled trials) into systematic reviews. The focus of the Collaboration is on health care in general, bringing to each field the same rigor employed in the generation of the *Oxford Database of Perinatal Trials*. The Collaboration has drawn expert participation by researchers in countries around the globe, and the McMaster University researchers are important contributors. The Cochrane Controlled Trials Register provides a database of trials and relies on an international team that hand searches the literature to make the registry more comprehensive and accessible to anyone wanting to conduct a systematic review of an area. In turn, these reviews are published in a database of reviews.

The Cochrane Collaboration drew its inspiration from a number of sources, but the name honors the work of Archibald (Archie) Cochrane. Cochrane developed a passionate interest in the eradication of bias in a series of studies of lung disease in Welsh mining communities (Cochrane et al. 1952). In the process of conducting these studies, Cochrane became convinced that the health services provided to these communities were inadequate, beset as they were by inconsistencies in both diagnosis and treatment. What was required, Cochrane argued, was a research method capable of assessing the achievements of health services in meeting community needs.

Cochrane saw the randomized controlled trial as a prime means of analyzing medical care in the community. He, in turn, drew on the work of the statistician Austin Bradford Hill and the application of the trial design to the post–World War II evaluation of streptomycin treatment for tuberculosis (Medical Research Council 1948). He went on to argue that each clinical specialty should collect and synthesize all trials conducted in its field and then issue regular updates and critical summaries. Cochrane's work predated the developments at McMaster University, but the two developments were independent and different. Cochrane's major commitment was to creating an effective National Health Service in which ineffective procedures would be identified and eradicated. The financial savings could then be used to fund more effective forms of care. McMaster University's major commitment was to the practicing clinician.

Cochrane's emphasis on conducting trials and synthesizing evidence was the inspiration for the Cochrane Collaboration, where, over time, his political commitments have been sidelined. There was a clear overlap between his interests with those of the researchers at McMaster University. Underlying the initiatives of both was the age-old problem of uncertainty in clinical care, made all the more important from the 1960s onward by concerns about rising costs in health care that were not reflected in improvements in health status.

Uncertainty and the Clinical Task

*The clinician is the doctor at the sufferer's bedside, the doctor who
accepts responsibility for the life entrusted to him by the patient,
the doctor who plans the strategy and executes the tactics of
therapeutic care.*

Alvan Feinstein, *Clinical Judgment,* 1967

When people are faced with serious illness, they struggle with uncertainty
about what is wrong and whether anything can be done about it. When
they turn to medicine for help, they expect clinicians to listen attentively
to their problems, to diagnose the illness and then, where possible, to rec-
ommend interventions that will be effective in treating the illness or alle-
viating distress. It helps if patients believe that clinicians are able to make
these judgments with certainty, based on their training in the various sciences that underlie medical care. This is what enables us, as patients, to
accept the intrusion of doctors into our bodies and into our personal lives.

Unfortunately, the certainty of conclusions in clinical care is elusive.
Much of our belief in scientific medicine stems from research done in the
laboratory where experiments are conducted on animals, organs, tissues,
cells, and molecules, all isolated to exclude extraneous factors and studied under controlled conditions. Laboratory medicine, known as biomedicine after the advent of molecular biology in the 1950s, became the
basic science of medicine and dominated medical education. It produced
new forms of diagnosis and the cure of some serious diseases, as well as
the alleviation of illness. In the process, it diverted attention from the
problem of applying biomedical knowledge to the problems of live
patients in the clinic.

The scientific certainty of the narrow, focused science of the laboratory
is experienced as elusive when any new clinician enters the complex
world of the clinical consultation. Despite significant advances in treatment and cure of disease, clinicians make clinical decisions in the midst of
residual uncertainty. They are unsure about the extent to which they are
up-to-date with medical research, but they also know that medical knowledge is constantly evolving, often contradictory, and thus casts doubt on
current practice. When that knowledge has to be applied to patients, no
two patients are the same, nor are their complaints. The abnormalities in
patients' bodies often cannot be displayed but have to be inferred from
patient accounts or from diagnostic tests. There may be doubt about the
best management for a particular patient's problem. Patients may have

preferences or prohibitions that preclude certain interventions. They work in social settings that may contribute to their disease or serve as an impediment to recovery. Giving the patient's problem a disease label can, in itself, have social and economic and legal repercussions. In order for new clinicians to deal with such problems, they have traditionally been inducted into the art of medicine.

The art of medicine is the traditional medical response to uncertainty. It comprises a knowledge base derived from the clinician's own individual clinical experience interpreted in the light of the collective experience of the profession, learned through apprenticeship to eminent practitioners, usually in technically sophisticated teaching hospitals. Young physicians are trained to observe, gather information from patients and tests, and make judgments about prognosis and the extent to which a particular procedure is suitable for a specific patient. When cure fails, they are trained to provide comfort and care. Clinical skill rests on the authority of senior clinicians, and it reduces but cannot finally resolve uncertainty (Fox 1979). So clinicians have to learn to act with certainty in the midst of imperfect information, making black-and-white decisions when the field is gray, committing themselves to procedures that may carry some risk when they judge the risk to outweigh the benefits. Clinical socialization into firm decision making in the midst of uncertainty is seen as a professional prerequisite of benefit to the patient.

The art of medicine has to be flexible and responsive to the individual patient's problem. It is difficult to encapsulate the art of medicine in defined procedures that can be tested and shown to be effective in terms analogous to the science of the laboratory. While the art of medicine has served clinicians well, generating a coherent and disciplined profession, it is also true that the considerable social status that the medical profession enjoys derives from its public face, one that represents the profession as possessing scientific expertise in effectively dealing with the illnesses that beset us. Until the 1970s, these two aspects, the art and the science of the medical enterprise, coexisted, if not always peacefully.

A number of criticisms were leveled at clinical care in the 1960s and 1970s, both internally and externally, aggravating uncertainty. Doctors were treating patients with the same diagnosis in different ways, raising controversy about internal medicine (Ingelfinger et al. 1966) and contributing to regional variations in practice (Wennberg and Gittelsohn 1973). R. M. Magraw (1966) saw medicine as being in turmoil and beset by change, and called on his colleagues to redefine the core tasks of the profession. An influential voice in the debate was that of Tom McKeown

(1976), who produced evidence showing that reductions in mortality rates in the last two centuries were more attributable to improved environmental factors than to medicine. From the margins, Ivan Illich (1976) argued that medical care was doing more harm than good. Consumers who wanted an increased role in developing health policy criticized medical care (Riska and Taylor 1979). Feminist analysts described gynecology as sadistic (Daly 1979) and reproductive technologies as unethical (Corea 1985). In 1984, the Boston Women's Health Book Collective produced *Our Bodies, Ourselves,* intended to help women take health care "into their own hands" (1998, p. 15). Such critical accounts grew in significance in light of rising health care costs.

In the United States the cost of medical care was escalating, and the sense of crisis was particularly acute. D. W. Shapiro and colleagues (1993) provided a telling summary of concerns at the time. They drew attention to "stunning" figures: the share of gross national product consumed by health care rose from 7.3 percent in 1970 to 12.2 percent in 1990, with a projected cost for 1992 of more than 13 percent, totaling U.S.$809 billion. Health care spending by business exceeded corporate profits. There was no evidence that this expenditure was making much difference to health status as measured by infant mortality or life expectancy. The challenge, as they saw it, was to concentrate expenditure on necessary care while reducing services of little benefit to patients, and for this purpose they needed accurate data on costs, service use, and outcomes. Small area variations in the utilization of services not related to prevalence of disease provided an obvious target. They cited the analysis of John Wennberg and colleagues (1982) showing that the variation seemed greatest when there was professional uncertainty about the best approach to care. Thus their emphasis fell less on direct controls over medical expenditure and more on profiling and practice guidelines that clinicians could use to review and improve their own patterns of practice.

It is in this context, with growing interest in ways of enhancing health without increasing cost, that the emphasis fell on evaluating the effectiveness of health care. However, scientific evaluation of clinical practice outcomes proved to be a difficult task.

Science and the Clinic

Evidence-based medicine, a term both evocative and trite, evokes our belief that medical practitioners base their clinical decisions on evidence — as we expect them to do. If we include in our understanding of this term the idea that clinical decisions should be based on the application of scientific method to the problems of patients, then this is still no more than we expect from medical practitioners, given their years of scientific medical training. On familiar grounds such as this, evidence-based medicine equates with trust.

But the definition of evidence-based medicine that grabbed the attention of policy makers in the 1990s was more specific. The focus was on integrating *better* evidence into decision making — that is, evidence of the effectiveness of clinical interventions, together with procedures for incorporating this evidence into practice. This initiative placed a new responsibility on clinicians to seek out and use this kind of evidence in clinical decision making. While it resolved some questions, it raised others.

The new approach to evidence required new research tools but left unclear who was to wield the new methodological tools. Was this still a medical enterprise, or could other researchers, or even patients, contribute their skills? It was also unclear who would be the beneficiaries of the new approach. Clinicians certainly would benefit, but so could patients; health care administrators and policy makers would have a live interest in finding out what was worth funding from the point of view of government, health funder, or community. More than a decade later, these issues remain controversial.

Central to the growth of interest in evidence-based medicine was the understanding that the new evidence was to be derived through scientific study rather than from fallible clinical authority. Science has provided the most important source of certainty in clinical decision making, and evidence was to be the practical form in which science entered into clinical consideration. The form of science that dominates medical training uses the equivalent of a microscopic lens, focusing on the selected aspects of a phenomenon and excluding anything extraneous from the field of vision, seeing the cell rather than the human body from which it was extracted. The method strips away context, producing evidence seen as objective and value free. The founders of evidence-based medicine argued persuasively that the science of the laboratory was necessary but not sufficient for making decisions about clinical care, but it was toward this version of science that evidence-based medicine turned in its early years.

As a research method for establishing the effectiveness of an intervention, the randomized controlled trial was seen as the gold standard. In design, the randomized controlled trial is a relatively simple but effective translation of the experimental design used in the laboratory to clinical populations. Its promise was that it would achieve the rigor, and certainty, of laboratory findings. As defined at McMaster University, it focused on the clinical encounter and then, more closely, on what researchers saw as the critically important aspect of that encounter, clinical interventions. It had the potential to serve as the foundation for a programmatic approach to developing a science of clinical care.

It is hard to see how a primary, narrow focus on clinical interventions, however valuable, could address the full range of issues encountered in clinical care. For example, if we analyze problems concerning how physicians and other health care practitioners interact with patients, we may need to recognize that these patients live in family, community, and political settings that impinge on their health and their actions. If we are to take these contexts into account in our research, we need a broader notion of science, allowing consideration of how different aspects of a problem interact, sometimes with surprising effect. Instead of excluding context, we make it central to the analysis. Various intellectual programs have taken on this task.

Health services research is a leading proponent of the broad approach to research. It addresses not only the outcomes of health services but also the provision and organization of services, including medical care. One anthology describes health services research as the relationship between populations and health resources and presents it as a "field" that synthesizes input from various disciplines, including clinical epidemiology (White et al. 1992, p. xv). The anthology attests to a long concern about variations in practice, starting from a 1938 study of tonsillectomy rates in schoolchildren by J. Alison Glover in the United Kingdom. There is detailed discussion of a variety of research methods suitable for evaluating medical care.

Two of the papers in the anthology are from the *Milbank Memorial Fund Quarterly*, which published two special issues on health services research in 1966 (volume 44, numbers 3 and 4). The papers in these issues were commissioned by the Health Services Research Study Group of the U.S. Public Health Service. A foreword sums up the issues as follows:

During the past few decades the problems involved in the provision of health services have become increasingly complex, for various reasons — the increase of medical knowledge and techniques, leading to more complex and more expensive types of care; the increased diversity of interrelationships in society; the increase of urbanization; the changes in the age composition of populations; and, perhaps most importantly, the growing belief that everyone has the right to the "best" health care. Clearly the only approach to such problems is research. But research in this area is very difficult and, although it has increased in amount and quality during recent years, it falls far short of what is needed.

The articles in these two issues cover a variety of topics, ranging from the different ways of organizing and paying for services to the relationship between research and policy. Methods of analysis range from direct observation to social surveys, as well as experimental designs and evaluation research. Health services research, argues Odin Anderson, rested on the belief that "all people should have relatively equal access to health services regardless of financial status" (1966, p. 39). Health services research was clearly and inescapably multidisciplinary, and contributors included administrators of hospitals and health departments, clinicians and medical academics, as well as psychologists, sociologists, epidemiologists, operations researchers, and biostatisticians.

The program claimed by health services research had much in common with Archie Cochrane's agenda. Names are deceptive. Health services research in the United Kingdom was augmented by another initiative, that of social medicine, later public health medicine. It drew on the work of Henry Sigerist (1941), John Ryle (1948) and Jerry Morris (1957). Tom McKeown, professor of social medicine at Birmingham, who questions the effect of medicine on the reduction in mortality over the last three centuries (1976), devised a program for medical care that incorporated environmental measures and defined the health and related social services needed to apply medical knowledge in populations with different health needs (McKeown and Lowe, 1974).

In evidence-based medicine, a narrow focus on clinical interventions assessed by randomized controlled trial was clearly an important initiative, additional to biomedicine. Health services research, public health, and social medicine are examples of a broader scientific approach to clinical care, additional to both biomedicine and evidence-based medicine. The question is whether the additional and sometimes divergent skills required by such programs can be incorporated into medical training to supplement insights gained from both biomedicine and clinical epidemiology/evidence-based medicine. Past evidence suggests that this is a difficult task.

Statistics played a central role in the emergence of evidence-based medicine. The use of statistics in studying the health of populations reduced uncertainty by establishing the probability of events. By the end of the nineteenth century, argues Ian Hacking, the statistical concept of chance had "attained the respectability of a Victorian Valet, ready to be the loyal servant of the natural, biological and social science" (1990 p. 2). Alvan

Feinstein argues that clinical decisions about diagnosis, prognosis, and therapy already involved an assessment of probabilities (1985, p. 3). It was therefore a simple extension to apply statistics to the study of populations of patients.

The most likely route for bringing statistics into medical training was through public health, which claimed epidemiology as its basic science and cultivated a range of statistical methods for studying diseases in populations; these could readily be extended to the study of patient populations. In 1938, John Paul, professor of preventive medicine at Yale University, advocated the application of epidemiology to clinical care, calling this venture "clinical epidemiology." His approach was to start with the individual patient and then focus attention on the population and settings where illness originated (1966). The name *clinical epidemiology* did not persist, and this initiative was absorbed into what became community medicine.

The problem was that, historically in the United States and to varying degrees internationally, public health was viewed with suspicion by both biomedical researchers and clinicians. Kerr White (1991) describes the separation between medical care and public health in the United States as being so wide that it constitutes a "schism." Medical students had long shown little interest in public health subjects or in pursuing a career in public health (Coker et al. 1959). This left them ill informed not only about the broad focus of public health but also about probabilistic thinking in general.

Differences in the interests of medicine and public health are not surprising. Clinicians faced with distressed patients were predisposed by their biomedical training to look for a diagnosis and a therapeutic agent. The uncomfortable implication in public health was that the real practice of health care was out in the community, where the damage was actually being done to people, and not in the doctor's clinic. If clinical medicine, like public health, focused on the community in which patients lived and got ill, it might find itself engaging with the long-standing concern in public health over issues of social justice, poverty, and the other social determinants of health. This would negate some of the benefits that biomedicine brought with it — that is, it would not focus on scientific knowledge seen as objective and value free, abstracted from social and political contexts. The broad view taken by public health does not articulate well with the narrow focus of biomedicine, which casts doubt on the scientific credibility of research using a public health perspective.

Given the diverging interests of medicine and public health despite their common task of improving health, some degree of schism was probably inevitable. In more recent times, the divergence between the two may have decreased, as epidemiology has come to be seen as addressing only the study of disease occurrences to the exclusion of traditional social concerns of public health (Susser and Susser 1996). In the 1970s, the randomized controlled trial provided a resolution to the problem of turning to public health for help.

By extracting from public health the research method that replicates an experiment in the field, clinical researchers aligned themselves with laboratory science, using statistical analyses of large numbers to reduce uncertainty. There was a clear advantage in this alignment with experimental science instead of with public health. The problem was that evidence-based medicine then became subject to the same criticisms leveled at biomedical science: that it lacked relevance to the complex world of clinical care.

If clinicians focus only on good, rational, scientific evidence of the effectiveness of interventions (narrowly defined), patients who do not follow prescribed interventions will seem irrational, and the costs generated by their medical care will seem wasted. This is the problem of noncompliance, identified early in the research conducted at McMaster University (Sackett et al. 1976). The problem of "intuitions we could not explain" is therefore transferred from the clinician to the patient. If patients are beset by the same apparent irrationalities that troubled clinicians in the past, then a further initiative is needed, one that generates evidence of effective interventions in the decision making of patients. This initiative would focus on producing high-quality evidence of interventions that persuade patients to act in a way consistent with the evidence. The problem is aggravated when the interventions devised largely turn out to be ineffective (as has happened in the case of research into interventions to reduce patient noncompliance — see Haynes et al. 1996; 2002). However, this points to the gap in knowledge about how patients actually live their lives and make sense of both illness and medication. A broader focus may hold the answers to why interventions fail (for further discussion of this issue, see chapter 9).

Psychology, allied with psychiatry, provides a potential source of understanding about patient decision making. These disciplines have been successfully integrated into medicine to some degree, contributing, for example, to research into health behavior's origins in individual patient characteristics. Unfortunately the problem of patient noncompliance resisted interventions based on a psychological understanding of patients' behavior. The answer seems to lie in the way patients experience illness and respond to interventions in the context of their social lives. But the problem of incorporation intensifies when we look beyond individual behavior and recognize social context. Disciplines that focus broadly on social and political influences carry assumptions far less compatible with the basic training of both medical scientist and clinician. Additionally, there is a limit to the number of divergent disciplines in which any one person can become expert or even competent.

Public health is closely allied with health services research and is comfortable with the idea that the complex determinants of health are best addressed in a multidisciplinary, cooperative way. Different disciplines focus primarily on circumscribed aspects of health, developing extensive expertise in limited fields. When addressing broad-ranging issues of health, cooperation between relevant disciplines ensures that the evidence under consideration has been generated in well-established areas of study after critical disciplinary reflection. It is a tall order to require medical researchers to become expert in these unfamiliar and divergent disciplinary fields. Indeed, even in multidisciplinary collaborations there are many opportunities for confusion and misunderstanding when bringing together disciplines whose primary assumptions are mutually unfamiliar or even incompatible.

Nowhere is this problem more intense than for disciplines addressing the social and political context of health. Here I include the social contexts within which patients live their lives and the social and political institutions that constitute medical care. I call these disciplines collectively the social sciences.

Some social scientists working in health have long focused on exactly the kind of issues that concern clinicians: drawing conclusions from the subjective accounts of patients, focusing on the patient experience of illness and medical interventions. These focused studies are supplemented by the broader examinations of social and political scientists analyzing, for example, systems of health care delivery and the effect of medical care on structural problems like health inequalities.

While at least some of the problems addressed in the social sciences are familiar to clinicians, the research itself takes them into unfamiliar disciplinary territory. Perhaps, then, the methods of the social sciences could be extracted from their disciplinary base as the randomized controlled trial was extracted from public health. This is exactly what happened with meta-analysis, a statistical method for synthesizing the results of various trials of the same intervention and a method that became increasingly important to evidence-based medicine as the number of trials proliferated. Morton Hunt (1997) demonstrates that the social scientists Mary Lee Smith and Gene Glass (1977) engendered crucial development of this method, although Tom Chalmers was simultaneously and independently developing a medical version (see chapter 7). The gap in communication between the disciplines meant that a mutually beneficial cross-fertilization of ideas was delayed. The question then is whether the communication of innovative ideas between disciplines is the only problem, or whether there are methods that cannot be excised from their parent discipline.

Many disciplines, including medicine and the social sciences, have placed their "trust in numbers" (Porter 1995) and have relied on quantification to produce objective knowledge and reduce uncertainty (Matthews 1995). Numerical and statistical methods provide a common language that allows translation between disciplines. This ease of translation does not apply to qualitative research methods. The well-established tradition of qualitative methods of research (see, for example, Silverman 1985) relies on narrative argument rather than statistical reasoning and bases analysis on small samples generating a large quantity of narrative data. Researchers often explicitly draw on social theory for the justification of their findings. Their scientific value is not assessed by tests for validity but by the convincing nature of the argument presented (Silverman 1989). A considerable methodological gulf exists between these qualitative methods and the traditional narrow focus inherent in biomedicine and evidence-based medicine (narrowly defined). Closing this gulf is of immediate interest to still another player in the modern field of health care: consumer organizations representing specific patient views or community interests.

If clinical researchers have traditionally lacked expertise in epidemiological methods and have remained substantially ill informed about the methods of the social sciences, evidence-based medicine has significantly extended their methodological skills, enlarging what is seen as scientific in clinical care and clinical research. The question, finally, is, what remains to be done?

Conclusion

It is the underlying assumption of this book that, in analyzing clinical practice, researchers ideally should have available to them a compendium of research methods, from the narrowly focused to the broadly based, and the capacity to be versatile in the methods chosen to address specific clinical problems — even if this can be achieved only through multidisciplinary collaboration. This allows researchers to focus on a significant problem and then select the research method that best fits the problem. In this approach, the research question rather than the discipline determines the research method selected.

There is a range of theoretical and methodological traditions relevant to clinical care. The argument here is not that initiatives constrained by a narrow focus are in any way inadmissible. Biomedicine has clearly been effective in producing a range of important health interventions. Evidence-based medicine has produced important new information about clinical interventions. The question is whether these approaches provide sufficiently versatile methods for resolving the range of problems found in clinical care. Have other, broader approaches been sidelined? If so, why, and what are the implications?

There is, however, a problem if the perceived or claimed achievements exceed what the narrow focus is able to deliver. This is, after all, the very problem that set in train the various initiatives that constitute evidence-based medicine and that posed a challenge to biomedicine as an adequate basic science for clinical care. However, evidence-based medicine also depends on a narrow reductionist science, embodied in the randomized controlled trial, and so is equally subject to the very criticisms that justified its inception. There is a more substantial problem if researchers substitute a simple, focused problem for a complex one so that the problem can more readily be addressed with methods using a narrow focus. Such sleights of hand undermine the knowledge base of clinical care.

While acknowledging the range of relevant disciplines and fields of study, I focus here on how other disciplines or programs intersect with evidence-based medicine. Biostatistics and epidemiology are clearly part of the picture, but I have selected the social sciences to represent the scientific disciplines marginalized in medical training, with substantial disciplinary differences. Social scientists using qualitative methods are at the outside edge of the margin and provide a challenging test case.

CHAPTER 2

Clinical Epidemiology

The Intellectual Heritage

I begin my discussion with two clinicians who trained in medicine in the United States in the 1960s, Suzanne Fletcher and Robert Fletcher. They represent those clinicians who believed they were not doing their best for their patients, and who turned to clinical epidemiology to resolve bothersome aspects of the clinical task. They also wrote the 1982 textbook *Clinical Epidemiology: The Essentials,* coauthored with Edward Wagner, the first textbook to draw together the arguments of this emerging field. The work of Suzanne Fletcher and Robert Fletcher serves also to introduce those who went before, providing both intellectual inspiration and a rigorous methodological base for the field. Alvan Feinstein in the United States heads the list, acknowledged for the strength of his analysis and the inventiveness of his solutions. Henrik Wulff in Denmark provided a similar but simpler approach, but with an emphasis on a broader social basis for analysis. Kerr White was active in the United States, attempting to bring about a rapprochement between medicine and public health. His keen understanding of the political problems that were involved helped to secure an institutional base for an international initiative supporting clinical epidemiology.

Concerned Clinicians:
Suzanne Fletcher and Robert Fletcher

Suzanne and Robert Fletcher both trained at Harvard Medical School and studied internal medicine at Stanford Medical Center and Johns Hopkins

University. As young internists in the 1960s, they had immediate practical concerns about how they were caring for their patients. In common with many of the other founders of the discipline of clinical epidemiology, they found biomedicine alone to be inadequate for answering the more complex, open-ended problems of clinical care. Robert Fletcher notes:

You see patients and you worry that the data are not good, not making sense, that a lot is at stake. And you want a different kind of approach that you can believe in for making clinical decisions. We grew up in a very biomedical era. We were trained at Stanford in internship and residency, where everyone was a laboratory scientist; and it seemed to me that the kind of science that they brought to bear on patient care, which was mainly logical argument from laboratory data on mechanisms of disease, just wasn't the best possible way of answering these clinical questions. But we didn't have any heroes or mentors there or anywhere in the country to encourage another way of thinking.[1]

Both Suzanne and Robert Fletcher had a population perspective, one absorbed, as the former noted, "by osmosis" from her father, who was professor of international health at the Johns Hopkins School of Public Health and Hygiene. They considered careers in public health but decided they wanted to be clinicians and work with patients.

A number of concerns about the direction of medical care were current in the 1960s. Alvan Feinstein at Yale University articulated his concerns about clinical research by analyzing the abstracts submitted to the yearly clinical meetings of the American Federation for Clinical Research, the American Society for Clinical Investigation, and the American Association of Physicians (Feinstein et al. 1967). Armed with evidence of the predominance of nonhuman, nondisease clinical research, he accused these institutions of an obsession with "rat turd grinding" in the laboratory; instead they should focus on live patients. Robert Fletcher saw that leading medical academics shared a similar if less spectacular sense of unease about the direction of medical care and medical training. He observes, "Subspecialization and the laboratory, with its mechanistic biomedical orientation, however valuable it had been, spurred by the National Institutes of Health and enormous funding, was getting to the point where it had to be counterbalanced by people with other expertise. They foresaw trouble, the very trouble which every developed country in the world now has with distributive justice, cost containment, and the like."

The start of the clinical scholars program launched by the Carnegie Foundation and the Commonwealth Fund in 1969 presented Suzanne Fletcher and Robert Fletcher with the opportunity to combine public health and patient care. Taken over by the Robert Wood Johnson Foundation in 1972, it was renamed the Robert Wood Johnson Clinical Scholars Program. To date, it has trained more than eight hundred scholars at fourteen sites.

There was a perception, argued Robert Brook, director of the Clinical Scholars Program, that American medicine had arrived at a "watershed," given rising health care costs, the concern about the doctor-patient relationship in light of increased patient activism, and the growing medical responsibility for both the social and the physical functioning of patients (1990). What was needed was to identify young clinicians at an early stage of their careers and to provide them with the skills needed to work on these problems, thereby diverting them from careers in the laboratory. The new leaders in internal medicine would need to be both "scholarly activists and activist scholars" (Eisenberg 1990, 19).

Scholars were trained in the nonbiological sciences, including epidemiology, biostatistics, health services research, and health economics to address socially important health problems like access to medical care for vulnerable groups (Shuster 1990). They had the opportunity to combine an interest in taking care of individual patents with public health training. In 1974, one of the training centers of the program was located in Alvan Feinstein's department at Yale University, and Feinstein served as its director. He saw the program's task as training a "new breed of academic clinician concerned with issues in the strategy, delivery and policy of health care" (1985, p. xi).

Support from philanthropic foundations with a long-established interest in health care was critical to the success of the Clinical Scholars Program. Robert Fletcher saw support from respected academics as essential in order for the program to promote, among clinicians, change from within. He says, "Part of the reason for the Clinical Scholars Program is almost subversive. Clinicians will not allow people to come from outside and tell them anything. They are very ethnocentric. And so the program was almost a conspiracy — we see medicine has got to change, and the only way to change it is from within. First you have to get their trust."

While the Clinical Scholars Program presented scholars with the opportunity to combine an interest in taking care of individual patents with public health training, it created tension between public health and clinical medicine. Medical graduates wanting to work in both fields were likely to find it difficult to straddle conceptual and political differences, as well as to encounter quite different career structures in the two fields. At Johns Hopkins University, however, Charles Carpenter, the chair of medicine, offered scholars in the program residency slots on clinical teams even though they were spending part of their time at the school of public health. This is where Kerr White was located. White understood the implication of the program and took the clinical scholars under his wing in the school of public health, facilitating the success of the program.

Suzanne Fletcher and Robert Fletcher's growing interest in the area was strengthened by the knowledge that these ideas were also being addressed in other parts of the world. They read Henrik Wulff's book *Rational Diagnosis and Treatment* (1976); Archie Cochrane's book *Effectiveness and Efficiency* (1972) was known in the program. Cochrane was invited to the United States to talk about the methods he advocated, notably the use of the randomized controlled trial. Edmund Murphy, also at Johns Hopkins University, published *The Logic of Medicine* (1976), a book that carried many of the same ideas. As Robert Fletcher puts it, "There were people all over the world who were thinking along the same lines. I think the time had come, and certain people had just come to see the world that way; and these individual scholars then were a lightning rod for folks like that. It was not so much that they created that interest but that they were able to crystallize it."

After Suzanne Fletcher and Robert Fletcher graduated from the program with master's of science degrees, they taught at McGill University. Here their new skills were put to the test when they were asked to teach one of the unpopular subjects, epidemiology, in the medical school. They agreed to teach it if they could do it their own way: as clinicians with white coats, stethoscopes, and patients. Suzanne Fletcher recalls, "We and Ed Wagner, who is the coauthor of our book, started pushing the clinical applications. That's the key. You know, you walk in with a stethoscope and you bring along a patient, and you ask the clinical question. And then you bring in the method you are going to use to answer the questions. But you lead with the clinical question. Pretty soon all the students were coming."

Later at the University of North Carolina, Michel Ibrahim, dean of public health, also encouraged them to "go ahead, try it." As they recognized in a practical way, stethoscopes and patients were the ideological markers of scientific clinical care. What they needed next was a textbook that set out the scientific basis of patient care, but all they could offer was a set of articles by Feinstein, Sackett, and others, all in different styles. With the new field showing great promise, they decided to write a textbook for their classes. In the Clinical Scholars Program they had heard Feinstein talking about clinical epidemiology, but this was not yet the generally accepted term, so they debated what the book should be called. Suzanne Fletcher notes, "The term clinical epidemiology means different things to different people. When we were writing the book, we had to decide what to call it. A lot of people said, 'You should not call it anything to do with epidemiology, because when clinicians hear *epidemiology*, it puts them to sleep. They hate it; they remember the courses. It's a liability; don't do it.' And right about that time, which was about 1982, the term *clinical epidemiology* became attractive, a good thing, a nice label to attach to something. I think at that point in time it had a very positive connotation."

Their text, *Clinical Epidemiology: The Essentials* (1982), epitomizes an uncomplicated and practical approach. There is neither commitment to esoteric mathematical modeling nor polemic. They describe how methods developed in epidemiology can be effectively applied to bring greater certainty to clinical decision making. The emphasis is on measurement, on indices of accuracy of clinical information, on recognition of what is and what is not reliable in the medical literature, and on epidemiological pitfalls encountered — such as the problems associated with populations of asymptomatic people recruited in community screening programs. Their book is now in its third edition.

Many of the graduates of the Robert Wood Johnson Clinical Scholars Program found their way into divisions of general internal medicine in academic departments of medicine. According to Suzanne Fletcher, general internal medicine flourished in the United States at this time and clinical epidemiology provided it with a disciplinary base:

When this began, the reason why chairmen of medicine were interested in these new divisions was that patient care was increasing and the load of teaching was increasing. Medical schools doubled in size in the United States from 1965 to 1980 or thereabouts. So they had more students to teach, and they needed more residents to take care of these sick patients. So that was the interest in having the young faculty, but it very quickly became clear that the only way they were going to succeed was if they did research. Now what was going to be their area of research expertise? Clinical epidemiology.

I think that in very few cases did clinical epidemiology begin from the top down, because a chairman or a dean said, "We must have a clinical epidemiology unit. We will hire a chief and he or she will recruit people to create this thing." Usually it spread from the bottom up, from young people who were excited about this way of looking at the world and then found ways of banding together. In our case the meeting ground was teaching clinical epidemiology to medical students. People from all departments and all divisions came.

In contrast with McMaster University in Canada, where clinical epidemiology was centered in one department, clinical epidemiology in the

United States was practiced by groups of people, often but not always concentrated in divisions of general internal medicine. At the University of North Carolina, clinical epidemiology was first located in the division of general internal medicine, but then it was taken up in cardiology, infectious diseases, gastroenterology, oncology, and other subspecialties of internal medicine — and in the Departments of Pediatrics, Family Medicine, and Psychiatry. Wherever it was located, it drew together people with a shared interest in clinical care, providing a disciplinary glue across subdisciplines. At the University of North Carolina, there were enough clinical epidemiologists to give the new approach visibility and legitimacy. Moreover, the Department of Epidemiology in the School of Public Health had a long history of being sympathetic to clinicians, and this, Suzanne Fletcher argues, made their task simpler: "Their point of view was, if you want to try it and it sounds like a good idea, try it. If you succeed, fine. That's not all that common."

In the United States, as in Canada, clinical epidemiologists found a role in advising other medical departments about questions of research method raised by funding agencies and academic journals: questions about bias, measurement, chance, and generalizability. While there was still suspicion about the value of clinical epidemiology, new opportunities were being created. The 1990 appointment of Suzanne Fletcher and Robert Fletcher as editors of the *Annals of Internal Medicine,* the journal of the American College of Physicians, provided an illustration of this change of heart. Robert Fletcher notes, "We had none of the traditional characteristics of the previous editors of the journal — we were general internists, not subspecialists, and had a strong interest in prevention as well as an intellectual base in clinical epidemiology. These were all a wrong set of credentials. But they decided it was the right set of credentials at this point in time."

After serving as joint editors, Suzanne and Bob Fletcher joined the faculty of the Department of Ambulatory Care and Prevention at the Harvard Medical School in Boston. Frank Davidoff took over as editor in 1995, and he stated his support for the next initiative, evidence-based medicine (Gesensway 1995).

The Godfather: Alvan Feinstein

Clinical epidemiology was born during a time of ferment in health care and amid uncertainty about the processes of clinical decision making. There was a significant exchange of ideas among the founders of the new discipline, but the most influential in the early years was Alvan Feinstein in the United States. It was Feinstein who determined that the answer to clinical uncertainty lay in science, but not the science of the laboratory. Instead he set about generating a new science, a science specific to the problems encountered in clinical care, a basic science which would challenge that of the laboratory. He articulated its principles, developed its methods, and conducted studies that addressed a wide range of clinical problems.

Feinstein's prodigious output and strong arguments provided the banner around which the new brand of clinical researcher could rally. Suzanne Fletcher describes "the Importance of Alvan" as follows: "He had a great *philosophic* impact. He is a teachers' teacher, and through them he has had a far greater influence than just his own work had directly with students." Robert Fletcher adds, "At any other time when you look back at history, you can say, 'This stuff does not look that new to me.' But at the time, he was the only person saying it. And he said it very forcefully, pugnaciously; and he made people believe that this is a thing that they could do and succeed." He defended clinical epidemiology from outside attack but also turned on those who failed to respect the basic aim of providing a scientific basis for clinical care. Fittingly, he is widely referred to as the godfather of clinical epidemiology.

Feinstein was born in Philadelphia. He trained in mathematics, then medicine, at the University of Chicago. Mathematics was to have a substantial influence on his later work. He had a restless, critical mind, and he found himself frustrated by the lack of application of theoretical mathematics. He shifted direction and, later, gave a self-deprecating explanation of this shift. His fear, he said, was that he would never be more than a second-rate mathematician: "I figured if I had to be mediocre, I might as well be a doctor and make a good living out of it, and it was with that noble motivation, that majestic concern for the sick and suffering, that I went back to school!" After training in internal medicine at Yale University, he turned to academic medicine, at that time firmly located in the laboratory.

The citadel of academic medicine, Feinstein believed, was the Rockefeller Institute in New York, now Rockefeller University. He went there as an assistant and was put in charge of metabolic balance studies for one of the laboratory groups. He liked academic medicine, but he was unhappy limiting himself to the laboratory study of urine and feces. He saw the leaders of academic medicine as having both feet and heads of clay, as not deserving of reverence; he resolved to give up being "somebody's lab boy" and turned instead to clinical medicine.

Feinstein's objective, at that stage, was to go into private practice in New York. After an additional year of residency, he became clinical director of Irvington House, a rheumatic fever hospital and convalescent home affiliated with New York University. Irvington House, Feinstein says, was a wonderful place that provided an outpatient clinic, as well as a convalescent home and school for children with acute rheumatic fever who could not be adequately cared for by their families. Researchers at Irvington House were conducting an epidemiological study of prophylactic treatment for prevention of a recurrence of rheumatic fever (Feinstein et al. 1959). Feinstein's task was merely to take care of the children and collect clinical data for the study, not to conduct the analysis.

Rheumatic fever, precipitated by a streptococcal throat infection, can damage the heart muscle and valves. Subsequent streptococcal infection can cause recurrence of rheumatic fever, further damaging the heart. At the time, the accepted treatment was prolonged bed rest to ensure that the heart had fully recovered. At issue in the study was whether antibiotics could prevent reinfection and the recurrence of rheumatic fever. Laboratory tests were used to demonstrate that streptococcal infection was present, but only a clinical examination could establish whether the child actually had rheumatic fever and could be admitted to the study.

This apparently simple process of diagnosis turned out to be more complex than at first thought. When the heart is damaged by rheumatic fever, causing the valves to leak, heart murmurs can be heard with a stethoscope. However, "innocent" physiological murmurs are also commonly heard in normal children. The clinical distinction between innocent and pathological murmurs required critical judgment of slight differences in the sound heard through a stethoscope. Learning to make this distinction forms part of the clinical training for this specialist area. Since he was not trained in this field, Feinstein had to rely on his own judgment, supplemented with what the textbooks said. He was immediately struck with the uncertainty of the area: "Fortunately, not having had any specific training in rheumatic fever or heart disease, I didn't know what I was supposed to hear. Eventually, when I looked at the literature I thought, 'What those guys are writing about is not what is going on! Either I am being deceived by the patients, which I doubt, or the writers have been deceived and are wrong.'"

The textbooks did not provide clear criteria for the distinction. An even bigger problem, he suspected, was that clinical training was based on the authoritative conclusions of clinical teachers, and that these had not been exposed to critical scrutiny. It was therefore not surprising that different clinicians made different diagnoses when examining the same child. Faced with substantive uncertainty, Feinstein decided to follow in the footsteps of Thomas Sydenham (1624–1689) and develop a careful analysis of what actually happened at the patient's bedside. The first task was to reach agreement between observers through classification. According to Feinstein, "The first step was to recognize what we heard. I'd say, 'Look, do you agree that what you hear sounds like *lubsshh, lubsshh, lubsshh, lubsshh?'* 'Yeah, that's what it sounds like.' 'Okay, then what do you think is the *lub* and what do you think is the *sshh?* Or do you agree that it sounds like *lp dp, lp dp, lp dp?'* 'Yeah, yeah.' 'Okay what do you think is the *lur, up,* the *dd,* and the *pp?'* This type of cardiophonetics led my colleagues and me to agree on what we heard. We could then go on from there."

The next issue was to develop criteria for the acoustic distinction between a leaking valve in a heart damaged by rheumatic fever and the innocent murmur heard in children with a normal heart. This work was then extended to cover the diagnosis of other important manifestations of rheumatic fever, such as the size of the heart, joint pains, and chorea (jerky movements related to rheumatic brain inflammation). Feinstein's clinical objective was to make diagnosis more consistent, to accurately identify children for the study, and to care for them. At the time, he was less concerned with what would become the task of investigating inter-observer variability: "We still did not think of these activities as being particularly scientific. We did them because our job was to make diagnostic decisions, and it was easier to settle our arguments with data and specific criteria than with dogma and authoritarian decree" (Feinstein 1967, p. 6).

Identifying consistent criteria for the diagnosis of disease was the first step toward increased certainty in diagnosis. It was also the first step in the development of a taxonomic, classificatory science of clinical care. The next step was to address the natural outcome of the disease, its progno-sis. Only then could the effect of treatment on the natural course of the disease be determined. Merely to diagnose a group of children as having rheumatic fever was therefore not enough. Feinstein further classified patients into subgroups based on various combinations of symptoms, signs, and test results. He found that overlapping circles were a conven-ient way of illustrating these subgroups: "I used a circle to represent patients who all had a single common property (such as arthritis) and another, overlapping circle to represent patients with another property (such as carditis). The overlap of the circle would denote patients with both properties; the non-overlapping sectors would denote patients who had one property or the other but not both" (Feinstein 1967, pp. 7–8).

For each of these groups, the investigators could establish a prognosis and test the effect of treatment. They showed that children with the first attack of rheumatic fever who did not have murmurs indicative of heart disease were not subsequently at increased risk from serious heart disease (Feinstein and Di Massa 1959). Feinstein concluded that tradition was misplaced and was harming these children: "Quit keeping them in bed, quit keeping them from athletics, quit keeping them from having children!" In children with heart disease, on the other hand, antibiotics were effective in preventing recurrence of heart disease. Feinstein had defined the spectrum of disease in rheumatic fever and tested the effect of various forms of treatment. As a result, clinicians could categorize patients, defining the place their illness occupied in that spectrum, and choose the most effective treatment for that patient.

Feinstein's work drew on the principles of bedside medicine, updated through modern mathematical skills. This was at odds with the way results were being analyzed in the Irvington House study. The statistician categorized the data according to demographic characteristics, relating recurrence of the disease to age and gender. However, that was not what Feinstein wanted to know. The clinical data that Feinstein saw as the key to prognosis had been *deliberately rejected* as unreliable: "That made me realize what trouble we were in intellectually." After discussion, Feinstein's clinical groupings were included in the analysis (Taranta et al. 1964).

Feinstein's studies had important implications for clinical practice. With a scientific basis for clinical care, he argued, the simple stethoscope could cure more heart disease than could the surgeon's knife. "If I died when I was about forty, or forty-five," he says, "I hoped that my epitaph might be: 'He got them out of bed.' The usual convalescent practice was to keep all rheumatic fever kids in bed for a period of two years. By lowering the convalescent period to about one month, and also by showing effective antibiotic prophylaxis, I was responsible for the closing of Irvington House, the place where I was working. They couldn't keep the beds full!"

Feinstein concentrated on clinical decision making, categorizing subgroups and studying the effect of treatment on each. Disregarding the lack of mathematical skills in clinical practice, he took the view that clinicians themselves should be doing this research, improving their practice in the process. The patients in the study were receiving meticulous clinical care, which included ensuring that follow-up appointments were kept so that children remained under observation. In one case the researchers even obtained the release from jail of the father of one child. If these efforts were essential to the study, why should they not be seen as essential to good clinical care?

Despite its obvious practical clinical importance, research of this kind was considered inferior to basic research done in a laboratory. Feinstein says, "I think that this whole concept of 'basic' and 'applied' is a fundamental screwup in human thinking. I will not give to anything the title of 'basic,' because there is no human intellectual domain that can arrogate the title of 'basic' unto itself. Everything you do in life is basic to something and applied for something else. The idea of 'basic science' really developed after World War II. What gave it all the impetus was the success of the United States in making the atomic bomb and showing that allegedly basic physics could be applied."

In 1962, Feinstein returned to Yale University. Here he extended his observations of the spectrum of disease to other diseases, including cancer (Feinstein 1964a). His aim was simple: to distinguish cancers that are lethal from those that are not. The methods he used were complex. Later, in *Clinical Judgment* (1967), he described how he addressed the problem of analyzing the overlap of clinical features that he had previously noted in the case of rheumatic fever. Here Feinstein, the mathematician, comes to the fore:

The problem was that every system of classification I had ever known in biology or in physical science was designed for mutually exclusive categories. A particular chemical element was sodium, potassium or strontium, but not two of these, or all three. An animal might be fish or fowl, not both. But a patient might have many different clinical properties simultaneously. I wanted to have mutually exclusive clinical categories for classifying patients, but I could not get the different categories separated. They all seemed to overlap, and I could find no consistent way to separate the overlap. I suddenly saw the solution for the problem: I did not have to remove the overlap; I could preserve and classify it. Boolean algebra and Venn diagrams were a perfect intellectual mechanism for classifying overlap; they were an ideal way to distinguish multiple properties that could be present or absent, alone or in combination. (Feinstein 1967, p. 10)

The draft paper in which he set out these arguments was not well received by clinicians, in part, he suspected, because they did not have the skills to specify and categorize disease. He decided to approach the problem from a clinical perspective, emphasizing the relevance of his work to clinical judgment:

Clinical judgment depends not on a knowledge of causes and mechanisms, or names for disease, but on a knowledge of patients. The background of clinical judgment is clinical experience: the things clinicians have learned at the bedside in the care of sick people. In acquiring this experience, every clinician has to use some sort of intellectual mechanism for organizing and remembering his observations. I had inadvertently worked out a rational description for at least part of this intellectual mechanism. The system of clinical classification was a coherent, logical technique for cataloguing the information used as a basis for clinical judgment. (Feinstein 1967, pp. 12–13)

Clinicians are aware that they think and reason in terms of patterns of symptoms and signs as well as laboratory results. They also take account of the stage of a disease, the sequence of events in which the disease manifests, and the coexistence of other disease. Developing a classification of all these variables required what Feinstein called a taxonomy of disease. His findings differed substantively from those of Sydenham, who observed and classified patterns of disease in the seventeenth century, because the "new" mathematics provided a way of formulating the classifications (Feinstein 1963a), and the computer provided the means for storing and using this "systematic clinical taxonomy" (Feinstein 1967, p. 155).

Feinstein's clinical science was based on the systematic study of signs, of symptoms, and of the patterns of disease observed by the clinician at the patient's bedside (Feinstein 1963b). Using these methods, he argued, could make clinical care into a gold mine for researchers, an alternative to the laboratory as a focus for the academic clinician.

In 1964, Feinstein published a series of four articles on "scientific methodology in clinical medicine" in the *Annals of Internal Medicine*. In an introduction, the editor invoked the scientific heritage of Francis Bacon to describe the importance of the series. *Clinical Judgment* followed. Feinstein saw the book as a "labour of love," unique in arguing that clinicians should not deny the heterogeneity of clinical practice, that they should instead observe it accurately, classify it, and use it to determine prognosis and guide treatment.

In 1968, in a series of three articles, he proposed a range of activities, which he called "clinical epidemiology." He argued that epidemiology could be seen as a set of quantitative methods that, allied with statistical analytical methods, provided a basic science for public health. These could also, however, be married to clinical reasoning to study clinical populations or subgroups under the rubric of "clinical epidemiology." This application of quantitative methods to clinical care constituted an *additional* basic science for clinical medicine (Feinstein 1983). In *Clinical Epidemiology* (1985), he developed and elaborated upon the quantitative methods to be used for the new discipline. *Clinimetrics* (1987) concentrated on defining, categorizing, and quantifying clinical information in a way that was responsive to the goals of the clinician.

Initially, when Feinstein spoke to nonmedical friends about his new interest, he found it difficult to label what he was doing: "Unlike all my colleagues, I didn't have an organ! I couldn't say heart, lungs, or liver. I would have to say, 'Well, I am interested in the quantification of diagnosis, prognosis, and therapy.' And they would say, 'Ah, isn't that what all doctors do?'" At Yale University in the 1960s, a visiting British epidemiologist asked Feinstein to give a talk about his work in "epidemiology": "I said, 'What do you mean, epidemiology? I am not an epidemiologist. Epidemiologists are people who go around collecting useless statistics about the incidence and prevalence of syphilis in Tasmania. I don't do that.' He said, 'Yes, you are; you study groups of people and apply statistics to them: that is what epidemiologists do.' And I said, 'Well, if I am, I am a *clinical* epidemiologist.'"

Despite this overlap in methods, Feinstein saw no need for a rapprochement with public health epidemiology. Although he was elected to the American Epidemiology Society in 1971, he believed they may have come to regret the move. He was critical of British epidemiologists for losing touch with direct patient care and no longer knowing "which end of the patient is up." Conventional clinical research was doing no better, since it had become more concerned with research on animals, and with parts of animals, than with the study of living patients. While animal research into disease mechanisms is clearly valuable, Feinstein argues, it does not address all the problems specific to clinical care, and some of its practitioners denigrate the kind of research that does. His aim was to reverse this trend, and he describes his early papers as hitting the foreheads of clinicians with a two-by-four stick and saying, "Pay attention!" In setting out the scientific basis of investigation of the clinical process of diagnosis and treatment, he provided clinicians with critical tools for analyzing their healing task. The same tools could be used to evaluate the medical literature. He believed that a two-way flow of information between clinicians and statisticians would benefit both: "If clinicians need to know about the mystic statistic, statisticians might benefit from discovering the clinical pinnacle" (Feinstein 1977a, p. 7). Feinstein's later books, however, are so mathematically sophisticated that they are of little direct use to clinicians. This is why Suzanne Fletcher sees him as being influential primarily as the teachers' teacher.

Feinstein was vehemently opposed to the uncritical borrowing of models from other disciplines and abhorred the overoptimistic use of the methods that have contributed to the development of clinical epidemiology. These include the randomized controlled trial and the emphasis on Bayesian probability (see chapter 3). And when randomized trials failed to provide a clear answer, researchers, instead of turning to their own devices, were seduced by the idea that the techniques of meta-analysis could "convert existing things into something better" (1995, p. 71). This, Feinstein calls "statistical alchemy," the lure of "getting something for nothing" (1995, p. 71). The unthinking, uncritical application of mathematical models to complex patterns of disease characteristic of clinical practice he dismisses as "the haze of Bayes, the aerial palaces of decision analysis, and the computerized Ouija board" (1977b). As a result of enthusiasm for these inappropriate distractions, clinical science confronted an intellectual crisis, and important clinical challenges remained unmet (1992).

The problem, Feinstein says, is that clinicians are "taught to be intellectual dunces who have no basic challenges of their own," and medical students are taught to see clinical medicine as being of secondary importance to the "basic" sciences; they end up with "intellectual lobotomy" (1996, p. 210). "The basic challenges of patient-care interventions in clinical medicine, notes Feinstein, "cannot be solved by alien models, by the blandishments or 'guidelines' of academic nannies, or by the specious fashions of mathematical mandarins. Clinicians should make use of all the effective, consultative help they can get, but should not abandon fundamental challenges that require direct clinical solutions from wise intellects" (1996, p. 210).

Public health epidemiology was another target for criticism. Although Feinstein recognized the substantial contribution of public health research to the control of disease, he saw little advantage in collaborating with public health epidemiology, given its lack of rigor. A particular target were those epidemiologic studies that link aspects of daily life with the rise of chronic diseases. He argues that the resulting "epidemic of apprehension" is often based on studies flawed by lack of specified hypotheses, lack of properly specified cohorts of subjects, poor quality data, unsound analysis of the attribution of cause, and bias in the detection of outcomes (1988, p. 1262). Of particular concern were case control studies and studies that draw on convenience cohorts. So, for example, he argues that bias in the detection of outcomes has been ignored in studies that have led to what he sees as the spurious association of breast cancer with alcohol:

The apparent association of alcohol and breast cancer could easily be explained if women who drink in moderate "social" quantities are also more likely than abstainers to maintain a medical "life style" that brings routine palpation of the breast and mammography. Many studies of breast cancer have shown that it is more commonly found in women of higher socioeconomic status, where social drinking and routine screening of the breast are also more common. Furthermore, women who drink heavily may develop alcohol-related illnesses that also bring increased medical attention and the opportunity to detect hitherto undiagnosed breast cancers. If these features of the increased detection process are ignored, the associated increase in breast cancer will be fallaciously attributed to alcohol. (1988, p. 1261)

Such problems could be avoided by using, where possible, an experimental study design — namely, the randomized controlled trial. On the other hand, the randomized controlled trial could itself be overused. Because of its scientific stature, it could distract clinicians from substantive problems in clinical practice that cannot be analyzed by trials. Feinstein himself believes that *Clinical Judgment* has been largely ignored because the randomized controlled trial offers an easier alternative for clinical research than the methods he proposed: "What I talked about in that book was a need for clinicians to develop a scientific taxonomy for what they do. The development of that taxonomy has been generally ignored during the infatuation with mathematical models. Which is why the randomized trial is so powerful: because if you don't want to think, the randomized trial is a perfect way to avoid thinking."

Feinstein's overarching view in *Clinical Judgment* was not controversial: the art of medicine should be submitted to critical scrutiny. "I have tried," he states, "with undiminished respect for the past, to separate archaisms, sustained only by the hoary custom of intellectual inertia, from the old cherished clinical activities that are still valuable and as modern as tomorrow." (1967, p. 15). In *Clinimetrics,* however, he argues that this is most appropriately done by quantifying the "crucial, uniquely human information" related to the humane art of healing. He recognizes that there might be considerable resistance to this proposal: "Many patients and clinicians may even become intensely distressed by the idea that the 'art' produces a 'measurement' and that the process can be given so formidable a name as 'clinimetrics.' The distress probably arises from the fear that formal clinimetric attention to these acts of measurement may threaten the few remaining features of humanistic clinical art that have managed to survive the technologic transformation of modern medical science" (1987, p. 1).

The basis of his argument was that medical care is dehumanized when "soft" clinical data like "anxiety, gratification, love, hate, sorrow, joy" are rejected in favor of "hard" technologic measures from "the patient's blood, urine, faeces, tissues, cells, films or electrographic tracings" (1987, p. 3). While acknowledging that some qualities like sensitivity or love may be too complex to quantify, what he failed to consider was that the process of quantifying the variables of the humane art could, in itself, contribute to the dehumanizing trend, limiting what is human to that which can be measured. He overlooked alternate ways of integrating the humane variables without quantification. This would require an additional step that Feinstein resisted: acknowledgment that nonstatistical methods of study should be seen as valid.

Feinstein's contribution to clinical epidemiology cannot be doubted. It took a person with his caustic turn of phrase to attack the citadels of clinical research. Perhaps this same critical capacity meant that he did not go into team research to the extent that the researchers at McMaster University did — and which they see as crucial to their success (see chapter 4). Instead he became the critical overseer of the discipline, its respected but feared gadfly. His criticisms could be devastating, and he had the capacity to coin new terms that captured the imagination and confounded his opponents. On the other hand, he has no sympathy at all for any radical proposals for revolutionizing medicine. Feinstein says, "I am in favor of reform, but medicine needs an establishment. We need a conservative establishment to keep us from shifting with every new wind. But an establishment that does not recognize and reform when it is confronted with problems gets overthrown by revolution. I don't want to see revolution."

The direct influence of Feinstein's work has perhaps been limited by its inaccessibility. His program was complex, requiring developed mathematical skills possessed by few clinicians. His program sets expectations of rigor that the ordinary clinician (even with the aid of modern computing facilities) would find difficult to satisfy. His contribution, as critic and source of inspiration, has been indirect. One of the places where Feinstein's influence was felt was at McMaster University in Canada, where the infant discipline of clinical epidemiology was being nurtured, though in a very different way. One person whom Feinstein influenced earlier, however, was Henrik Wulff in Denmark.

The Broad European Concept: Henrik Wulff

In Denmark, Henrik Wulff drew on Feinstein's work to develop his approach to the study of clinical care. His book *Rational Diagnosis and Treatment* (1976) predates the Fletcher, Fletcher, and Wagner textbook by six years and the McMaster University textbook by nine years; the Danish edition of Wulff's book was published even earlier, in 1973. The subject matter is the same as that labeled as clinical epidemiology in Canada and the United States.

Wulff trained as a gastroenterologist, and he undertook his early research in the laboratory. Austin Bradford Hill's two books on medical statistics (1937, 1962) convinced Wulff of the need for a statistical approach to the study of clinical care. Further impetus for his change of direction came from Feinstein's *Clinical Judgment* and from subsequent discussions with Feinstein in Copenhagen in 1970. Wulff says, "Feinstein's book reflected a certain discontent with clinical practice. We did so many things to our patients, and we didn't know what was good and what was bad. We were also a bit fed up with the research which was being done; it was so far removed from clinical practice. There was a critical attitude to medicine. That's how it started."

Wulff has argued that a more critical approach to clinical care started in the United Kingdom in the 1960s and spread from there to other countries (1986, p. 128). These new ideas were being discussed in more than one center in Denmark. He believes that ideas can disseminate rapidly in a small country like Denmark. Danish primary health care general practitioners were seeking an identity of their own, different from that of specialists. Primary care became the focus for reform, providing the impetus for general practitioners to conduct research in their own clinical settings. The Danish Medical Association sponsored postgraduate teaching courses in research methods, biostatistics, and randomized controlled trials. Wulff participated in these, as did Bjørn Andersen, a surgeon with the knack of teaching statistics to the uninitiated (Andersen 1990), and Povl Riis, editor of the *Danish Medical Journal*. Rigorous statistical method became a requirement for publication in this journal. It was, according to Wulff, an idea whose time had come. Unlike McMaster University, Wulff and colleagues did not seek to institutionalize the new approach but simply incorporated it into existing structures. It became not a new discipline but one ingredient in the production of good clinical care.

Wulff came to see the basic problem for clinical care as philosophical in origin. Biomedical science, which dominated medical care, was based on a realist perspective that emphasized a mechanical model of disease and assumed a clear pathway from dysfunction to cure. The aim of scientific medical care was, therefore, to identify the cause of the disease and treat the dysfunction effectively with appropriate therapy derived from the results of basic biomedical research. However, clinicians knew that the basic assumptions of this model were questionable: apparently secure and scientific biomedical knowledge frequently failed in clinical practice.

Faced with the individual patient, the clinician had to decide on the extent to which biomedical knowledge was applicable to that particular patient. Lacking an adequate scientific basis for making these decisions, clinicians fell back on a master-apprentice model of training that promoted uncritical imitation rather than evaluation. Thus, while the clinician could make good use of the results of biomedical research, the research did not provide a sufficient basis for clinical care. What was needed was a more detailed understanding of the principles of clinical decision making. Wulff uses the term *clinical decision theory* to describe this "missing subject" (1976, p. 2).

Wulff set out to define an alternative to the realist perspective. What he sought was the means for better exploiting laboratory progress by a rational scientific approach to clinical care, one that incorporated the complex realities of the clinical setting. In *Rational Diagnosis and Treatment,* Wulff provided a comprehensive discussion of scientific thinking in clinical care, nesting this discussion in a historical account of the development of disease classification and of methods of evaluating treatment. Acknowledging his debt to Feinstein, he saw his audience as being clinicians rather than mathematicians, and he guided readers through a simple, practical account of the statistical methods needed. His focus was not on research but on the need for clinicians to draw sound conclusions from the medical literature. On the other hand, clinical care represented as big an intellectual challenge as work in the laboratory. The book concluded with a discussion of the randomized controlled trial as an important research method for the evaluation of treatment. Wulff agrees with Feinstein that this research was best conducted by clinicians. This adds to his disquiet about the term *clinical epidemiology:* "I think it's a misnomer. The word *demos* in epidemiology means people or population. Epidemiologists study diseases in the population, and the term *clinical epidemiology* suggests that they are also qualified to analyze clinical problems as they present in the individual patient. They are not. We prefer the neutral word, *clinical theory.*"

Wulff calls his activity "rational diagnosis and treatment" and describes its adherents as members of the "critical clinical school." As part of this critical approach, he celebrates the contribution of the randomized controlled trial, but he also sees the need to study the role of statistical thinking within a more complex clinical framework: "You will have to take into account the humanistic aspects; then they will come to the surface much more. So the RCT [randomized controlled trial] doesn't stand alone; it requires other activities as well."

Wulff is unusual in considering humanistic aspects of care in their own right, without requiring that they be reduced to reproducible measures. This extends his approach beyond standard medical training, and thus it involves collaboration with other disciplines, an approach that Feinstein rejected. A second book, *Philosophy of Medicine: An Introduction,* coauthored with a philosopher and a psychiatrist (Wulff, Pedersen, and Rosenberg 1986), addressed the notion of the paradigm of medicine as a set of tacit beliefs that guide practice and research, examining its components in terms of underlying philosophical principles. The first component of clinical care is the biological component. From theoretical knowledge of biomedicine, clinicians infer what is the matter with the patient and what the rational treatment should be. Applying biomedical knowledge is, in itself, insufficient. The second or empirical component is inference from clinical experience with previous patients, ideally in the form of the results of controlled clinical research. This component, essentially what clinical epidemiology provides, is a necessary adjunct to biological knowledge. Bringing these two components together was the basic aim of *Rational Diagnosis and Treatment.*

Wulff was, however, dissatisfied with the result. There were two further components that he felt he had neglected in the book, ones neglected by clinical epidemiology in general. The interpretive component of clinical care concerns the self-reflecting doctor's empathic understanding of the patient. In this component, disease is not seen as a mechanical fault to be fixed; instead the focus is on how patients perceive symptoms in the context of their everyday lives. It is this patient perspective that the clinician has to understand. The fourth component is the ethical component: it concerns the value judgments of individuals and the moral norms of society, and it has to be incorporated into every consultation. In Wulff's view, economics is classified under ethics because it is concerned with distributive justice.

When Wulff revised *Rational Diagnosis and Treatment* for a second edition in 1981, he added a section on ethics. This proved to be a controversial decision:

In reaction to that inclusion, some scientifically orientated colleagues argued that ethical reasoning could not be called rational. I disagree strongly with that point of view, which seems related to the emotivist theory of empirical philosophers. Moral judgments may not be objectively true or false in the same way as some diagnostic statements and statements about the effect of different treatments, but they may be mutually consistent or inconsistent and they may be logically compatible or incompatible with certain fundamental moral beliefs. It may be expected of the clinician as a minimum requirement that he be able to discuss complex moral problems rationally, i.e., that he be able to express in words his own fundamental moral beliefs, to analyze in detail the problem at hand, and to defend his decisions in terms of both the facts of the case and ethical analysis (1986, p. 132).

This sets a high standard for clinicians, especially as Wulff requires ethical thinking to be integrated into clinical reasoning:

What I don't like today is that doctors reason scientifically and then, *apart from that,* profess an interest in ethics. The two things are not combined. I like to see ethics as part of humanistic medicine together with the hermeneutic aspect, understanding another human being; and I like to see clinical medicine as both a scientific and a humanistic discipline. Here we are back to Habermas's three fundamental interests. I also dislike that ethics today, especially in North America, is always reduced to the rights of the individual. Medical ethics also concerns our duties towards each other. That is, after all, the motive force of any health service.

Here Wulff refers to the work of a difficult-to-grasp philosopher and social theorist, Jürgen Habermas (1971), whose work is classified under the term *critical theory*. Habermas argues that there are three fundamental interests in social life. The technical interest is concerned with technical means of extending control over nature, the practical interest focuses on ways of communicating with people, and the emancipatory interest lies in freeing people from domination. Habermas's argument is that the technical interest is now dominant, distorting social life. It needs to be reunited with the practical and emancipatory interests. Wulff has applied Habermas's critical theory to clinical care, in the process expanding the technical interest into the first two components of his model. The practical and emancipatory aspects of care, appearing in Wulff's work as the interpretive and ethical components, have been neglected.

Wulff saw the need for a much broader paradigm of research in clinical care than that of any of the North American pioneers. While they saw the need to reduce uncertainty by analyzing the technical aspects of clinical care, Wulff saw the need to integrate the biomedical component and the empirical work that constituted clinical epidemiology with two other approaches — and, he believes, until this work is done, uncertainty will remain. An interpretive understanding of the social interaction between doctor and patient in the clinical consultation remains a substantive area of uncertainty, and medical ethics can be the source of contention. Wulff argues that recognition of the need for this additional work represents a European initiative: "In continental Europe, the importance of the statistical approach is appreciated among critical clinicians everywhere, but, at the same time, there is a much greater interest in medical philosophy and the humanistic aspect of clinical thinking than in North America."

Wulff's work is important in two respects. His early work provides an accessible interpretation of some of the major points being raised by Feinstein. His later work presents a clear contrast with that of Feinstein: Feinstein proposed to quantify the humane aspects of clinical care in order to produce "hard" data; Wulff proposed, in addition, a quite different critical and interpretive form of knowledge. While this more philosophical approach is made explicit only in his later work, it underlies his approach to the science of clinical care. Together with Feinstein, Wulff provided an important focus of interest for young clinicians embarking on their training in the 1970s before the McMaster University version of clinical epidemiology had attained general currency. His work remains current. The third edition (2000) of *Rational Diagnosis and Treatment* is coauthored by Peter C. Gøtzsche of the Nordic Cochrane Centre and is subtitled *Evidence-Based Clinical Decision-Making*. Now available in seven languages, it retains its criticism of a narrow statistical approach to the analysis of clinical care.

The Internationalist: Kerr White

The account of Suzanne Fletcher points to the watchful eye that several philanthropic foundations maintained over health care in the United States. In this context, Kerr White played an important role in nurturing the new discipline. His approach represents two strong commitments. The first is to exemplary clinical care as it affects the health of both individuals and populations. The second is to recognizing the political context of health and health care, so that the opportunity can be found to implement unpopular ideas. Like Feinstein, White casts a long shadow because of his passionate commitment to the field. Starting in the 1950s, he pursued the critical appraisal of medical care. His agenda, unlike Feinstein's or Sackett's, was its reintegration with public health. John Evans, founding dean of the McMaster University medical school and chair of the Board of the Rockefeller Foundation (1987 to 1995), sees White's influence in many areas: "If you scratch almost anywhere, in my opinion, you find Kerr White's beneficial influence in the development of this area, what I call health of the public, to distinguish it from the narrower view of public health. Brilliant mind! He sampled a variety of the academic perspectives but, I think, never found any academic perspectives that were very satisfying for the vision he had."

White's initial training was in economics and political science at McGill and Yale Universities; after graduation he worked in the personnel department of a factory. He recalls with pride that, concerned about the rates of pay and conditions of workers, he helped organize a successful strike to improve their status. After World War II, during which he had served in the Canadian army, he decided to study medicine and specialize in public health. But public health was preoccupied with "building privies," and the power lay with those specialties that dealt with patient care. He turned to internal medicine. Says White, "I saw that general practice was on the wane, and was denigrated, and the internists seemed to be in control, so I thought, 'Well, I am going to get training in internal medicine.' This seemed to me where the power was, the intellectual power and also the academic power. The surgeons had it in the past, and now the internists had it."

White says that he grew up with an international perspective. His mother was English, and his father a newspaper journalist, and White attended schools in Los Angeles, Ottawa, and London. After the war, he planned to spend a year at Oxford University with John Ryle, who was appointed as the first professor of social medicine in 1943. Ryle died in 1950, before White could fulfill this plan, but he was influenced by Ryle's dissatisfaction with medical schools (see chapter 6). Like Ryle, he saw the promise of working with other disciplines to produce a broad program of research in community health.

White moved to the University of North Carolina, in Chapel Hill, in 1953 and started doing research on the multifactorial nature of chronic illness, working in a team made up of clinicians, epidemiologists, sociologists, statisticians, and social workers. They conducted a three-pronged investigation of cardiac failure, including clinical, laboratory, and population-based research (White et al. 1959; Martin et al. 1959; Klainer et al. 1965). Their laboratory studies on the effect of perceived traumatic events on cardiovascular function confirmed what they observed in patients: "We followed up hospitalized patients with cardiac failure and found that virtually all of them had experienced separation of some kind; either the dog had died, a son had gone off to the wars, a spouse had died, they had lost their home, there was a financial catastrophe, or something. Now, sure enough, they had organic heart disease, no question about that, but you always have to ask, why they go into failure on Tuesday at four o'clock in the afternoon? Why not Monday, and why not next week?"

He recalled that such insights were becoming increasingly popular with some colleagues and students but were regarded as "outlandish" by the biomedical establishment. When he attempted to evaluate the efficacy and appropriateness of care for hospitalized patients by analyzing hospital discharge data, he came up against resistance from clinical colleagues who saw the university hospital's major task as the setting of "gold standards" for clinical care. Kerr White would not compromise: "I said, 'Well, maybe so, but wouldn't it be nice, as Alice in Wonderland said, to do all this in writing and with figures; then we could be a little bit more certain about it.' But no, they wouldn't have any truck with this. I said, 'Well, that's too bad.' So we assessed the medical care in the outpatient department which we controlled. We found all kinds of loopholes: tests overlooked, things not followed up, neglect, omission, and other errors."

The problem was an uncritical acceptance of biomedical science as the only scientific basis for evaluating the benefits and risks of clinical practice, and it derived, White argues, from the historical dominance of laboratory science in hospitals. He notes:

The laboratory became the focus for research, and the laboratory moved into the hospital next to patients. Increasingly the laboratory became the principal source of information for purposes of diagnosis and the main source of understanding of the nature of disease. The population outside the hospital gradually was shifted aside, and observational methods went into disrepute. Now, after World War II, with the laboratories having produced sulfonamides and penicillin, this seemed the most promising way to go. It was quite reasonable; there are no villains in this thing! But it led to a narrow paradigm — diseases have single causes, and they are mostly "bugs." What I call the Big Bug Hunt was under way: we have got to look for bugs everywhere. Meanwhile, the hygienists who looked at the environment, including the social scene, poverty, economic conditions, and occupational hazards, were cast aside by the biomedical establishment.

In 1959, White went on sabbatical leave to the United Kingdom to work with Jerry Morris in the Medical Research Council's Social Medicine Research Unit at the London Hospital. He studied statistics and epidemiology at the London School of Hygiene and Tropical Medicine under Austin Bradford Hill and Richard Doll. White credits Morris with most of the ideas he pursued upon return to the United States (Morris 1957). He also found he had concerns similar to those of the British epidemiologists Archie Cochrane and Tom McKeown (Cochrane 1972; McKeown 1976). McKeown, he found, had also decided that clinical medicine was not achieving its potential and had turned to public health for a more critical perspective on medical care. White learned a great deal from the studies that Cochrane was conducting in Welsh mining valleys, including those of large populations, intensively examined, from which samples could be drawn for further research (see chapter 6). White concluded that epidemiological methods might be applied to the study of patient care to develop something called "medical care research." In the process of setting up these links in the United Kingdom, he became one of the conduits through which the ideas of the British epidemiologists were to flow to the United States.

When White returned to Chapel Hill, he found that the medical hierarchy still saw the future in laboratory research: "One day, after an unsatisfactory discussion with the acting head of the Department of Internal Medicine," he says, "I got really mad: 'These biomedical types just don't understand what the people's problems are!' I sat down, took the data from our patient referral study, data from censuses in the U.K. and U.S., and wrote our paper on the 'Ecology of Medical Care.'" In this 1961 paper, he and his coauthors analyzed the huge number of people in the community with symptoms, a large proportion of whom were treated in primary care; only one in a thousand adults reached one of the academic medical centers where most medical education was conducted. White was starting to conceptualize his "broader view of medicine." Like Feinstein, he recognized the need to analyze clinical care in all its subtle complexity. He too drew on a biological analogy, but, significantly, he speaks not of a "taxonomy" but an "ecology" of care. Traditional epidemiological methods were not adequate for this ecological task, according to White and colleagues: "The traditional indexes of the public's health, such as mortality and morbidity rates, are useful for defining patterns of ill-health and demographic characteristics of populations who experience specific diseases. They are of limited value in describing actions taken by individual patients and physicians about disease and other unclassified manifestations of ill health. It is the collective impact of these actions that largely determines the demand for and utilization of medical-care resources" (1961, p. 885).

What was needed, says White and colleagues, was an overview of the health of the community: "Each practitioner or administrator sees a biased sample of medical-care problems presented to him; rarely has any individual, specialty or institution a broad appreciation of the ecology of medical care that enables unique and frequently isolated contributions to be seen in relation to those of others and the over-all needs of the community" (1961, p. 886). Evaluating the quality of hospital care therefore required a focus on the place of hospitals in the health system as well as on the patients and the community from which they came. According to White, "Our approach had to be population-based if we were really going to find out what was going on for the whole population. We set about trying to find out how hospitals were linked to the population, and what the patients were like when they come into the hospital and when they left. It is only on that basis that we can really have comparisons among hospitals and populations. *There is no denominator otherwise*" (emphasis added).

White found that population-based surveys of issues such as the reasons for referral to hospitals had clinical significance. They provided clinicians with a more detailed understanding of problems of categorization or "labeling" and of problems of communication between patients and doctors and among doctors: "We studied a stratified random sample of physicians in North Carolina and their patients. We found that patients were frequently referred by their physicians for one reason while the patients thought they were being referred for a second reason. The students would identify a third problem; the intern would feel a nodule on the thyroid and say that that was the problem. And this would go on and on. There would be about four or five different agendas being pursued. There was total confusion." His views brought him up against intense opposition: "When proposing a population-based study of hospitals, for example, I was called before the local medical society and accused of trying to mount a communist plot! I said, 'Well, this idea comes from Florence Nightingale; it is not new with me, and she recommended the use of hospital discharge abstracts back in the 1860s.'"

Unlike some of the British epidemiologists whom White admired, he was not attracted to communism. His concern was the renaissance of the generalist working in "primary medical care." White believed that, in order to understand the phenomena of health, disease, and healing, researchers needed to draw on the full range of health-related disciplines, including the use of the quantitative methods of statistics and epidemiology, and the observational methods of the social sciences. The question of what to call such research was approached pragmatically: "One has to start where the profession and the people are," he notes. Thus he used the term *health services research* to describe efforts to improve identification, labeling, and measurement of patients presenting problems, and "outcomes research" to describe the evaluation of interventions designed to ameliorate these problems.

By 1964, at Johns Hopkins University, White was founding chair of what became the Department of Health Policy and Management in the School of Public Health. Among other initiatives, he attempted to bridge the gap between the medical school and the public health school "We had a hell of a time doing that," he says. "The two schools had different calendars, different parking lots, different secretarial salaries, and different times to start to work. I think we violated every rule in the book. But at Hopkins you can do that sort of thing; that is why Hopkins is such a remarkable place to work. They have only one rule that can't be broken and that is: 'There are no rules that can't be broken!'"

It was here, in the Clinical Scholars Program, that Suzanne Fletcher and Robert Fletcher met Kerr White the teacher. White's concern was to link the academic medical center to public health but also to encourage cooperation with other disciplines and other ways of thinking. One of his students at Johns Hopkins University was the radical physician-sociologist Vicente Navarro. White recalled with pride that the Marxist-oriented *International Journal of Health Services* was conceptualized in his department.

White, like Feinstein, accepted the need for using rigorous statistical methods, but he was also concerned with the use of epidemiology as a fundamental science for health services research (White et al. 1976). His major concern was the political realities of changing practice and changing health policy. While some of his colleagues continued to view his approach with considerable suspicion, the political context shifted and health services research became increasingly important to government and charitable institutions with an interest in health. According to White:

Of course in the sixties you had the Berkeley phenomenon and the free-speech initiatives; you had the uprisings of the blacks and the downtrodden. You had Mr. Nixon in charge, and I think that the major motivation of the government at that time was in containing costs. That was not my motivation. I didn't think that cost was basically the problem. I felt the problem was the medical profession's unnerving failure to respond to the people's needs: they were not responding to the needs of individual patients, on the one hand, or collectively to the needs of communities, on the other.

Determined to broaden the ideas and methods underlying clinical epidemiology and health services research, White moved to the position of deputy director for health sciences at the Rockefeller Foundation. After John Evans left McMaster University to become president of the University of Toronto in 1972, White asked Evans to conduct a review of schools of public health for the Rockefeller Foundation. His review concluded with "some endorsement" of clinical epidemiology (Evans 1981). Evans saw the commitment of the Rockefeller Foundation as encompassing research into major health problems but also the provision of "compassionate and efficient services" (Evans 1981). This was a supportive environment for implementing White's strategic plans. According to Evans, "The steam was there from the day Kerr White entered the doors." White's message was that something had to be done about the split between public health and medicine in order to bring the population perspective back into the heart of clinical medicine. Encouraged by Evans's accounts of the new medical school at McMaster University, White visited it and concluded that the schism could be alleviated by locating clinical epidemiology units in departments of medicine. After a slow beginning, the Rockefeller Foundation decided to throw its weight behind the new initiative.

White acquired some notoriety as a critic of public health and for favoring clinical epidemiology in recommendations for funding. His says that his criticism was aimed neither at public health itself, at the great bulk of faculty in the schools of public health, nor at the students. His target was the institutional format that isolated public health from medicine and that institutionalized the dominance of medicine. His preference was for broad-based schools of health sciences that would integrate the two. Failing that, clinical epidemiology had the potential for an integrative function. White had some difficulty with the term *clinical epidemiology* but used it for pragmatic reasons to reflect the aim of involving clinicians in the planned activities. As he explains it,

You had to have some kind of label, and we had to call it something. "Health of populations" was a bit confusing. "Public health" we didn't want — we wanted something broader, and that term would turn off the clinicians. We wanted the word *clinical* in our program because we wanted to appeal to clinicians. We wanted to train clinicians in the concepts and methods of epidemiology, the object of the exercise being twofold: One, we wanted to make them more critical of the interventions that they apply, questioning whether they did more good than harm. Two, we wanted to *take them gradually out into the community*. (Emphasis added.)

As part of the Rockefeller Foundation's response to international health concerns in 1978, White devised the International Clinical Epidemiology Network (INCLEN). Its aim was to support clinical epidemiology worldwide, especially in developing countries, by providing training and support to build up clinical epidemiology units in each participating medical school. Each unit would have a critical mass of clinical epidemiologists, together with statisticians, social scientists, and economists. Initially the Rockefeller Foundation funded three training programs: at McMaster University in Canada, at the University of Pennsylvania in the United States, and at the University of Newcastle in Australia; later the Universities of North Carolina and Toronto were added.

White was inspired by what he saw as "the sea change that swirls about us" (1988, p. 86) and by the dissatisfaction of some practitioners — especially general physicians — with the prevailing medical paradigm. His aim was to generate a dialogue among critics from various disciplines with a view to broadening the conceptual base of medicine. The directions he favored are evident in the summary of a meeting he recounts in *The Task of Medicine: Dialogue at Wickenburg* (1988). In the introduction to the volume, Alvin Tarlov, then president of the Kaiser Family Foundation, argues that improving health and enhancing the effectiveness of physicians require a "revised intellectual foundation for medicine" that recognizes the influence of social, cultural, and economic factors on health (White 1988, p. x). This echoes the social reformers of the last century. There was a plea for more attention to the phenomenology of illness (Schwartz and Wiggins 1988). Thus White saw the need for a rigorous scientific understanding of the communicative interaction between doctor and patient, contesting Feinstein's belief that clinical "soft" data of this kind should necessarily be quantified: "Not everything that is measured is important and not everything that is important can be measured" (1988, p. 16). White called for a paradigm of medicine, both scientific and humanistic, guided by a broad view of science characterized by a critical attitude rather than merely by quantitative precision and exactitude.

Conclusion

Suzanne Fletcher and Robert Fletcher saw the need for a new approach to clinical care and recognized that such change would need to involve clinicians. Their focus was on establishing the essential constituents of a scientific way of thinking about clinical care. The intellectual inspiration for their program came from a number of sources representing ideas current at the time. These sources represented considerable variety, but all provided broad and challenging approaches to research. Alvan Feinstein drew on his clinical commitment and on his mathematical skills to develop, first, a program for taxonomic study of clinical care, later extended into a formidable body of methodological work. He sought to devise a comprehensive set of methods for generating a science specific to clinical care. Henrik Wulff in Denmark emphasized the need for critique in addition to the search for a more scientific approach to research into clinical care. Wulff's model encompassed the early taxonomic work of Feinstein but, for Wulff, the new, additional science of clinical care was not enough. Clinicians also needed to understand how doctors and patients communicate about disease, and the ethical dimension of care. These were new uncertainties requiring new alliances with nonmedical disciplines.

Kerr White had an international perspective and pursued an eclectic research career in internal medicine. His broad program of research was more ecological than taxonomic. He saw clinical epidemiology not as a means to greater clinical certainty but as a means of healing the schism between clinical medicine and public health, and he was responsible for founding INCLEN.

There was clearly a need for an additional science specific to clinical care. These various intellectual strands served as sources of inspiration for the development of this science. One of the products of the interplay of these intellectual strands and circumstance was called clinical epidemiology. Not surprisingly, there was a variety of interpretations of what clinical epidemiology actually was. Clinical epidemiology was developed as a specific medical discipline at one center only. That was McMaster University in Canada.

Notes

1. Unless otherwise noted, all quotations come from personal interviews.

CHAPTER 3

The Discipline
of Clinical Epidemiology

By the 1970s, clinicians concerned about the uncertainties of clinical practice could draw on a number of different perspectives designed to address their specifically clinical concerns. The intellectual ideas and practical concerns that inspired the rise of clinical epidemiology had their most concrete effect at McMaster University in Canada, where clinical epidemiology emerged as a full-fledged discipline. John Evans and Fraser Mustard developed an innovative curriculum for the new medical school at the university and established the first Department of Clinical Epidemiology and Biostatistics. David Sackett, the department's first chair, gave clinical epidemiology an institutional base and developed its practical potential as an evaluative tool for clinical practice.

The model of clinical epidemiology institutionalized at McMaster University owed much to Feinstein's work. Feinstein's program focused on developing a range of methods to be used in the research process — and this was a considerable task. His aim was to improve patient care by these means. He paid little attention to the world outside of clinical research and to how the researchers using these methods would interact with the medical school, university, and health care system. In contrast, Kerr White focused on the difficulties of implementing change in existing academic structures. McMaster University started a new medical school, and the founders clearly saw this as an opportunity to introduce changes that might never see the light of day in established academic centers.

The advantage of studying the McMaster University model is that it permits identification of its original objectives and how it diversified over time. Successive leaders within the department have brought a variety of skills and talents to strengthen the department. Mike Gent, the second chair, was a statistician, and his appointment attests to the central role of statistics in the new department. George Torrance was an early recruit who helped develop a component of the research program to address evaluative processes involving health economics.

Central to the success of the new discipline were its methods of dissemination. A key initiative was locating one of the International Clinical Epidemiology Network (INCLEN) training programs at McMaster University. Given the differences between Canada and the less industrialized countries from which the INCLEN fellows were drawn, it is important to assess the relevance of the program in these settings. Arturo Morillo gives an account of the perhaps counterintuitive way in which clinical epidemiology was useful in bringing about change in Colombia.

McMaster University's model of clinical epidemiology is renowned for its articulate spokespeople and the quality of their research and methodological development. Their methods are persuasively presented in person to international audiences, but the McMaster University textbook, which sets out the basic principles of their approach to clinical epidemiology, has been another major means of communicating their ideas. Chapter 4 of this volume discusses the practitioners who carried the banner into the next stages of development as clinical epidemiology diversified, mutated into evidence-based medicine, and disseminated worldwide.

The Founders: John Evans and Fraser Mustard

John Evans of the University of Toronto was appointed as the first dean at the new medical school set up by McMaster University in the mid-1960s. Evans argues that the 1960s were characterized by prosperity and the belief that the burden of disease would be relieved by greater access to medical care. The latter required new medical schools and an enlarged medical workforce. Evans himself had trained in internal medicine and then in cardiology. At the University of Toronto, he became concerned about the direction of Canadian health care, particularly the lack of understanding of disease in the community and the decline of primary health care. Canada had before it the example of the United States. In Canada, primary health care was still valued, and there was, Evans believed, an opportunity to halt its decline. In 1964, Evans was part of a committee that proposed that the University of Toronto set up a training program to strengthen primary care: "We looked at patterns in the United States," he recalls, "and saw the progressive rush to specialization and the vacuum appearing at the primary care end. We saw the subdivision of primary care. We saw the patient really becoming the primary care triage person and selecting among specialists. We did an analysis and found that about 50 percent of our practitioners were still general practitioners in Canada. Instead of thinking about that as an embarrassment, maybe it was a resource. Maybe one ought to build on it."

Toronto University, he says, saw this proposal as "an unconscionable breach of academic faith." A year later the decision was taken to set up a new medical school at McMaster University. When Evans was appointed as dean, he had an unusual opportunity to implement his vision. He appreciated the need for good scientific clinical practice, but his focus was considerably broader and he presented it in simple language. His arguments were aimed not at patients but at primary care physicians, who were at risk of being excluded from the complex scientific deliberations of academic medicine. The fundamentals, Evans says, can be boiled down to common sense and "the kind of questions that you would ask about your garden": "First, you've got to know what the most important problems are, and secondly, you've got to make sure that your limited resources are being applied to the most important problems where you can make a difference or are likely to be able to make a difference. The third thing is, you had better check whether you are making a difference. So it isn't very complicated. But then, when you try and classify the research effort in relation to those three objectives, it is less than 5 percent."

Fraser Mustard was appointed as the chair of pathology six months after Evans's appointment. David Sackett refers to Mustard as "the platelet genius" in recognition of his pioneering biomedical research. But Mustard was also a committed clinician. At the University of Toronto, where he trained, he saw the culture of the physician as dominant in the medical system and as containing the notion of responsibility to society, but this culture was shifting. Driven by a belief in medical science and technology, medicine was losing a "sense of the human subject." Instead of finding refuge in the rewards of his laboratory research, Mustard turned his attention to medicine's overall lack of achievement. He says:

You cannot be trained as a health professional, particularly as a physician — if you are open and honest — and not understand the limits to medicine. And if you have a social conscience, the limits to medicine bother you. If you looked at the hard evidence as to why certain beliefs were there in medicine, you found that nobody ever sat down and asked the hard questions about what is the most appropriate way of doing things. It became pretty apparent that you had to have a better way to assess it than just simply the beliefs of physicians.

So, if you were going to start a new school, you wanted medicine to prepare physicians to fulfill their real role in society as caring professionals. You have to bring them up in a world which blunts their confidence and comfort in simply just mastering technology and applying it without any sense of what it's doing. It's extraordinarily wasteful. It's bad for patients. You know, I've always been antsy about even labeling people whose blood pressures are different from the so-called "normal" when I'm not sure what normal is. You only have to look at the labeling impact on people and what it does to their behavior to understand the importance of very critical assessment of procedures: to make sure they do more good than harm.

The new medical school could have provided a key setting for implementing a new program for the scientific study of clinical care. Evans and Mustard both had a clear focus on clinical care, but they included care in the community as part of their vision: the burden of disease in the city of Hamilton created the need for good primary care. The two men were disenchanted with public health, which they saw as moribund, but Evans wanted to teach public health skills and methods: "We decided, instead, that public health was everybody's business, and preventive strategies were everybody's business, rather than the terrain of a single department of a medical school, and that, indeed, it would be counterproductive to let everybody else off the hook by having a department for that area. So we said we would set up a department that deals with the skills and the methods."

Here Evans is echoing the much earlier views of John Paul, professor of preventive medicine at Yale University. It was Paul who first used the term *clinical epidemiology* (1938). He argued that disease rather than health was the motivating force for clinicians (Viseltear 1982a), and he advocated extracting from public health some of its methods, notably epidemiology, and incorporating these into medicine. Clinicians needed to use epidemiology, but only to the extent that they needed to know about the setting (family or community) in which the patient became sick. Thus clinical epidemiology would teach medical students about preventing as well as treating disease. He opposed setting up separate departments of preventive medicine, because, he argued, this would let internal medicine off the hook: it would then confine itself to therapy (Viseltear 1982b).

In Evans's vision, the new department would do research and act as a methodological resource for the whole medical school. In addition it would give family physicians the confidence to reason clinically and critically. According to Evans, they would learn to answer such questions as:

"How do you know what you are doing? What is the measurement? What is the burden of illness that is neglected? How many cases are there? You've seen Pap smears on twelve patients; how would you know how many you are missing? What would be the predictive factor? And so on." Even with these modest proposals, they were pushing against the dominant paradigm. Evans remarks:

When you talk to some people in the biomedical area, they say, "Well, that really isn't science!" These were people of goodwill, and bright and able people, but the blinkers had gone on in areas that were reductionist in nature, as opposed to population-based, expansionist, and multivariate. Eliminating variance was the goal, not entering into areas that had more variance.

At first, I must say, one personalized this and said, "These people are nerds, intellectually dull, they can't understand." But then the more you thought about it, the more you began to understand that there were very important fundamental differences in paradigms of thinking. To expect people to understand this and to be at ease with it was really the error, not faulting them for not understanding. And once one got that view, *it became a bit like spreading religion.* (Emphasis added.)

Evans was invoking an evangelical approach. He and Mustard needed a charismatic leader to preach their message and make converts, not in the populace but in academic medicine.

Prophet and Disciples: David Sackett and the McMaster Team

Under the guidance of Evans and Mustard, the McMaster University medical school set about creating what would become its trademark: a medical program based on self-learning, without examinations or grading, and on problem-based instruction conducted in small groups of students meeting with a tutor. The excitement of establishing a new and different medical school created a rare opportunity for trying out radical new ideas. David Sackett became its prophet.

Sackett believes that clinical epidemiology originated as a North American phenomenon because insightful individuals took advantage of a combination of circumstances. He credits Feinstein with doing the pioneering work, but this work was extended by keen young clinicians in Canada and the United States, of whom Sackett was one. Sackett was born in 1934 in Chicago, and he trained in internal medicine and nephrology at the University of Illinois College of Medicine. When he was drafted because of the Cuban missile crisis, he was placed in the U.S. Public Health Service. He was dismayed because he saw epidemiology and public health as boring and irrelevant, but it brought him into contact with some of the leading epidemiologists of the time, including Abraham Lilienfeld and Warren Winkelstein. They were all physicians who had moved into careers in public health, and they gave Sackett enormous encouragement. Alex Langmuir was most closely involved with the draftees:

> Alex Langmuir was just an outstanding charismatic sort of person. He took these very, very bright young clinicians, who didn't want to do epidemiology and biostatistics and [who] wanted to get back into clinical or research careers, and put them through a crash course in epidemiology as it applied to understanding disease outbreaks.

> I was in a terrible outfit called the Heart Disease Control Program, and most of its posts were awful. But I happened to have been assigned to an outstanding public health epidemiologist named Warren Winkelstein Jr., at the State University of New York, Buffalo, and had to start doing community surveys. I had to start learning epidemiology and biostatistics for the first time for these surveys. This was the fall of 1963. And in my despair, as I was reading through my clinical journals, I came across an article that was written by Alvan Feinstein, called "Boolean Algebra and Clinical Taxonomy." As only Alvan can do it!

For Sackett the only viable alternatives in medicine at the time were laboratory research or clinical medicine. This changed after he wrote what he calls a "fan letter to Feinstein" (2002). Feinstein invited him to the spring clinical meetings of the societies of academic internal medicine and also to join him at the Sydenham Society, which met the night before the clinical meetings. Feinstein explained that the society was named after Thomas Sydenham in recognition of the latter's attempts to assemble and analyze groups of individuals with common presentations, like gout. The aim of the Society was to focus on empirical patterns of disease and issues of prognosis and therapy. Sackett decided his future lay with intact patients, and he became coorganizer of the Sydenham Society with Feinstein and Tom Chalmers. He reviewed his career options:

> Towards the end of my two years in the Public Health Service, I became interested in whether you could work at the interface between clinical medicine and epidemiology and biostatistics. Although I recognized the enormous need for major public health activities and movements and pushes, I still regarded myself as a clinician, one-on-one. That's where I had the most enjoyment, and that's where I wanted to stay. It seemed to me that the laboratory work I was talking about doing, while it might be fascinating, had very low utility. Although it might help us to understand a bit more about how the kidney worked — and that is a fascinating organ — it lacked for me a relevance and an immediate payoff in terms of doing something for patients.

Sackett realized that he had to gain additional epidemiological skills for this task. With support under the GI "Bill of Rights," he went to the Harvard School of Public Health to develop these skills. Here Brian McMahon was his mentor. As Sackett recalls:

He said, "If I were you I wouldn't take any of the public health subjects, but I would take all the methods subjects. And then you might want to go across the river and do demography, and you might want to go to MIT and do some computers." He saw that I wanted to do public health, but that I wanted to do it in a medical school, not a school of public health, and he thought that that was the sort of thing which someone ought to do. He didn't want to do it himself. The careers of those epidemiologists were just like the careers of bench scientists: clinical practice interfered with their careers.

In 1967 Sackett was back at the State University of New York, Buffalo, establishing himself in the department of medicine. Evans and Mustard invited him to McMaster University for an interview. At that stage they were still of two minds about a public health department. Sackett recalls the interview as follows:

The first question was, "What sort of Department of Social, Community, and Preventive medicine should we have at this Medical School?" I said, "None." Unless the clinical departments each took on the aspects of social and community medicine that related to their disciplines, no one would pay any attention to it. The second question was, "Then what sort of course should we have in epidemiology and biostatistics?" Again I said, "None." Unless it was integrated with courses in pathophysiology and clinical skills, et cetera, it would be just as bad as it was everywhere else, and the students would hate it and the faculty would not enjoy it and it wouldn't work.

They mistook a novice for a sage and asked me to come and help them do this. We hit upon the idea that you might have a department that would be a resource, — that it might do some of its own research but also serve as a statistics and design resource for people doing bench research and animal research, that it could serve as a similar resource for people wanting to do studies on patients, and that it could serve as a similar resource for those in the clinical departments who were oriented towards social, community, and preventive medicine and might be wanting to do health care research and public health research.

Evans and Mustard were persuaded that David Sackett was energetic, enthusiastic, and innovative. McMaster University appointed him to chair the Department of Clinical Epidemiology and Biostatistics.

Sackett was warily treading a path through the maze of academic medicine, alert to the political pitfalls of alliances. He would not align himself with public health, nor would he engage with patients in community settings. What he did was align the new department with clinicians in the academic faculties, borrowing methods from public health and using these in such a way that he was able to forge an alliance with dominant laboratory research. From the outset, one focus of the department was therefore inward, toward clinical medicine, introducing clinicians to the methodological tools of public health in order to apply them to clinical questions. It is this aim that Sackett defined as clinical epidemiology: "the application, by a physician who provides direct patient care, of epidemiologic and biometric methods to the study of diagnostic and therapeutic process in order to effect an improvement in health" (1969, p. 125). Sackett later extended the definition to include all clinicians. The other focus of the department was still community care, reflecting Evans's concerns. Sackett turned away from the "external public health orientation," but the department did offer methodological support to encourage clinicians in the community to conduct their own research (Sackett 2002, p. 1162).

The relationship of the new discipline to public health epidemiology was an issue for debate. In 1968, in the first of his series of papers on clinical epidemiology in the *Annals of Internal Medicine,* Feinstein describes clinical epidemiology as including "the occurrence rates and geographic distribution of disease; the patterns of natural and post-therapeutic events that constitute varying clinical courses in the diverse spectrum of disease; and the clinical appraisal of therapy." Sackett describes these as including "elements of 'big E' epidemiology and public health," merely enlarged to include clinical decision making (2002, p. 1162). In Feinstein's view, Sackett was the one who remained too close to the public health origins of the methods he proposed to use. Says Feinstein:

And what is fascinating, if you have read those papers — I mean if you are actually doing more than just traveling around gathering tape recordings and have actually read those papers — what Sackett proposed and what I proposed were utterly different, completely different. I was proposing a *specific intellectual domain* and trying to define its contents and challenges with clinical people. What Sackett proposed was that clinical epidemiology was classic public health epidemiology done by someone who happened to be a clinician. I thought that was idiotic. Nevertheless, he had used exactly the same title that I had, and Sackett and I somewhere met, having realized that we were both poaching in the same turf.

Faced with such differences, the McMaster University department invited Feinstein to visit them in Canada. Sackett recalls:

And we got into a big fight, as everyone does who works with Alvan. Towards the end of the fight, I can remember we were sitting in my MG, outside the motel at about two A.M., and I said to him, "If you're so damn smart, why don't you come up and teach us how to do research better?" And he said to me, "If you're so damn rich, why don't you pay me?" The Canadian federal government provided the funds for two years, 1971–73, making an enormous difference. Feinstein set up the program for continuing education in methodology for people in the department and just pushed us and cajoled us and harassed us, and then helped us put much more science into the sorts of studies which we were then beginning to do.

Continuing education remains an important feature of the department, and the clinical epidemiologists honor the requirement that they remain active, part time, in clinical practice.

The McMaster University model spread, in part because Sackett traveled the world, spreading the word in workshops and lectures. Six years after the McMaster University program started, the University of North Carolina started a similar program; other centers followed. The ideas proliferated, Evans argues, as a result of the same "concatenation of events" that precipitated the McMaster University department: the need to get public health skills and methods incorporated into all departments of the medical school. Sackett adds, "Then it became apparent to the most powerful people at most medical schools, namely chairmen in departments of medicine, that clinical epidemiology would allow them to do exciting stuff, build up their departments, get interesting things going. And also, increasingly, being able to justify themselves to the public, to their universities, and to funding agencies as doing things with direct payoff to patients." Sackett points out that, in the United States, clinical epidemiology was taken over as the scientific discipline of general internal medicine that, in the United States, is a combination of primary and secondary care. This gave it a prominence it otherwise would not have had. In addition, training programs proliferated, providing training in clinical epidemiology and biostatistics to supplement clinical training. These were funded by the Robert Wood Johnson Clinical Scholars Program, the Kaiser Family Foundation, and the Milbank Memorial Fund.

Summarizing the activities at McMaster University at this time, Sackett says, "A group of us came here in the late sixties, rebels with a cause. We set this thing up. We said, 'We know a lot of stuff about medical education (we think it's crap) and we ain't going to do any of that.' We had an idea about how it might work. We got it all done." This statement ignores the careful planning that went into recruitment. Sackett's first aim was to establish biostatistics in the department. The first three members of staff appointed were a computer analyst and the statisticians Mike Gent and Charles Goldsmith.

MICHAEL GENT AND CHARLES GOLDSMITH

Mike Gent was born and educated in the United Kingdom. In 1969 he was senior lecturer in statistics at Bradford University, when he decided to move to McMaster University: "The single thing that moved me here was Sackett. I couldn't believe Sackett! He actually interviewed me lying on one elbow on the floor. He had outrageous ideas, half of which would never work, but if only 10 percent worked it would be fantastic. All the concepts about clinical epidemiology were there, including getting together a group that was really going to shape the thinking of medical colleagues."

Charles Goldsmith, born in Manitoba, did his postgraduate training at North Carolina State University. His work on experimental design included pioneering work on multivariate analysis, an increasingly important tool for handling the complexities of clinical research. He too was impressed with the opportunities presented by the new medical school. Together with Mike Gent, he developed the new department's biostatistics courses. In order to model the wide range of variables encountered in health care, they needed a good computer, and this was one of the first major purchases of the department. Goldsmith recalls, "We had an IBM 101, a machine in which you had to wire the board so that it would add up a column of numbers and put a total at the bottom of it! You had to feed cards in on one side. We had one of the few rooms that had air conditioning, because this machine had to have a stable temperature."

Both were excited by the opportunity to be part of what was emerging as central to Sackett's vision for the department: a collaborative team. Gent notes, "Most statisticians try to change your problem to one that fits into their formulae. What we were doing was shaping people's thinking a little bit, bringing a fresh perspective, shaping your own ideas a little bit more." With the methodological skills in place, the department needed support from clinical faculty. The team approach needed close collaboration with and integration with clinical departments. The chair of medicine at the time was Jack Hirsh. Says Gent, "He came along and said, 'Do a few sums for me.' I did. And then we started doing a few things together; then we started going off to meetings together. He was learning a little bit more about the way in which I think, and I was learning a little bit more about biological issues and the problems he was working on." Gent and Hirsh developed a relationship in which "Jack and I can just fire off at each other," but Hirsh came to play a centrally important role as clinical mentor to new members of the department.

JACK HIRSH

Jack Hirsh trained as a hematologist in Melbourne, Australia. His research focused on thrombosis, coagulation, and the function of blood platelets. Further training in the United Kingdom, Canada, and the United States turned out a product characteristic of academic medicine in the 1960s: a clinician who was also trained in experimental pathology and biochemistry. When he returned to Australia for three years, he changed the direction of his research to focus on the clinical management of thrombosis. In keeping with the clinical research of the late 1960s, the research was mainly descriptive, with rudimentary attempts at randomized clinical trials. He was then recruited to the newly established McMaster University, where his research focused on the important clinical problems of venous thrombosis and pulmonary embolism, including its diagnosis, prevention, and treatment using anticoagulants and thrombolytic (clot-dissolving) agents. When he went to McMaster University for his interview at the invitation of the founding professor of medicine, E. J. Moran Campbell, he also met with John Evans, David Sackett, and Fraser Mustard. Hirsh was swept away by their enthusiasm and creativity and decided to join these "crazy, maverick, exciting people" setting up the new medical school.

Hirsh continued to study unresolved problems in clinical thromboembolism both in the clinic and in the laboratory. When he presented the study design of his work evaluating optimal heparin doses in the treatment of venous thrombosis to the department in 1970, David Sackett and the other members roundly criticized the study design. Hirsh recalls:

They said it was the wrong design. I was really upset. Where they fell down was that they could have told me what the right design was and how to perform the study. They were showing off. At that stage, no one was doing the correct studies, and I thought they were just using words that they didn't even understand. So it was somewhat intimidating. But anyway, we did the study (and it turned out to be quite revolutionary and still sets the standard for current practice in 2002). Some time later, I presented the results of the study at their regular weekly meeting. They were quite impressed, but I remember Alvan Feinstein saying that the tables were presented in the wrong way. I didn't know what he was talking about. Once again they did not explain it. At that time the clinical epidemiologists were an exclusive, rather arrogant group.

In a move that was to become characteristic of his operating style, Sackett went with Gent to visit Hirsh in his laboratory to explore the possibility of cooperative work. So persuasive were they that Hirsh became a student again and enrolled in the department's master's course in 1975. Convinced that clinical epidemiology presented a complementary activity to basic science for the training of medical practitioners and researchers, Hirsh started teaching in the department.

The lasting research relationship within the new department between Gent, methodologist and statistician, and Hirsh, the clinician-researcher, is testimony to the sustained team approach. They have worked together for decades on research in which either Hirsh or Gent could be principal investigator. Says Gent, "I don't try to replace Hirsh; I couldn't. I can't see patients; I'm not a physician. But I have come to know a bit about the biology and what he's doing. I know a fair bit about the clinical problems like stroke and heart attacks. I can use their language; I can understand everything they say. What you're trying to do is to communicate information, but you have to develop knowledge and a language base, which makes communication so much better."

Gent and Hirsh went on to found the Henderson Research Centre, with its commitment to large clinical trials and basic science research. The center, has four programs and a staff of over 150 people. Charles Goldsmith continued to do collaborative work in the department, including work with a group of surgeons to develop a series of articles on evidence-based surgery.

The fact that Gent, the biostatistician, became the second chair of the department, in 1973, was a tribute to the growing multidisciplinary nature of the department. The target for the departmental activities was changing, as Sackett explains: "The initial targets for research were other clinicians, so we drew on the best clinical medicine, epidemiology, and biostats to generate results that we saw as referable to frontline clinical medicine. Some results immediately got applied and some didn't. The problem, we were told, was, 'We are unable to put you guys' work into terms which could be understood by administrators, hospital boards, the sorts of folks that have to free up resources.'" Their response was to diversify further.

GEORGE TORRANCE

One of Sackett's recruits was, at first sight, quite startling for a medical department. George Torrance was an engineer doing operations research and teaching in McMaster University's business school. In the late 1960s he enrolled as a doctoral student with Warren Thomas, chair of the Department of Industrial Engineering at the State University of New York in Buffalo. He was investigating a dissertation topic related to manufacturing methods, inventory control, and production line scheduling when Warren Thomas suggested that he talk to Sackett, whom Thomas had met during Sackett's time in Buffalo. Torrance went to see Sackett "out of courtesy to Warren." Torrance recalls, "I was just blown away by a whirlwind of creativity and ideas, energy and enthusiasm. We talked about decision making in the health care system, and I was amazed to find that they did not have a systematic way to evaluate what they were doing, to determine if they were doing more good than harm, if things were being done cost-effectively, if they were allocating resources in the best way, if they were getting the most health benefit for the resources at their disposal."

Sackett's focus was shifting from investigating individual clinical practice to health care in general, including health policy. If interventions could be compared in terms of their effect on mortality and morbidity as well as their costs, this was clearly going to be useful to health policy makers, and this, in turn, would earn additional credits for the new department. The problem was that health economists were still primarily concerned with large-scale health economic problems such as hospital funding and taxation. Torrance was persuaded that his dissertation should focus on health services at the level of the intervention itself, a view strengthened after a one-week course in health services research with Kerr White at Johns Hopkins University. His dissertation, presented in 1970, developed the method of cost utility analysis — although, in the thesis, he called it "generalized cost-effectiveness analysis" — and further developed the method of cost-effectiveness analysis. These remain the basic methods of health economic evaluation. In this way, George Torrance, the engineer–operations researcher, became the pioneer of health economic evaluation. It is now a burgeoning international field.

Torrance's work turned out to be critically important in the department that he joined formally only in 1989, after early retirement from the business school. Clinical epidemiologists needed to measure the health outcomes of interventions as endpoints for trials, but this task turned out to be so difficult that it limited the use of trial methods. If an intervention saved lives in comparison with a control group, measurement was relatively straightforward. Most medical interventions, however, only reduce morbidity, and not all patients show the same improvement in health. Clinicians could describe the changes in health state expected from interventions — for example, reduction of pain or increased mobility. The economist's contribution was to attach a value to these outcomes.

Torrance obtained brief scenarios from clinicians of the various health states that could result from an intervention. He then applied decision theory and utility theory to methods for measuring the value attached to each health state (its utility). His teaching commitments in the business school gave him the opportunity to try out his theories on these students. He asked his students to indicate what risk of death they would be willing to take to avoid a particular bad outcome. This was the first use of the standard gamble in health (Torrance et al. 1972). He also asked them to indicate how much time they would be willing to give up at the end of their life in order to avoid a lifetime in a particular bad health state. Thus was born time trade-off, one of the methods for measuring the utility or worth that the public attaches to a given health state (Torrance et al. 1972; 1982; Torrance 1976). Torrance recalls:

I had given my students a number of health states, and I'd asked them to rate the degree of dis-utility — that is, the degree of badness associated with these health states. And I remember there was one quite bright student in the class who was kind of argumentative and very thoughtful, and he kept struggling with this. He kept saying, "What do you mean, how can I know, how am I to feel what it is I'm rating? How do I know one thing is twice as bad as something else?" So we got into a discussion in class, and somebody — I think it might have been him — said, "Well, if it's twice as bad, then I should be willing to spend only half as much time in that one as the other one." And I said, "Yeah, I think that is a helpful way for you to get your mind around it. Think about how much time you would trade off from one to the other." The whole class agreed.

At the heart of his methods, Torrance says, are simple processes: "I keep counting people and adding them up." Torrance's emphasis on measurement of health outcomes from interventions is what makes his work highly compatible with the McMaster University approach, but what marks his work as exceptional is the careful attention to what is measured. When working on a trial of neonatal intensive care, George Torrance became concerned that some of the children whose lives were saved by the intervention, especially those with very low birth weights, had such serious chronic health problems that the public scored their health states as worse than death. Clearly, the outcome measure of lives saved should allow for the quality of the life saved (or its utility). By 1970, there were a number of other economists in the United States and Britain who, with Torrance, were measuring health outcomes in terms of their equivalent in years of healthy life (Bush et al. 1972). This measure became known as the quality-adjusted life year (QALY). It then became a relatively simple task to calculate the cost per quality-adjusted life year gained from a procedure. In the case of neonatal intensive care, this showed that, for infants with very low birth weight (below one thousand grams), the net economic cost per quality-adjusted life year gained was 17.5 times higher than that for infants with slightly higher birth weights (one thousand to fifteen thousand grams; Boyle et al. 1983).

Such rigorous measures of health outcome were time-consuming, especially if they were specific to a particular intervention. Multi-attribute scales of health sought to overcome this problem by developing measures that could be applied across a wide range of interventions with different health outcomes. This approach defined the fundamental attributes of health (physical function, role function, social-emotional function, and health problem) and used these to define a health state for which the utility could then be calculated (Torrance et al. 1982). The utility is the value of that particular health state. This, in turn, is used as the quality weight to determine quality-adjusted life years for use in comparing health interventions and, particularly, for use in cost-utility analyses.

These universal health-outcome measures were compatible with the research directions of the department. It was also central to research about the broader issues of resource allocation in health care. At the simplest level, they could now assess whether funding "more community nurses on scooters" was going to be more worthwhile than funding new diagnostic technologies in hospitals. Part of the reason for the increased emphasis on this kind of evaluation was the looming problem of rising health care costs. Says Torrance, "I think the other part of it was probably the beginning of the funding problems, funding crises, budget crunch, and so on, where people were starting to look more critically at what is done in the health care system: what we can afford to do and how we can sort out what is really very valuable and what is quite marginal."

Later, as part of the Centre for Health Economics and Policy Analysis in the department, Torrance turned to critical reassessment of the field, including problems of equity. The basis of utility measurement is that people are the best judges of their own welfare, but it is unclear whether patients or the community should make this judgment and who is to make the judgment on behalf of the mentally ill, the old, and children, groups at risk of being disenfranchised. It is difficult to factor in the potential of a life lost when evaluating alternative scenarios for the outcome of interventions like abortion following fetal screening programs.

There is also the difficulty of knowing what is a fair distribution of health resources. Torrance asks, "How can we measure if we are now more fair than we were before, if this particular allocation of resources is more fair, more equitable, and therefore better for us to do? If we can answer that, then we know how to do resource allocation. I think that what everybody is realizing is that all these different approaches we have been using have got sort of hidden equity statements which have never been very well articulated, laid out on the table, and compared to each other." The problem of measuring "more abstract concepts of a community's sense of itself, its healthiness as a community" is more difficult and, at present, "just not in our concept."

PETER TUGWELL

Under the influence of a diversified team, the department grew rapidly and generated a multimillion-dollar research program. This program started recruiting graduates from the university's undergraduate program. In addition, it provided a home for a steady stream of what Sackett refers to as "brilliant young minds" that had been radicalized during the protest movements of the late 1960s. What Sackett was interested in was their capacity to think critically about clinical medicine rather than about issues in the community. Says Sackett, "That was also a time when medical students, although not central to this movement, were clearly affected by it and began to concern themselves about issues outside their own narrow professional interests. They therefore began to turn away from traditional academic medical careers in which their research would necessarily be at the bench. They were beginning to see that as insufficient, or inadequate, or inimical to what they wanted to do. So these were very, very bright, very effective folks who were really raising very serious questions about the role of medicine and about traditional medical education."

Under Sackett's charismatic leadership, they were forged into a group of committed disciples who further promoted the Sackett vision of clinical epidemiology. Sackett is lavish in his praise of their "breathtaking" pioneering achievements (see chapter 4). One of these new recruits was Peter Tugwell. He was to become the third chair of the McMaster University department. As chair, he took the department in new directions, strengthening its position by making it one of the training centers of INCLEN funded by the Rockefeller Foundation and taking on the training of students from less industrialized countries. He also negotiated the difficult and controversial link with health economics.

Peter Tugwell came to McMaster University by a circuitous route. He grew up in the United Kingdom and received his medical training at London University. He then spent some years in Nigeria, where he became interested in doing clinical research. Here, in 1974, he first heard visitors from McMaster University talking about an unusual curriculum with problem-based teaching in small groups. After returning to the United Kingdom, he explored opportunities for doing research into the relationship between clinical problems and the health needs of populations. This implied an epidemiological focus, so he went to talk to Jerry Morris at the London School of Hygiene and Tropical Medicine about health services research. Tugwell remembers:

He told me it was amoral to combine seeing patients with being involved in epidemiology where you are looking at populations. He said I had to make a decision; he just didn't believe you could change hats. He said, "You will not be able to be true to yourself in the clinical environment, in talking to a patient, when you know from a population perspective that they shouldn't be availing themselves of high technology and various other resources — in terms of the greatest good for the greatest number and the kinds of decisions you should be making as an epidemiologist." It just rocked me back on my heels!

Discouraged, he decided to train as a rheumatologist at McMaster University. On his first day there he was converted: "There was this big guy with this white beard, a bit weird, in shorts and a long white coat, and it looked as if he was wearing nothing underneath! He picked up my English accent, and he came across and was his usual friendly self. I said I was going into private practice as a rheumatologist, and he was polite about that. He said he was doing clinical epidemiology, and I said, 'What is that?' By the end of lunch, he had got me to agree to take his master's course."

This was David Sackett. He persuaded Peter Tugwell that clinical epidemiology combined clinical and epidemiological thinking. After Tugwell completed the master's course in 1977, he joined the department but continued working half-time in rheumatology. Two years later Sackett suggested Tugwell as the new chair of the department: "Another of his wild ideas!" says Tugwell. "But he gave me fantastic support throughout."

Tugwell was interested in quality-of-life measurements, and early research involved a pilot study in which all conversations with heart attack patients were audiotaped from the point of entry to the hospital, through the clinical process, and after their return home. It became clear that medical records did not capture the factors that determine whether a patient does well or badly after a heart attack. The analysis of the tapes, however, turned out to be complicated and expensive, requiring a research team to contribute the necessary analytical skills. The alternative approach was the one promoted in the department: to conduct studies using the randomized controlled trial, a method with established processes and proven reliability.

The department's reputation spread. John Evans was researching a report that would be published in 1981 by the Rockefeller Foundation: *Measurement and Management in Medicine and Health Services: Training Needs and Opportunities.* He drew the foundation's attention to the potential of clinical epidemiology to strengthen research in medical schools. Kerr White, deputy director for health sciences at the foundation, took his own direction, changed the focus to students from the developing world, and started negotiations with Peter Tugwell. Recalling White, Tugwell says:

> He came from the public health, population health perspective but he was obviously quite intrigued with what was going on at Mc. He said he would like to support a program. So he went away and called us up a couple of months later, saying he'd got a little bit of money out of the Rockefeller Foundation. He wondered if we would take some international students for six months and train them in clinical epidemiology. We said we would be very interested in taking them, but we were not prepared to do it for six months because, if Canadians took a minimum of one year, maybe two, we didn't think it was fair to people doing it in six months, with the culture shock, et cetera.

Tugwell had in mind an initial small enrolment, but White wrote to medical schools throughout the world listed by the World Health Organization, inviting senior medical academics to a conference to discuss how clinical epidemiology might be developed at their medical schools. Two hundred applied, fifty were chosen. They were "locked up" for a week at Cambridge University (U.K.), where they were trained in critical appraisal by David Sackett, Peter Tugwell, and Mike Gent and persuaded to develop clinical epidemiology in their medical schools. In return, they were asked to identify promising young people for the McMaster University program. Seven from seven different sites were chosen for the first intake. This was the start of the INCLEN program.

As part of the INCLEN initiative, White wanted the department to provide more public health epidemiology as well as health economics and policy. In 1984, a departmental review found "a superb department with problems resulting from its too-narrow mission," and with epidemiologists, economists, and biostatisticians expected to serve the needs of the clinical epidemiologists and to conduct randomized controlled trials.[1] These were some of the stimulants that lead to changes in the department. Introducing classical epidemiology created some resistance, since it took the focus of the department away from the clinical interface. Allowing an independent research role for health economics and policy studies was challenging. Economists had proved their worth in developing methods for assessing the cost-effectiveness of care. Quite another matter was the role of economics as a social science. Addressing policy issues like resource allocation in health care was even more unfamiliar. Tugwell's lasting achievement in ten years as chair of the department was that he steered the department through these changes, creating a more diversified but still highly productive team of researchers. In recognition of these skills, Alvan Feinstein describes him as a "supreme manipulator and a wonderful politician."

In parallel with these activities, Tugwell worked with George Torrance and Katherine Bennett to develop utility measures of health-related quality of life in rheumatoid arthritis (Bennett et al. 1991), and then used quality-of-life measures to estimate the effect of arthritis on population health (Tugwell et al. 1993). This work was anchored by always "going back to the patient." At the end of his term as chair, he moved to become chair of the Department of Medicine at the University of Ottawa. Here he encountered real resistance to this outcome-centered approach from clinicians, one of whom complained to him, "Outcomes, outcomes, outcomes! God damn it, you guys, all you want to talk about is outcomes. We spend more time looking at outcomes than we are treating bloody patients!" The challenge, as Tugwell saw it, was to persuade colleagues that the measurement of outcomes was one step along the way to studies that could ultimately lead to patient benefit.

Disseminating the Model I:
INCLEN and Arturo Morillo

The McMaster University model of clinical epidemiology seemed, at this time, to be spreading by osmosis to any area where it was needed. This model was developed in an advanced economy, but it was seen as also relevant to less industrialized countries. Sackett's leadership attracted medical rebels, but it was not yet clear what their cause was to be. My interviews with the "brilliant young minds" recruited by Sackett (see chapter 4) show that they were attracted to the discipline because it was iconoclastic: it allowed them a way of questioning the pervasive authority of leading clinical teachers. Certainly, this was relevant to less industrialized countries, where clinical teachers trained in Europe or the United States could exercise considerable clinical power. INCLEN was set up to disseminate clinical epidemiology internationally. But how did it fare?

Arturo Morillo was executive director of the INCLEN program from 1991 to 1996. He was located at the University of Pennsylvania, which ran one of the INCLEN programs. His saw clearly the difficulties of implementing White's vision in the setting of a less industrialized country. Morillo came from Colombia but worked for many years at the National Institutes of Health in the United States doing experimental physiology. When he returned to Colombia in the 1960s, he found that some of his colleagues exerted a strong influence on health policy and stimulated research, but medicine was dominated by private practice:

The country was following a French tradition. Our traditional professors went to Paris, and they came back very elegant, with a dictator kind of power, all important, walking along with everyone behind. The professor would come three times a week, eight o'clock in the morning, go to the ward and say, "Is there anything interesting here?" "Interesting" would be the case you would probably never see again. He would pronounce, impress the people with how clever he was. The next Wednesday he would come again: "Is there anything wrong here?" Forget about what happened to the last man! He would make a long speech about the twenty-five possible diagnoses — he was so erudite; he knew everything. He would not have anything to say about what was actually happening in Colombia. And then, when the university was founded, they said, "This is a famous clinician; this is the professor." But, of course, they were not interested in any research. They would say what they saw in France and keep repeating that. Some would come with new treatments from France to put into practice there. So the famous doctors of our old generations were famous because they first brought the treatments or the surgery from France.

Public health epidemiology was in disrepute because of the tension between clinicians and public health doctors trained at Johns Hopkins University, at Harvard University, at the London School of Hygiene and Tropical Medicine, and in Chile. Says Morillo, "They were talking to the Ministry of Health but not to the school of medicine. They were making the whole health policy of the country, setting priorities. We must vaccinate, garbage disposal, and so on. The medical profession was not prepared to think of itself as having that responsibility."

There was no tradition of research. As professor of physiology at Pontifica Universidad Javeriana, Morillo decided to put his efforts into training students to recognize the importance of research. As a first step he had to break down their confidence in the authority of their professors trained at prestigious foreign universities. Morillo recalls, "I used to keep challenging the students, trying to make them realize that what they were expecting from the class was wrong. I said, 'Listen, if I tell you what the books are telling now, or the journals, I give you the impression that this is *the* knowledge, forever. And I want you to realize the knowledge in science has a determinate kind of life expectancy. Like a radioactive material, it fades out eventually. Listen, ask questions, don't believe anything that the books are telling you. Try to do experiments.'"

These ideas were also put to use in a journal club, the aim of which was critical presentation of selected articles from medical journals. In a bookshop he discovered a little green book, the text by Fletcher and colleagues, *Clinical Epidemiology: The Essentials*. It gave Morillo a name and a focus for his efforts. In contrast with the Feinstein and Sackett approaches, and in agreement with White, he saw it as a way of instituting a critical approach to clinical care. Once this first step was taken, it might be possible to lead students back into questions about the community. Morillo recalls his thoughts at the time: "This is what I have been missing. We need to get people into clinical epidemiology! Let us, at least in this university, try to see if we can guide the people with a different approach: they have to do research to increase their knowledge, they have to do research into the people they have to serve, they are not to think anymore as a doctor who is going out into private practice."

In 1984, representatives from the Rockefeller Foundation came to the university, and Morillo was introduced to them: "And they came to tell the people what clinical epidemiology was. I suppose they were surprised that somebody already had some idea. So later came a letter to the university from the Rockefeller Foundation to say could they be involved in this program." The foundation proposed setting up a clinical epidemiology unit of six clinical epidemiologists and one biostatistician, later to be joined by a social scientist and an economist. These individuals would be trained to apply the methods of clinical epidemiology in clinical and teaching work. Their influence would change clinicians' attitudes to research and promote a new philosophy of medical care. Morillo already knew who the candidates should be: aggressive, intelligent, well-prepared, and academically respected young clinicians from a range of departments. They went for training to Pennsylvania, North Carolina, and McMaster, and to Newcastle in Australia. On their return they were located in the clinical epidemiology unit, attached to the dean's office, at Pontifica Universidad

Javeriana. The university strongly supported this program, ensuring the success of a unit equipped with computers, fax, e-mail and other facilities paid for jointly by the university and the Rockefeller Foundation. Morillo became dean. Suddenly he had a journal club of the sort he had always wanted, one engaged in critical appraisal of the literature and the development of shared research interests.

Gradually, from this small start, he saw change being effected in medical training. Attitudes to medical authority changed as students started asking their teachers, respectfully, "Why are you doing this with this patient? What is the evidence you have for this?" With about half to two-thirds of medical training based on clinical epidemiology, the aim was to reinforce the clinical abilities of students to make them less dependent on medical technologies that tie them to practice in cities. This training made them susceptible to arguments about the significance of community efforts. Morillo recalls:

I said to a [specialist]: "I cannot believe that an intelligent person like you would want to set up a large emergency room for trauma because trauma has increased so much in the city, and training more and more people in traumatology, when you should be trying to find out why the people are coming with so much trauma, and trying to find out how to decrease the trauma." "But I am not a public health man!" I said, "You are a public health man, and sooner or later you will discover that you are responsible for that. You are not going to tell me that, because the people are consuming more and more cocaine, you are going to solve the problem just by discovering how to treat the addict. You have to discover [how] to get the people not to get addicted." So this is the fight. They are the product of the education they receive. Through continuous education, the fellows in clinical epidemiology realize that they have a social responsibility that goes beyond the personal relationship with the patient looking for their service. They are making a difference, and they are influencing health policies, research, and training.

Morillo accepted that fellows trained in clinical epidemiology should do what might be seen as esoteric research with little direct relevance to community health. However, in his view, change comes through the gradual evolution of new practice and not by brute effort, a lesson he learned many years earlier as a rural doctor. As Morillo tells it:

I was young and enthusiastic. I had this project of having the campesinos build latrines. I was fighting with them; they did not want to build them. This was a coffee-growing country where you had this worm in the foot which produces anemia. So I was teaching them how to build them; I was very strong! Finally I got almost all the guys of the region, and we had a meeting with the leaders. And they said, "You know, Arturo, you are a fool!" "Why?" "You are happy because we have built the latrine. You could oblige us to build that, but you can never oblige us to use it." I was fighting the social issues behind it, the values, the strategies. So, was I a failure or a success?

Disseminating the Model II: The Textbooks

Arturo Morillo's account bears witness to the importance of textbooks in preparing the ground into which clinical epidemiology could then be transplanted. There is still sustained interest in the textbooks written by Fletcher, Fletcher, and Wagner (1982) and Wulff (1976). The textbook written by members of the McMaster University department similarly became a classic text. It captures the essence of their approach. *Clinical Epidemiology: A Basic Science for Clinical Medicine* (Sackett, Haynes, and Tugwell 1985; Sackett, Haynes, Guyatt, and Tugwell 1991) is a commonsense, accessible discussion of the scientific principles underlying clinical medicine. It addresses the clinical processes of diagnosis and management, presenting a critical, science-based approach to the techniques of patient care. Reflecting the emphasis in the department on techniques of critical appraisal, the book devotes a section to methods for a clinician to use when critically assessing the medical literature and then applying this evidence directly to clinical problems at the bedside. This extension of critical appraisal to the bedside has subsequently been substantially elaborated under the rubric of "evidence-based medicine." However, as is characteristic of most of those who call themselves clinical epidemiologists, the emphasis is on scientific rationality: understanding clinical processes, critically evaluating the evidence, and applying it to clinical decision making. The expectation is that this rational process will override the largely unconscious way that expert clinicians would otherwise make their decisions about diagnosis and treatment. Thus clinical intuition associated with the art of medicine will be made rational. As noted in the textbook:

Our underlying assumption, once again, is that medicine is rational and so are you. That is, your clinical acts of diagnosis and management reflect your assessment of the evidence that this or that diagnostic test is valid and will do more good than harm. If this view of clinical practice is correct, then you should constantly be seeking evidence, not just conclusions or, worse still, authoritarian opinions. Just as your ability to achieve accurate diagnosis and efficacious therapy determines your clinical effectiveness today, it is your skills in self-assessment and in tracking down and assessing biomedical knowledge (most of which resides in the journals) that will more and more determine your clinical effectiveness tomorrow. (Sackett, Haynes, and Tugwell 1985, p. 246)

The focus is on comparative studies to measure the accuracy of a diagnostic test, cohort studies to establish prognosis and case-control studies to determine the risk inherent in an intervention. The randomized controlled trial is presented as the best method for comparing the effectiveness of interventions in achieving a specified health outcome. From such studies, clinicians learn about the probability that an intervention will achieve its purpose. The apparent advantage is that they know what is likely to happen with a particular patient without needing to go into the fine detail of Feinstein's program based on the use of a clinical taxonomy and specifically clinical models in analyzing the case of each individual patient. The Feinstein agenda did, however, contribute ways of measuring specifically clinical outcomes for these comparative studies.

The use of probabilistic reasoning to improve diagnostic decisions is an important feature of the McMaster University text. Approximately one-quarter of the book is devoted to the application of Bayes' theorem, named after Thomas Bayes, an English clergyman and mathematician of the eighteenth century. In simple terms, Bayes' theorem is a mathematical model, technically no more than a formula for transposing conditional probabilities. In clinical decision making, the theorem provides an estimate of the probability of a particular diagnosis based on a given sign, symptom, or test result, by making allowance for how common that disease is in the population from which the patient is drawn (Last 1995). In the McMaster text, it serves as one of the cornerstones of thinking about clinical evidence, providing insight into important clinical errors such as false-positive or false-negative results.

An example of the value of Bayesian probability to diagnostic interpretation is provided by exercise stress testing for coronary heart disease. In a young woman with atypical chest pain who is unlikely to have coronary disease, a negative test result provides good evidence that coronary disease is not present. In the same patient, a positive result is very likely to be a false positive, hence potentially misleading. Caution is advised. In contrast, in a middle-aged man with a convincing history of angina pectoris (chest pain), a negative exercise test is probably a false negative result. These are important theoretical insights for the clinical practitioner. A detailed and clear, well-illustrated exposition on this subject is one of the strengths of the book, with scales (nomograms) provided for the use of clinicians. Essentially, Bayes' theorem shows how the accuracy of a diagnostic test is in practice highly dependent on the kind of patient, clinical problem, and context of use.

Bayes' theorem contributes to improved clinical decision making, warning of the risk of error in certain clinical situations. There are, however, problems in advocating its direct application to clinical decision making. The formula quantifies the independent contribution of each piece of clinical information. In practice, various kinds of diagnostic information are considered together and may be interdependent. When they are linked as pieces of a pattern, a clinical picture in which the pieces interact, their contribution to the diagnosis may be greater than their sum, taken in isolation. Often multiple diagnoses are considered at the same time, and these may be related to important information about a patient's social circumstances in a way that is not readily quantifiable. Such concerns lead Feinstein to dismiss the routine application of Bayes' theorem to clinical decision making as the "haze of Bayes'" (1977b).

The use of the results of randomized controlled trials as clinical evidence also has its critics. Again Feinstein counts as a leading voice, arguing that this method is misapplied if it serves merely as a shortcut to understanding clinical care. The method offers control over potential sources of bias comparable with that of the laboratory experiment, and it has acquired an aura of scientific infallibility for studying clinical practice. But this degree of control exacts its price in problems of generalizing trial results to individual patients and to similar but not identical interventions. As another by-product of the emphasis on the randomized controlled trial, the art of medicine has increasingly been seen as so profoundly fallible that it has to be replaced by rigorous evidence from trials. What then is the clinician to do when there is no evidence from trials?

Conclusion

McMaster University's Department of Clinical Epidemiology and Biostatistics owes its success to a number of factors. There was the foresight of its founders and their commitment to improving community health. David Sackett was an articulate proponent of a different direction based on the new discipline of clinical epidemiology. His inspirational leadership gathered around him insightful researchers with complementary skills who were dedicated to similar ideals. What developed was a team approach to research in which biostatisticians worked collaboratively with leading clinical researchers and health economists.

At the time of the new department's inception, its first objective was to support research into clinical care, with the aim of bringing about improvements in health. This aim has clearly been achieved. While the quantity and quality of the research is evident in international publications, the focus of the research program has been a narrower one than that set out by the founders. It is arguable, however, that this contributes to its success. The narrower agenda is simpler, it is easier to capture in directives that practicing clinicians can incorporate into their daily tasks, and the processes for doing so are clearly articulated in the textbook. The limitation of this approach in addressing the problems of clinical care has drawn substantive criticism of the department's agenda (see chapter 5). Without the second objective, the department might not have achieved its preeminent position.

The second objective set out for the new department by Evans and Mustard was to encourage clinicians to participate in research in the community. This objective has been met in an unexpected way, not by addressing the needs of local communities, but by taking on a much broader perspective, that of research into health services with the aim of persuading policy makers. The move of the department into addressing issues of health policy took it still further from Feinstein's central concern for the development of a complex "taxonomy" of clinical care. This was not a narrow focus on practitioners in the community, but a broad focus on policy.

There is a possible disjunction between how the department has developed and its incorporation into INCLEN. In a country like Colombia, there would seem to be an urgent need for research that addresses health issues in the community. Morillo, however, points out that the critical attitudes engendered by processes of critical appraisal are essential, the first step of drawing practitioners into a program of reassessment of clinical teaching and its legacy of authority. This resembles the argument of Robert Fletcher in the preceding chapter, that change has to come by stealth, through the involvement of clinicians.

From these early foundations, clinical epidemiology developed as a phenomenon of Canada and the United States. The discipline was not static, and there were further developments and new agendas in the content and goals of clinical epidemiology. The most striking change was the development of evidence-based medicine.

Notes

1. Site visit and departmental evaluation, Department of Clinical Epidemiology and Biostatistics, July 11–13, 1984, Thomas Chalmers, Byron Brown, Robert Evans, and Byron Spencer, McMaster University papers.

CHAPTER 4

The Rise of Evidence-Based Medicine

Despite local success, clinical epidemiology had gained only a tenuous position in medical schools in Canada and the United States by the late 1970s. This position was, however, consolidated by the next generation of clinical epidemiologists — those who were trained in the discipline, who did not have to invent the concepts de novo, and who styled themselves after powerful role models from the first generation. The most charismatic of the founders, David Sackett, served as mentor and inspiration for generations of McMaster University staff, a prophet for the disciples of the discipline. This evangelistic style of leadership has been the subject of considerable criticism (see chapter 9), but it served an important role in establishing clinical epidemiology as a discipline.

The idea of charisma and charismatic leadership deserves a closer analysis than can be provided here. The term *charismatic leadership* derives from the work of the sociologist Max Weber (1864–1920). The charismatic leader can be endowed with superhuman powers, but the term can also be applied to leaders with heroic or specific exceptional capacities who are persuasive visionaries (Weber 1947). Charismatic movements, argued S. N. Eisenstadt (1995), bring about institutional change by undermining existing institutions and suggesting creative and innovative alternatives. While charismatic leadership is essentially based on nonrational motives, in religious as well as scientific movements, there is the promise of rational answers that will resolve a source of stress in existing arrangements.

Charismatic movements are sustained and perpetuated by endowing disciples with the same charismatic aura. At McMaster University, this is given explicit consideration. When the medical school was established, careful attention was paid to recruiting people with insights and leadership capabilities. Once the school was well established, the focus shifted to internal recruitment: students with talent were carefully identified and nurtured to produce the next generation of what Sackett refers to as "brilliant young minds." This new generation emulated the "laid back" style of Sackett's verbal presentations, and they are renowned for the incisiveness of their critiques. They have played a critically important role in spreading the message, traveling widely, delivering keynote speeches, and running training workshops. An important distinction here concerns the activities of Kerr White. The McMaster University team concentrated on spreading their message from the charismatic hub. White was instrumental in providing a conduit back, introducing new ideas from other countries to Canada and the United States.

In 1993, Sackett himself argued that these recruits to clinical epidemiology were part of an enterprise that resembled a social movement. His tendency to label new recruits to clinical epidemiology as brilliant minds (perhaps the equivalent of Great-Men-in-the-making) may have enhanced the prestige of the group, except that outsiders could very well see the claims as self-aggrandizement, in which case the effect would be counterproductive. Nevertheless, claims play an important role in forging the social movement that is clinical epidemiology. When the potential of promising new recruits was identified, they gained entrance into an exclusive group, where their talents were nurtured and their interests promoted. As Sackett clearly recognized, this profited the young researchers, providing a benefit they would not have enjoyed in mainstream science. Sackett notes, "It will be interesting to see what happens to them over time. Established science that is seen as totally legitimate and mainstream is populated by people who are extraordinarily bright, but a lot of them are not very nice, and at times they are certainly not very nice at all to each other. They certainly do not rejoice in one another's success. That hasn't happened in clinical epidemiology. There have been battles and exchanges and bad feelings between clinical epidemiologists and classical epidemiologists, but within clinical epidemiology we rejoice in each other's success. There is enormous camaraderie, enormous mutual support."

It should be noted that in turn this support forged a strong commitment to clinical epidemiology, as well as the risk that clinicians could become uncritical of its directions. On the positive side, there is the clear need to acknowledge the importance of the intellectual mentoring that Sackett provided. There is a story told repeatedly about how Sackett used evidence to resolve professional disagreement. It concerns a consensus conference where it was difficult to reach agreement because authoritative clinical experts saw their own clinical views as definitive. Unable to persuade them otherwise, the McMaster people at the conference sent for Sackett. He proposed that experts be encouraged to make any recommendations they chose, but that they also rate on a scale the quality of evidence to back the recommendation. If a recommendation was based on evidence from randomized clinical trials with sufficient power, it would head the list. If the evidence was a case report, the recommendation would still be accepted, but it would be rated as a lower grade of evidence. Thus was born the hierarchy of evidence.

The hierarchy of evidence had important consequences in narrowing the focus of research done in the Department of Clinical Epidemiology and Biostatistics. If experimental designs are seen as the apex of the pyramid of study designs, then attention is diverted from the many study designs that constitute the more lowly rated base of the pyramid. It should be noted here that the hierarchy of evidence applies only to study designs for evaluating the effectiveness of interventions — that is, the technical aspects of care. But once it is recognized that the randomized controlled trial effectively persuades by producing evidence about the effectiveness of clinical interventions, why not focus on those topics that are appropriate for study using this design? This illustrates Henrik Wulff's concern about how the technical interest comes to dominate a field, shifting attention away from interpretive studies of communication and social context.

In the department itself, the mantle fell on a new generation of researchers, including George Browman, Brian Haynes, and Gordon Guyatt. They were to play a key role in further developing the apex of the pyramid of studies to include "N of one" studies, or single patient trials, and meta-analyses. They were all clinicians whose clinical skills were essential to the central role of clinical epidemiology in the department.

The New Generation: Generating Evidence-Based Medicine

GEORGE BROWMAN

After Peter Tugwell, the next chair of the department was George Browman. Trained at McGill University, Montreal, he was a specialist oncologist and appreciated the need for good drug trials. Says Browman:

Cancer therapies are very toxic, and we're constantly thinking of the bounds between good and harm. So as a cancer physician I was always very concerned about whether I was doing the right thing for the patients. . . . I started doing clinical trials to test a drug interaction that worked in animals and worked in the lab but didn't yet work in people. I developed the clinical drug, and we were halfway through the trials and we were getting positive results. Jack Hirsh, who was chairman of medicine at that time, had established a weekly seminar in which people presented their research, and there were methodologists and plenty of comments. So I presented my study. They commented on the work, and I found I had done a lot of things right and I had done quite a few things wrong. I just liked the people, and I eventually started to attend every week.

George Browman turned his attention to methodological develop-ment in guideline development for cancer care (see Browman et al. 1995; Browman et al. 1998) but remained active as a medical oncologist, a fac-tor that Jack Hirsh describes as central to his success as a clinical epi-demiologist. Says Hirsh, "I believe that if someone has in-depth knowl-edge either in basic science or in a subspecialty of medicine, they are much better methodologists than the undifferentiated academic, who can be very naive." If we bear in mind that McMaster University clinical epi-demiologists see it as essential to maintain their own clinical practice, and to get training in epidemiology and biostatistics, then this makes clinical epidemiology an exclusive specialty inaccessible to the undifferentiated academic trained in only one discipline. It also has implications for the nonmedical members of the department, who cannot achieve these goals.

Browman distinguished himself during eight years as chair in the care-ful consideration that he gave to the political realities facing the depart-ment during a time of economic cutback. The view of one anonymous critical colleague still committed to the art of medicine was that some cli-nicians remained unconvinced that clinical epidemiology was the answer to all their problems:

There are some traditionalists who believe in the art of medicine who feel that what a very experienced clinician can bring to decision making is a very unique, intangible kind of expertise that cannot be generalized — that every patient is different, they would say, and you can't generalize findings from one patient to another patient. Of course we agree that every patient is different, but they are similar enough that we can have policies and study them. I think the point of view is one that we have to take into account, because it's what limits people from accepting the clinical epidemiology approach.

There is no doubt that more traditional practitioners can wield a con-siderable degree of control over clinical care; they have a unique clinical knowledge base that enables them to make decisions about patient care. It was when some of the more traditional clinicians found the department helpful in solving methodological problems that they were converted. What the department contributed was methodological innovation to help clinicians solve their research problems. This service role, central to the department's original objectives, was somewhat in conflict with its traditional academic role. What was needed was a fine balance between the two. The demand for expert methodological advice from other faculty and community organizations had, however, created a fiscal burden, and the pursuit of academic prestige proved to be a safer option for academic staff. According to Browman:

When they get evaluated at tenure and promotion time, nobody is interested in the service work they've done with the university. They're interested in what they've published. You can be so good and so helpful, your product can become so marketable — which our product is — but you have to remember that you're in a university. What are the values of a university? On the one hand they want us to act like a business in order to bring in money, but on the other hand our faculty members, if they wanted to be in business, would have consulting firms; they wouldn't be at the university.

Here Browman reflects a common complaint of all academics, one from which they may have been protected during the early years of a new medical school.

BRIAN HAYNES

Browman's preference was for a smaller department that would be judged on the quality of what it produced, not on the size of its research grants. However, when Brian Haynes, the next chair, took over in 1998, the department had entered a growth phase with annual research funding of CA$10 million and with expanded epidemiology and social science sections. As Sackett foresaw, deans of medicine saw the department as willing to participate in teaching and research in addition to maintaining their commitment to clinical care. Clinical epidemiology had produced a steady stream of good research and a veritable avalanche of articles on the methods of critical appraisal.

Haynes emphasizes that the rigor with which clinical epidemiology can assess clinical practice contributes to this success, and that its achievements are particularly impressive in comparison with those of public health epidemiology, which has been driven by hope rather than evidence. There was success with prevention of infectious diseases, and prevention programs in the early years of life have clearly succeeded. But Haynes sees mass trends in society, like the cessation of smoking, as unexplained and casts doubt on the achievement of disease prevention programs:

If you try to prevent disease in the population, an awful lot of people may have to receive the intervention so that one can benefit. At least in the treatment of established disorders, you know who's got the problem and you deal with them directly. Most of prevention until relatively recently has been a pipe dream. It would be nice to prevent. We all want to prevent. We wouldn't want somebody to get sick. But the means aren't there. We don't have an effective means that's inexpensive, that doesn't have adverse effects, that can be applied to the mass of the population to prevent them from getting disease.

Haynes has a keen appreciation of the role of the team approach. There is a clear competitive advantage in having a critical mass of researchers from various disciplines collaborating on a variety of projects. He is, however, uneasy about collaborating with some qualitative social scientists. From his perspective, their methods lag twenty years behind in terms of addressing issues of reliability and generalizability. He believes that qualitative researchers must "beware of taking their observations solely from talking to people, and must check them out against some other way of looking at what is going on. Because many people do simply tell you a tale." He finds perplexing the idea that knowledge is culturally specific: "It leaves most scientists wondering what the hell's going on." These views stand in direct contrast with the emphasis of Henrik Wulff on a more theoretical and interpretive understanding of clinical care, and they relate in part to Haynes's experience in one of the most difficult areas of clinical practice, patient noncompliance.

Early in his medical training in Toronto, Haynes wondered how much of what they were being taught was based on myth and how much on fact. When challenged about the evidence for their assertions, his teachers would become uncomfortable and resort to authority. He decided that he had to get training in "some scientific area" that would help him better understand evidence. Despite what he saw as an anti-clinical bias, epidemiology seemed to offer a systematic approach, and he enrolled in a course for physicians in the University of Toronto School of Public Health. David Sackett came as a visiting lecturer to give a talk titled "Is Health Care Researchable?" What Haynes heard was "just music." In 1972, he moved to McMaster University to do graduate work on the "most perplexing problem" of patient noncompliance. Compliance is defined as "the extent to which a person's behaviour (in terms of taking medications, following diets, or executing lifestyle changes) coincides with medical or health advice" (Haynes et al. 1979). Initially, his focus was on high blood pressure, one of the first chronic diseases for which there was effective treatment. Patient noncompliance was a major barrier to achieving health benefits, but the problem turned out to be much more difficult than anticipated (see Haynes et al. 1978, 1979). According to Haynes:

In the first studies, we tested ways of giving patients better information about their treatment because we thought that might help them. We also wanted to include some measures of adverse effects. We did find that giving them instruction increased their knowledge of the treatments, but it didn't improve their compliance with the treatments and there were adverse effects. The people — these were steelworkers — missed more time from work after we gave them instruction in comparison with a group that did not get the instruction. Over the next five years they had fewer job promotions. They had more marital stress. They didn't earn as much money. They didn't get as many raises as their colleagues who had not been given the instruction. Of course, when we first presented these results, they were regarded as heresy, and in fact one notable cardiovascular researcher with a public health orientation felt that we shouldn't publish the information.

Their findings raised concern about the effect of some media-based health promotion campaigns. Haynes notes, "There's the cholesterol monster, the shark in your blood stream — if we are talking about hypertension, with people who are anxious to begin with, they may become so anxious that they just become dysfunctional." Given these problems, it was important to develop interventions to improve compliance, but to focus on those interventions where there was clear evidence of health benefit. In 1991, he argued:

So now we are seeing doctors being a bit more aggressive and calling up patients. I think the patients are easily able to rationalize: "Well, if the doctor didn't call me back, maybe it's not very important for me to go." Whatever is going through their heads, I am not sure. But anyway, they don't come back if you don't call and tell them that things go wrong, and they get sick. So I think we are understanding gradually the sorts of steps for changing doctors' and patients' behaviors to get better mileage out of the treatments that are now coming out at a great pace.

The immediate aim was to change patient behavior rather than understand "whatever is going through their heads." With a proliferation of exactly this kind research in the 1980s, there was the need to collect the literature and submit it to critical review. In 1987 Haynes and coworkers decided to collect and review all published trials of interventions to improve compliance with medication. The development of online index-ing services greatly facilitated this task. Medline, for example, the National Library of Medicine's database, carries 11 million references to articles in the health sciences. They selected those trials that met specific methodological criteria; these criteria included having both compliance and treatment outcome as endpoints in the trial. Among interventions offering short-term treatment, only two trials met the study criteria; most studies failed to report whether patients were better off as a result of com-plying with the recommendations for medication. No single intervention was effective in the long term. Most of the interventions tested involved practitioners and were technical (long-acting intramuscular injections, specialized medication dispensers) or behavioral (information provision, cues and rewards, counseling), but it was recognized that social support from a spouse or partner could be beneficial.

Haynes and his coworkers were engaged in the first steps of what became known as evidence-based medicine. In 1979, Archie Cochrane in the United Kingdom had called for each medical specialty to collect and prepare critical summaries of all trials relevant to their field of practice. The purpose was to inform practitioners of the overall conclusions to be drawn from the literature. By 1996 Haynes and coworkers had found 1,553 studies of interventions to improve compliance, but only 13 trials were methodologically defensible and even fewer showed some positive health effect. Their article concludes with a call for innovative approaches to the problem of "adherence." A later review in *The Cochrane Library* (Haynes et al. 2002) explains that "adherence" had become the preferred term; it was synonymous with compliance but without overtones of blame. This later review found little improvement in outcome. The next step in the process of synthesizing evidence from the literature was impossible: the trials were so disparate that it was impossible to combine their results using a statistical analytical process called meta-analysis with the purpose of producing an aggregate result.

Clearly, with respect to noncompliance, evidence of the effectiveness of interventions is elusive. In 2002, the authors called for collaboration across "clinical disciplines" to resolve this important problem. This accords with the emphasis in this body of work on the concerns of the practitioner. Excluded from consideration in the trials and the overviews are those issues of culture and interpretation of patient views that could generate a different understanding of the problem — and different inter-ventions (see, for example, the argument by Trostle [1988] that compli-ance is an ideological preoccupation of medicine and does not reflect patient interests). Given Haynes's view of qualitative social science research, these options are closed. Technical concerns with noncompliance have obscured the necessary, additional understanding that comes from communication and interpretation.

When the problems with noncompliance research first became evident, Haynes concluded that this work was "a bit nihilistic," that it unsettled clinicians without giving them a sound alternative basis for clinical decision making. He changed the focus of his research: "When we did the early study," he says, "we found that practitioners did not know enough about prescribing antihypertensive medications for compliance to be a safe thing to do. For example, a doctor could be prescribing a tranquilizer like Valium, and we knew that that wasn't going to lower the blood pressure but would have other adverse effects. So if we encouraged the patient to follow that treatment we were actually doing the patient a disservice. That set me off on a different tangent — that is, we have got to fix the docs first, because they are not following current best knowledge."

The exponential increase of good trials of therapeutic practice provided part of the solution, but there was still a time lag of about ten years in disseminating the results of trials into practice. Haynes's next focus was therefore on continuing education for doctors, but they supplemented this with initiatives like mailed reminders as a way of improving practice (Evans et al. 1986). At the time, the techniques he favored somewhat resembled techniques for improving patient noncompliance. According to Haynes:

We know that sending them stuff in the mail doesn't work, but you can take a leaf out of the pharmaceutical companies' operations book and send an academic detailer, somebody who has not got a vested interest in the product but who's working through, say, a pharmacy at a university hospital, to go out and tell practitioners about new products and maybe give them some samples or whatever. Audit and feedback in general are the most effective ways to do that. That's where you look at a person's practice, the records, and you compare what they do for patients of various types with standards of care that are established on the basis, hopefully, of good evidence. And give them a report card.

With increasing numbers of studies being published, there was a problem of overload: "Clinicians get so much information thrown at them, and so many claims, only some of which are actually valid and true, that they are not in a very good position to sort out the information in the first place," says Haynes. Information technology provided ready access to a condensed presentation of medical knowledge. Clinicians would no longer need to make decisions by "the seat of the pants" or on the basis of an out-of-date textbook. Instead, they could draw on an electronic resource with up-to-date, sound information on what worked and what did not work: "Instead of every clinician having to go through 170 different journals to keep up to date," says Haynes, "we go through those journals by explicit criteria — the critical appraisal criteria that we try to teach people — and pick out the articles that are directly relevant to internal medicine and that meet the criteria for validity. And then we do a structured abstract from that, with commentary, and dish it out as a supplement to the *Annals of Internal Medicine*. The feedback from that has been overwhelmingly positive. I think what it's done is, it's allowed clinicians to heave a sigh of relief."

Condensing good information from the medical literature to make it readily available to clinicians represents one of the contributions of McMaster University to what became evidence-based medicine. A team of researchers reduces the mass of selected published material down to the 2 percent of articles "that are both valid and of immediate clinical use" (Sackett et al. 2000, p. 3). Nine research assistants and four editorial assistants prepare abstracts of relevant articles selected for their quality on the basis of explicit criteria of critical appraisal. Abstracts are sent to clinical epidemiologists for editing and to a clinical expert commentator, who points out strengths and weaknesses and places each abstract in the context of other studies and clinical practice. This is the evidence that clinicians need for decision making. The first publication developed to present this evidence was the *ACP Journal Club*. The team now also produces *Evidence-Based Medicine, Evidence-Based Nursing, Evidence-Based Mental Health,* and a section of the *Journal of Bone and Joint Surgery.* The accumulated contents of the *ACP Journal Club* and *Evidence-Based Medicine* are produced as an electronic database, *Best Evidence* (now www.acpjc.org). Together with the Cochrane database and Medline, this is now available on the information service Ovid. Other ventures have also been stimulated to similarly amass information in a number of specialized areas and translate it into a range of languages. Haynes now hopes that it will become increasingly embarrassing for clinicians not to use this extensive and growing service.

Even with these publications, there has been no guarantee that the evidence would get to those clinicians who most needed it. In parallel, Haynes is now developing information technologies to take this evidence into clinic settings. After reviewing trials of computerized decision-support systems for doctors, he decided that they failed, for the most part, because the computer programmers produced systems that reflected neither the complexities of the clinical condition nor current best practice. At any rate, says Haynes, "the whole notion of an expert trying to tell someone what to do seemed like a wrongheaded one from the perspective of somebody interested in research transfer and getting research into practice." The Health Information Research Unit set up by Haynes is now developing its own information systems that assemble evidence on a disease (with online access to the *ACP Journal Club*) and make recommendations for care based on that evidence. The challenge is to make the system accessible in clinic settings. One possibility is to locate computers with touch-sensitive screens in doctors' waiting rooms so that patients can directly supply answers to about ten minutes' worth of questions. The computer would then deliver recommendations in lay language for patients and in medical language for their doctors, "hopefully getting everybody on the same wavelength," says Haynes. While most doctors' offices may not have computers, they do have fax machines. These could be used to send a one-page fax of patient responses to the computer to read from a mark-sensitive form; the computer would then fax back the recommendations. He admits, "Patients like it better than doctors, partly because it forces the doctor to spend more time with patients implementing the recommendations or forces the doctor to explain why the patient represents an exception. So, they're mad at us!" The focus of this intervention on explicitly involving consumers has some resemblance to the activities of the Cochrane Collaboration, with which Haynes is associated (see chapter 7).

Haynes has maintained the department's commitment to making presentations at conferences and workshops at home and around the globe. Modeled on David Sackett's charismatic and influential presentations, these have proved to be a highly effective mechanism for spreading the word. Another major contributor to this effort is Gordon Guyatt.

GORDON GUYATT

While Brian Haynes has been developing technological systems for delivering evidence to clinicians and patients, Gordon Guyatt has concentrated on methodological development and direct education of clinicians both at McMaster University and in external training courses in clinical epidemiology. The term *evidence-based medicine* sprang directly from his need to justify the training program in the medical school.

Guyatt was an early graduate of the Department of Clinical Epidemiology and Biostatistics and one of those politically aware recruits treasured by David Sackett. After studying psychology and English, Guyatt looked for something to do that was concrete and politically effective. A summer holiday in South Africa inspired him to study medicine. Since he lacked a background in the natural sciences, only the McMaster University medical school would accept him, remarkably without requiring him to take any further science subjects before admission.

After graduating, Guyatt first tried respiratory medicine with a focus on occupational health but found the area boring; then he tried general internal medicine. While waiting for a hospital opening, he was advised to do the postgraduate program in clinical epidemiology. Says Guyatt:

I remember I went and talked to Peter Tugwell, and he said, "How much research do you want to be doing?" Well, the true answer was zero, and to be polite, I said, "Oh, maybe 25 percent." And he said, "Well, don't say that during your interviews; you won't get in." So, when I had my interviews I appropriately said 50 percent. So I started. Very quickly Jack Hirsh got hold of me, and I remember his making this pitch to seriously try some research. Well, he was the chairman of medicine, and I knew I wanted an academic job.

Guyatt's feeling of insecurity about his career rapidly dissipated under the mentorship of Jack Hirsh, Peter Tugwell, and David Sackett. He says, "Whereas, among the chest physicians, I was never appreciated at all, these guys made me feel like somebody special. There was just a tremendous amount of support. So from then on, I just took off like a rocket!'

Clinical epidemiology offered Guyatt a team approach, the opportunity to do research, and a chance to develop his skill at writing. He has produced a range of research output, from the treatment of heart and lung disease (Guyatt and Canadian Lung Oncology Group 2001) to the evaluation of health services (Molloy et al. 2000), but he has limited interest in large trials funded by drug companies. He sees his major challenges elsewhere. As a result, his focus has been on methodological innovation. An early focus was on the development of the quality of life as a clinical outcome measure (Guyatt et al. 1993), with the early studies addressing the treatment of chronic lung disease (Guyatt et al. 1987). Guyatt recalls, "I knew that I wanted my outcome measures to be quality of life and some functional exercise measure. We had the six-minute walk test, where, as an alternative to putting people on a cycle or a treadmill, you get them to cover as much ground as they can in six minutes. Nobody had ever studied the properties of this test: how reproducible it was, how it could be influenced by things like encouragement, by the person telling them what to do." He needed to make a bridge between the psychological concepts and clinical applications: "All the psychologists' thinking had been about using instruments to discriminate between individuals. In other words, to detect differences between people: who's more intelligent, who's less intelligent, who likes blacks, who hates blacks, that sort of thing. What we were using these instruments for was for clinical trials, for an evaluative purpose, to detect change." Any measure insensitive to change over time would underestimate health outcome. He conceptualized the problem as one of signal and noise. The signal is the difference between individuals at a point in time and the change in an individual over time. Measurement error is the noise that obscures the signal. The issue is the ratio of signal to noise. In this endeavor, Guyatt was pursuing a clinimetric approach similar to that promoted by Feinstein (1987).

A further example of interdisciplinary cross-fertilization was the development of the "N of one," or single patient trial. It was developed in response to the concern that the results of a trial might not readily apply to the particular characteristics or circumstance of a particular patient, so that a treatment shown to be effective in a population was not necessarily the best option for an individual patient. Guyatt and colleagues (1986) introduced a variation on trial procedure, in which a single patient was given a random sequence of alternative treatments and the outcomes of these were compared. The treatment with the best outcome defined the best treatment option for that single patient. While the use of single patient trials was new in clinical epidemiology, such trials were well known in psychological research, hence were familiar to Christel Woodward, a psychologist in the department. Guyatt recalls:

Periodically Chris would say, "Oh, this would be good for a single case design," and we'd all say, "Thank you, Chris, now let's move onto something that makes some sense!" And she'd said this, I think, three, four, five times in various discussions, and suddenly — actually about the same time — it twigged to Sackett and to me that this had potential application. Sackett was getting up in public at the departmental round presenting the idea when it was still very half-baked. But it was the smart thing to do. I remember going down to him at the end of that round and saying, "You know, whatever you do with this in the future, I'd really like to be involved in this." So what happened is, I ran the first N-of-one study in town. There was a guy with bad chronic asthma who had had all sort of medications, everything I could think of. The first try was testing whether theophylline made him better or not, whether it made any difference. It made a difference all right: he was a lot worse. I took him off it, and he was a lot better. It had quite a profound effect.

Here the strength of this department is evident in the ferment of ideas, followed by implementation. The critical contribution of Sackett, however, was to ensure that their methodological innovation received early and full recognition (Guyatt et al. 1986): Guyatt says, "The way I was thinking of going about it was doing fifty of these studies and then publishing our experience, which we eventually did. The paper appeared in the *Annals of Internal Medicine*. Not Dave; he wanted to write up the idea and send it to the *New England Journal of Medicine*. It would never have occurred to me to take that approach, but we did; the *New England Journal* published it, and it was my first *New England Journal* publication."

Inspired by Feinstein, Guyatt and colleagues had been keenly aware of the terminological packaging. David Sackett popularized "critical appraisal" to describe the process of assessing the literature according to explicit rules of evidence. When applied to clinical practice, this was "bringing critical appraisal to the bedside." Guyatt took the next crucial steps in naming an approach in which clinical decisions were justified by reference to a systematic assessment of the medical literature. In 1990, as director of the internal medicine residency program, he focused on training practitioners in a "new brand of medicine":

What we talk about is applying certain rules and concepts of science to clinical experience and systematizing it. "How do you know that treatment X works?" "Well I gave it out and the person did well." OK. And then you say, "But to what extent can you be confident?" You find out very quickly that you can't be confident at all. And then you say, "OK, well, how can I be more systematic in my accumulation of clinical information to strengthen my inference?" And if you push it, you end up with a double-blind randomized trial as a systematic way of accumulating clinical experience. The problem isn't clinical experience: the problem is that we were so unsystematic, intuitive, and with no notion of scientific principles in our accumulation of clinical experience. And now, is clinical experience worthless? No, but you need the appropriate level of skepticism and knowing how things go wrong.

Guyatt refers to "scientific medicine" as a paradigm shift in clinical thinking:

What were the assumptions of the old paradigm? First, that clinical experience was a valid way of obtaining knowledge about prognosis, the value of diagnostic tests and therapy. Second, that one could work out the appropriate way of treating people just on the basis of physiology and physiological principles. If you knew the physiology, and you knew how the drug affected the physiology, you could predict its clinical effects. The third assumption is the high value on authority, and the fourth is that good medical training and common sense allow you to be appropriately critical about the medical literature. Those are the four assumptions of the old paradigm.

The assumptions within the new paradigm are different in all four. The new paradigm suggests that clinical experience has severe limitations as a guide to understanding the properties of diagnostic tests, whether treatment works, or prognosis. Second, medical training and common sense are very inadequate guides to deciding whether something is scientifically valid. One needs rules of evidence that are, essentially, clinical epidemiology. Third, reasoning on the basis of physiology often proves misleading without empirical testing. And, fourthly, following from all this, a much lower value in authority and, in fact, a sort of iconoclasm.

At the point where you say I'm going to be tremendously rigorous and systematic in my accumulation of clinical evidence, you're into the new paradigm and you're into doing science.

A new way of seeing things needs a name. Guyatt used the term *scientific medicine* to describe what they were doing. The term drew strong criticism from colleagues who saw it as implying that what they were doing was unscientific. He then called it "evidence-based medicine." The term is a trifle mischievous, carrying the implication that clinicians who did not subscribe to the "new paradigm" were basing their decisions on intuition rather than evidence. It repeats the argument of the McMaster University textbook, that clinicians should rely on evidence rather than authoritarian opinions when making decisions (Sackett, Haynes, and Tugwell 1985, p. 246). Since evidence is what clinical epidemiology produces, evidence-based medicine is the practical application of clinical epidemiology in patient care.

Guyatt first used the term in 1990 in an information document for residents to describe the principles outlined in Sackett and colleagues (1985). The following year he defined it as "the application of scientific method in determining the optimal management of the individual patient" (Guyatt 1991). Guyatt played a key role in the Evidence-Based Medicine Working Group where, he says, they came to see evidence-based medicine as "a new paradigm" and "the way of the future." At the time of interview he offered the following as his preferred definition for evidence-based medicine: "Evidence-based medicine is an approach to practicing medicine in which the clinician is aware of the evidence in support of her clinical practice, and the strength of that evidence."

The new name *evidence-based medicine* proved irresistible to some (and aggravating to others). A textbook, *Evidence-Based Medicine: How to Practice and Teach EBM,* includes Sackett and Haynes among the coauthors. They celebrate the fact that the number of articles on evidence-based medicine grew exponentially, and six new evidence-based journals had a combined circulation of over 175,000 (Sackett et al. 2000, p. 2). The textbook, one of many, was first published in 1997 and revised in 2000. It sold upward of seventy thousand copies total and was reprinted three times in 2000.

The idea that clinical care requires a scientific base is not new, but evidence-based medicine has reactivated these concerns under a catchy title. Training workshops have disseminated the skills required by this approach, and these have been very well received. These shifts articulated well with the Haynes initiative in secondary publication and electronic accessibility. Sackett and Straus (1998) went one step further and proposed a cart or trolley with electronic resources to ensure instant access to evidence during clinical rounds.

Perhaps reflecting the evangelical origins of the Department of Clinical Epidemiology and Biostatistics, Guyatt acknowledges that belief in evidence-based medicine is "an act of faith"; but it is also "aesthetically more appealing" and defensible on a priori logical grounds. A physician who knows the properties of a diagnostic test, for example, should perform as well or better than a physician who does not. Changes in paradigm are not based only on rational evidence, let alone faith, but also on shifts in the social fabric, and Guyatt recognizes the importance of personal charisma in the success of the McMaster team as role models: "If we convince people, it is through a host of personal and social factors and our effectiveness as sales people and our attractiveness as role models." It could be argued that this is exactly how traditional clinical experts achieved their authority, and this puts clinical epidemiologists in conflict with traditional experts. However, Guyatt and colleagues see the resolution of this conflict as resting not only on their charisma but also on the scientific legitimacy of their views.

In recent years Guyatt has seen his primary contribution as educational. His talent as an educator has contributed to his capacity to "indoctrinate clinicians with the appropriate attitudes, to promulgate the philosophy of evidence-based practice, and to give clinicians the necessary tools for the task." He conducts intensive workshops attended by leading health researchers, practitioners, and administrators from around the world. He chaired the Evidence-Based Medicine Working Group, which produced a series of twenty-five articles in the *Journal of the American Medical Association* that set out guides for clinicians interested in practicing evidence-based medicine (see Guyatt and Rennie 2002, pp. xi–xiii). This has been produced as a textbook with an attached CD-ROM (Guyatt and Rennie 2002).

Sackett and colleagues (2000) emphasizes a step-by-step "cookbook" approach to doing evidence-based medicine, with the implication that anybody can do it (although busy people may prefer the easy fast-food option). In contrast, Guyatt has changed his mind about the central task of evidence-based medicine:

When I started, I thought we were going to turn people into evidence-based practitioners, that they were really going to understand the methodology, that they
were really going to critique the literature and apply the results to clinical practice. I no longer believe that. What I believe now is that there will be a minority
of people who will be evidence-based practitioners, and that the other folk will
be evidence users who will gain a respect for the evidence and where it comes
from and a readiness to identify evidence-based sources which summarize the evidence for them. But they are not actually expected to read and understand the articles and really be able to dissect the methodology.

Some members of the Evidence-Based Medicine Working Group saw
this idea as elitist; one described it as "evidence-based capitulation."
Guyatt and colleagues (2000) published an editorial setting out these
views after "a year of agonizing." Clinicians who are not interested in
acquiring the skills for synthesizing the primary literature or who lack the
time to apply these skills are referred to secondary sources such as the
ACP Journal Club and the Cochrane Library.

Another new development, in Guyatt's view, is the understanding that
clinical decisions are not made on evidence alone, that value judgments
mediate the shift from evidence to implementation. He argues that only
a small minority of people have been aware of the importance of value
judgments that he sees as lying outside science. These values have to be
made explicit to ensure that decisions do not simply reflect the values of
a dominant group. Researchers at the methodological frontier must now
build on the work of the health economists in measuring patient preferences, so that these are incorporated into clinical decision making
through, for example, the decision aids devised by Brian Haynes. Importantly, doctor preferences also need to be explicated. The next challenge
will be to devise ways of incorporating the evidence produced into actual
clinical decision making. Doing so will further undermine clinician
autonomy, but Guyatt takes the argument still further, calling into question the biased role of "advocate clinicians" in making policy recommendation for their own areas of practice. With his fine focus on generating evidence that will produce more effective practices, he does,
however, ignore evidence from social science that identifies the structural
and professional determinants of clinical decision making.

Guyatt's major research commitment is to clinical practice, but he also
has a strong political commitment to equity of access to effective health
services, and he sees this as separate from his research. He was a founding member of the Canadian Medical Reform Group, which, he says, promotes analysis of "the social, political, and economic forces shaping

health and health care in Canada." He also writes a biweekly column on health policy in the *Hamilton Spectator*, where he promotes, among other issues, the sustainability of public, universal health care. According to Guyatt, "There is no doubt then, that Canadians will be spending more on health care in the future. The question is, who will benefit from the increased spending? If we go the American private route, the affluent private health insurers and private companies will be the winners. If we see through the false arguments about 'sustainability,' we will put the increased resources into public health care, and all Canadians will benefit. Let's hope we blow away the smoke screens and make the right choice."

Guyatt is reluctant to address such issues directly in his research, as it would require him to make a difficult disciplinary move into health policy. He has, however, ventured into the academic field with these views in an editorial in the *Canadian Medical Association Journal* addressing the structural changes necessary to sustain public funding for equitable health care (Guyatt et al. 2002). It was coauthored by an economist, Armine Yalnizyan, from the Canadian Centre for Policy Alternatives, Ottawa, and P. J. Devereaux, a new member of the McMaster team. Devereaux has been anointed as "the one who's really got it" in the latest generation of McMaster researchers.

P. J. DEVEREAUX

In common with many McMaster University academics, P. J Devereaux followed a circuitous route to medicine. He went to Dalhousie University on a military scholarship to study biology, then worked as a diving officer in the Canadian navy. During placement in a hospital in Moose Jaw, Saskatchewan ("the coldest place on earth"), he changed to medicine and chose McMaster University for its problem-based approach. Within the first month of training, even at McMaster University, Devereaux was struck by the conflicting information given to students. In the navy Devereaux had experienced blind obedience to orders from a superior and had disliked it. Fortunately David Sackett was his student adviser, and Sackett introduced him to evidence-based medicine. Devereaux saw evidence-based medicine as a way of empowering young clinicians, freeing them from the dictates of "some staff guy who's been around for twenty years." After training in cardiology elsewhere, Devereaux returned to McMaster University as a research fellow to do research into evidence-based medicine. Gordon Guyatt was his mentor. Devereaux says, "I have met some of the most unbelievably brilliant people, but of everyone I have met, Gordon is light-years ahead of anyone. Gordon is incredibly brilliant in a number of ways. Not only is he a person who has original, intuitive ideas, he is a great communicator and he is a great writer. You can be brilliant and a great scientist but still have little impact because you are not a good communicator. He is just phenomenally gifted; he has the three."

Despite this lavish praise, Devereaux is committed to taking a critical, reflexive approach to evidence-based medicine so that he does not contribute to the creation of "a new monster." The double-blind randomized trial could become a "rubber stamp" for validity, despite the fact that there is remarkable variation in the interpretation of blinding in trials (Devereaux, Manns et al. 2001). Uncritical acceptance of trial results is especially likely if the results match doctors' clinical preferences: "If physicians' preconceived views agree with the results of a study," he says, "there is never any question; the results are true. If they disagree with the results they frequently go back and nitpick things that may well be irrelevant. They want to find something to discredit it. Instead the more rigorous way is to say, before even looking at the results, I will make a decision about the validity and recognizing validity as a continuum; I will make a decision about whether to accept whatever the results show."

Physicians have also been shown to be inconsistent as a group in terms of the choices made on the basis of the same evidence (Devereaux, Anderson et al. 2001). Devereaux argues that such variation highlights a point central to evidence-based medicine — that is, evidence does not tell us what to do; rather, it allows us to make more informed decisions. Beyond considering evidence, there is also a necessity to incorporate patient preferences and values into medical decision making. All medical decisions involve a trade-off between a potential benefit versus a potential harm, cost, and inconvenience. Individuals can consider the same valid evidence but make very different decisions because of variations in their individual values and preferences. To date, evidence-based medicine has primarily made advances in influencing the medical profession to obtain and identify valid evidence. However, there is now a need to advance evidence-based medicine beyond "the evidence," to take it to the next level by incorporating patient values and preferences. In his research Devereaux is committed to devising ways of ensuring that patient values, rather than physician preference, determine the choice of intervention.

Devereaux shares Guyatt's political commitments. He too is a member of the Canadian Medical Reform Group. Given the collaborative style at McMaster University, it is difficult to establish individual research territory, but he feels the need to do this: his research is not simply the result of academic commitment. For example, one project involves a critical analysis of the introduction of private, for-profit health delivery systems in Canada.

What was needed was a "systematic, comprehensive, and unbiased accumulation and summary of the available evidence" comparing private for-profit hospitals with the private not-for-profit system that operates in 95 percent of Canadian hospitals (Devereaux et al. 2002). Based on a meta-analysis of fifteen observational studies with a combined total of twenty-six thousand hospitals and 38 million patients, all in the United States, Devereaux and his colleagues showed that private, for-profit hospitals were associated with an increased risk of death. This adds weight to the argument that Canada should retain its not-for-profit hospitals, a conclusion that sits well with Devereaux's political views. He says, "I am doing this research because it represents who I am. I probably would not take on research like this if it were not for my political views. Our political views can drive the research we do, but we can do it in an evidence-based fashion utilizing systematic reviews. There has been a paucity of such studies."

It remains to be seen if such political commitment will alter the research base of the department. Certainly both Devereaux and Guyatt are pushing the paradigm to its limits. What they have not done is to step outside it and forge substantial allegiances with other disciplines except where it is integral to the research problem, although Devereaux is collaborating with John Lavis from the Centre for Health Economics and Policy Analysis in the systematic review of private for-profit and private not for-profit health care delivery systems. It would seem obvious that this is the group at McMaster University with whom both Guyatt and Devereaux have the greatest affinity. Health economists and policy analysts here have excellent international reputations and a commitment to extending the measurement task initiated by George Torrance, but also to engaging in a broad-ranging approach to research. In this sense they represent those social science disciplines that have not been sufficiently integrated into the clinical research task. Their relationship with the other members of the Department of Clinical Epidemiology and Biostatistics is therefore well worth analyzing in detail.

The Centre for Health Economics and Policy Analysis

GREG STODDART

George Torrance, Greg Stodddart, and Jonathan Lomas started the Centre for Health Economics and Policy Analysis in 1988. The founding coordinator was Greg Stoddart, who trained in economics but turned to health economics because "you hung around people instead of commodity exchanges." At that stage, in the late 1960s, the focus of much of health economics was at the level of specific services or procedures, and it often involved no more than costing exercises; he was more interested in evaluations that examined clinical effects as well as costs. Dissatisfied with his early experiences with public health epidemiologists, Stoddart joined the Department of Clinical Epidemiology and Biostatistics at McMaster University, at the same time becoming an associate in the Department of Economics.

In 1978, together with George Torrance, he devised a health economics course for health science students, which focused on cost-effectiveness, cost benefit, and cost utility analysis. The course generated a textbook, which they cowrote with colleague Michael Drummond: *Methods for the Economic Evaluation of Health Care Programmes* (Drummond, Stoddart, and Torrance 1987). It is now going into its third edition, has been translated into several languages, and is still the standard graduate-level text on the subject used internationally. Stoddart and Torrance saw their approach as being more appropriate to the health field than the standard economic techniques. But these methods were still focused on the evaluation of specific services. In his continued work with his economics colleagues, Stoddart applied economics to health care at another level, that of the health care system, or the "market." He saw the need for clinical information on effectiveness as well as efficiency at this level also. Debates about user charges were one example. According to Stoddart, "People were thinking about user charges in a way that was intuitive pop economics: you charge people, they stop using the services, and they stop using the least necessary item first, so you can eliminate the frivolous care. Boy, either way you win; charges are the answer! The only problem with that is it's wrong. It sounds good in theory, but it turns out, of course, that for lots of reasons, charges actually deter people from using services regardless of the necessity of care."

The health market, he argues, should be organized first on the basis of technical efficiency and cost-effectiveness analyses, and not simply by controlling the supply of services. Thus health economics and clinical epidemiology are highly compatible both at the level of the evaluations for specific services and at the level of entire health care systems. In 1993, he became interested in well baby examinations. Stoddart states:

We know we do far too many well baby examinations; we've got a randomized trial to prove that from years ago. But we still pay for ten or twelve in the first two years of life, when we know that four or five would suffice. Then at the market level, there is what economists would call allocative efficiency: are we producing the right products, in the right mixes, and distributing them in a way that society deems to be OK? And at that level you say, "Well, folks, look, we've got clinical epidemiology information that says public health nurses do well baby exams as well as anybody else. General practitioners certainly do them as well as anybody else, and pediatricians can do them, but it seems like a hell of a waste of talent and training. We've got information that says too many are being done anyway, so here's what we're going to do, folks. We're going to use a little bit of pricing here. If you really want your well baby examined by a pediatrician: $500 surcharge, or $150, or whatever you want to say. If you want it from a general practitioner, that's fine: there's only a $10 surcharge. But, you know, where public health nurses exist, you can get it free from them." That is using information from clinical epidemiology at the market level to tie in with the economist's view of efficient allocation.

This program fitted well with the vision of David Sackett that clinical epidemiology should be used not only to change practice but to generate health policy. However, it should be noted that the Sackett program required a narrow focus on the clinical encounter, whereas Stoddart was turning to macroeconomic issues of health policy. At first the distinction was not obvious. Greg Stoddart thinks that people were amused by this approach until the late 1970s, but then they realized its potential for health policy: "I think that people thought, 'That's nice stuff; I'm glad Greg's having fun in the economics department.' But as the health care system evolved, and as the policy issues became tighter, I think people realized, first, that these are important issues, and second, that there was a lot of scope at the market level for the application of economics to health care beyond clinical epidemiology and biostatistics. And there was a fair amount of support then, all of a sudden; and I was saying, 'Take it easy, I'm already stressed out here!'"

As a result the number of economists in the department grew, and in 1988 they set up the Centre for Health Economics and Policy Analysis. The aims of the center are to develop and apply appropriate methods for the economic evaluation of specific services, to design and evaluate systems of health care delivery, and to study decision making in health, including that of consumers, providers, and policy makers.

Stoddart then also turned his attention to the big picture in the economics of health rather than the economics of health care. He says:

Let's be clear. If your objective is to improve health and you have 5 million dollars, should you be putting that into a social assistance program targeted at the homeless in Toronto or, say, unemployed youth in Hamilton, some kind of social program. Should you be putting it into health promotion activities — you know, let's all get out and jog — or should you be putting it into trauma care units in the major urban hospitals? That's a type of resource allocation decision. It's the analog of what we were doing here in 1975 about how to produce health *care:* should procedure A or procedure B be done? I see those as intellectually similar methodological questions. We are still talking about comparing something with something else.

Some health care providers are threatened by thinking like this, yet I wonder if it's a good use of scarce research skills to keep doing only health care cost-effectiveness comparisons. Instead of comparing different frequencies of reuse of dialysis coils, why don't we compare renal or other health care programs to income support or programs to reduce family violence?

In this enterprise, Greg Stoddart argues, it was not clear whether they should focus on health itself or a higher concept of well-being to which health, narrowly defined, is but one contributor:

I observe behavior every day, as a social scientist, which indicates that most people don't think health is everything. If you think about it for a minute: if I was sixty-five years old, and I was retired and I loved going to museums — and I derived utility from them, of the kind that George Torrance measures — if somebody said to me, "Well, you know, you're going to lose your left arm in an accident for which you will get $2 million and a free airline pass." If I was right-handed, I'd say, "Mmm, look at all those museums; I've still got life, mmm . . ."

Stoddart finds it understandable that middle-class people have a greater sense of well-being and a more optimistic concept of the future. Health-detrimental behavior is, however, rational among people "who don't want to look forward to their future because they don't have anything to look forward to." Unless larger issues like this are understood, resource allocation is extremely difficult.

At the same time that Stoddart was founding the Centre for Health Economics and Policy Analysis, he was approached by Fraser Mustard to help begin a program in population health for the Canadian Institute of Advanced Research, joining Robert Evans and Ted Marmor. The deceptively simple question that this new program sought to answer — Why are some people healthy and others are not? — encouraged Stoddart to continue his broader examination of health and its determinants. Among other activities, Evans and Stoddart synthesized existing research on the individual and societal determinants of the health of populations and questioned whether the existing allocation of resources in most industrialized countries was producing as much health as it could (Evans and Stoddart 1990). The institute's Population Health Program has grown considerably and continues to attract international attention, especially for its work on early childhood development and income inequality as social determinants of health. The most recent turn in Stoddart's career has taken him deeper into the field of knowledge up-take and research transfer. Throughout his research career, he has at-tempted to inform policy makers and the policy process about relevant research findings. Now, he is part of a research program at McMaster University (www.researchtopolicy.ca) that seeks to understand how and why evidence gets used in policy making, as part of an overall objective to improve the use of evidence.

JONATHAN LOMAS

In 1982, Jonathan Lomas joined the Department of Clinical Epidemi-ology and Biostatistics. He points out that, by this time, the department was no longer seen as renegade. It had joined the mainstream. Lomas recalls, "Having gone from basic science to applied clinical epidemiology to health economics with cost-effectiveness, there was some interest in the next stage: health policy including both clinical and administrative-man-agerial and public policy, government policy. But even then, when I came in 1982, we weren't allowed to talk about policy. We had to talk about evaluation. We talked about evaluation of health programs. We did not talk about policy, because it was not considered kosher, in this environ-ment in particular, to deal with such a squishy and disrespectful kind of thing as health policy."

Lomas's background is in political science and social psychology, the latter giving him, he says, an excellent training in research methods. It also prepared him for a role as critic and innovative thinker in the department. He had been working on physician and manpower policy issues with Greg Stoddart and had a link to Fraser Mustard and what was to become the Canadian Institute of Advanced Research. He was employed at McMaster University, he believes, as part of the department's drive under Peter Tugwell to continue with its radical program, doing things that other medical schools were not doing. And indeed, his output has been challenging, ranging from consideration of the effect of nurse prac-titioners on the requirements for physicians in general practice (Lomas and Stoddart 1985) to a reflective article on the difficulties of moving from practice guidelines to clinical policy (Lomas 1993a) and analysis of the possibility of public input to health care priorities (Lomas 1997).

From his perspective, clinical epidemiology is a two-edged sword. A technical-scientific view of the world, in which treatment X is evaluated for its effectiveness in treating presentation Y, is necessary in order to secure public funding and public support for the medical system. However, this has to be balanced against claims to having an art of medicine that is the basis for the discretionary judgments the profession is allowed to make, Lomas says, "in order to justify why our algorithms and practice guidelines can't apply to me in my situation with this patient." Systematic evaluation of clinical practice, especially when that evaluation shows that certain treatments are *ineffective,* can destroy the fine balance between the science and art of clinical practice.

By the early 1990s it was clear to Lomas that "medicine is no longer in the driver's seat." Health policy makers determined the allocation of resources to health care or to alternative ways of achieving health in the community. The medical profession could no longer stand aloof but had to engage in the health policy debate. Superficially, clinical epidemiology provided an important means of arguing that funds should be spent on medical care rather than alternative ways of improving health. According to Lomas, "If none of the other disciplines — whether it be social work or whether it be psychology or whether it be public health nursing — have acquired any of these skills of clinical epidemiology, they will be at a severe disadvantage in the public policy forum when arguing for allocations of resources to their programs against a medical community which can turn around with all of the evidence out of clinical epidemiology and say, 'We know that this program does good, because we have done our randomized controlled trials.'"

Evidence of effectiveness is, however, not an easy matter. There are, Lomas argues, serious theoretical problems with the measurement of utilities. Utilities may not adequately capture the individual experience, but more seriously, the aggregated individual experiences may substantially misrepresent societal values. As Lomas puts it, "We are, as societies, more than the sum of our parts." Judging the value of a health state may itself be an art rather than a science. In Lomas's view, utilities are therefore not the magical panacea that will allow policy makers to decide where to allocate funds within the health care system. They provide no guidance at all for decisions concerning the allocation of funds between the health care system and other areas of government expenditure, like social welfare, highways, or the environment: "It is no longer a question for us of whether or not you can demonstrate your service is effective," he says; "it's what the degree of its effectiveness is worth relative to other potential expenditures, the expenditure in the societal sense. Never mind the issues of the patient preferences!"

Conclusion

The Department of Clinical Epidemiology and Biostatistics at McMaster University has been home to some of the most energetic and prolific researchers in the field of clinical epidemiology and evidence-based medicine. Like David Sackett, these researchers overpower both active and passive opposition. Their major focus has been a relatively narrow one: producing a highly polished and refined set of techniques for the study of the effectiveness of clinical care. Central to this focus was a move away from the Feinstein agenda and an endorsement of the randomized controlled trial as rating higher than other designs rated on the hierarchy of evidence. This thrust, more than anything else, gave the department its focus and its international stature.

Activities in the department did diversify. Apart from methodological development, there was mutual reinforcing of activities. Gordon Guyatt produced the notion of evidence-based medicine, and this linked directly to those researchers who were producing a steady stream of evidence of the effectiveness of care, and to Brian Haynes's systems for disseminating this evidence in a synthesized form. The Centre for Health Economics and Policy Analysis allowed input into macroeconomics and health policy. George Browman signaled a move to greater multidisciplinarity; but at least from an external perspective, the degree to which public health disciplines and alternative research methods have penetrated into the research activity of the disciples is small.

As with most such endeavors, it is possible to stand back from the enthusiasms of the proponents and assume a more critical stance. When we do so, three issues seem to require further analysis. It is necessary to address the claim that evidenced-based medicine represents a change in focus that constitutes a new paradigm. In addition, it is necessary to reexamine issues of expertise and authority. If clinical authority has been challenged, is there not here a suggestion that these new forms of knowledge have, in turn, lead to a new authority? In this respect, it is relevant to bear in mind the evangelical origins of the evidence-based-medicine movement in Canada. The third issue relates to the role of economics. As the social science that has achieved the highest degree of integration with clinical epidemiology and Canadian evidence-based medicine, it was well placed to generate policy initiatives resting on good evidence of the effectiveness of clinical interventions.

Lastly, it seems necessary to comment on the issues raised by Jonathan Lomas, who now heads the Canadian Health Services Research Foundation in Ottawa. There are clearly broader issues of health policy at stake, but the main proponents of the McMaster University model appear to see their enterprise as being much like the objective production of truth in a laboratory. Thus their political judgments and commitments appear to be part of their lives outside of the research. P. J. Devereaux suggests that the potential exists for a new approach to this problem, perhaps a next generation of politically committed disciples. This might raise the opportunity for collaboration with disciplines better versed in the study of the social and political context of life and health. However, as Lomas makes clear, such issues have been considered, and while there has been some limited engagement, they have not been taken on.

CHAPTER 5

An Appraisal, with Critique

There is no doubt that clinical epidemiology injected specifically clinical scientific thinking into clinical care. Clinicians became more aware of the uncertainties of practice, and the validity of clinical authority was called into question. The focus shifted to the technical aspects of care. The reliability of clinical signs and of test results was questioned, and terms like *sensitivity, specificity,* and *predictive value* became more familiar, at least in the academic world of clinical practice. The medical literature could be submitted to critical appraisal, and studies to establish the effectiveness of treatment modalities were reviewed with appropriate skepticism.

A series of textbooks made the ideas of clinical epidemiology accessible in publications aimed at practicing clinicians. In more recent years, a spate of books on evidence-based medicine has appeared. A collaboration among Canadian, American, and British authors produced *Evidence-Based Medicine: How to Practice and Teach EBM* (Sackett et al. 2000). The Evidence-Based Medicine Working Group chose the title *Users' Guides to the Medical Literature: A Manual for Evidence-Based Clinical Practice* for their 2002 publication. The aim was to help clinicians and practitioners draw conclusions from the medical literature. In his foreword, Drummond Rennie (deputy editor of the *Journal of the American Medical Association* [JAMA]) extols the virtues of "the brilliant group at McMaster," whom he met when JAMA began publishing this series in 1992: "Like Sackett, their leader, they tended to be iconoclastic, expert at working together and forming alliances with new and talented workers, and intellectually exacting" (Guyatt and Rennie 2002, pp. vii–viii).

With its activities extolled in this way, it would be surprising if the McMaster University Department of Clinical Epidemiology and Biostatistics did not become a target for criticism. In the early 1990s, when it began to speak of evidence-based medicine as the practical application of clinical epidemiology in patient care, McMaster University was subjected to considerable critical scrutiny. The term *evidence-based medicine* is, in part, a response to this critical appraisal. Evidence-based medicine presented a much smaller target — who can be against it? — and has proliferated in a way that clinical epidemiology did not. The topic of evidence-based medicine elicited a sharp rise in articles after 1995, but another set of criticisms arose in tandem. Some of these criticisms are now aimed specifically at the version of evidence-based medicine that appeared in the United Kingdom; however, the distinctions are blurred because, after 1994, David Sackett was located at Oxford University, where the 1997 book by Sackett and his colleagues originated. I address the criticism directed at this broader collaborative effort involving the Cochrane Collaboration in chapter 9. Here I cover the criticism directed primarily at clinical epidemiology and evidence-based medicine based at McMaster University.

I add a word of caution at this point: What this chapter records is critical comment, but comment that has a constructive purpose. It should not be viewed in isolation; some of the people who stood back and reassessed their views were instrumental in the genesis of evidence-based medicine and clinical epidemiology as a discipline and remain strongly supportive. In general the criticisms are directed at the narrow focus of the discipline but offer varying views on the direction in which it should be extended.

A Science of Clinical Care?

The most immediate question is whether clinical epidemiology provided a secure scientific basis for clinicians making decisions at the patient's bedside, replacing the more intuitive aspect of the art of medicine. Undoubtedly Alvan Feinstein is the person who articulated the most comprehensive program for this new science, which was based on the generation of new methods of analysis and developed by clinicians for clinical study. His program did not take hold. This could be because it was too complex for the average clinician, drawing as it did on mathematical concepts outside medical training. In contrast, McMaster University proposed a more selective approach, one that drew on a limited number of methods from epidemiology to provide clinicians with an accessible set of tools for use in critically appraising the literature and applying it to their own practices. Even this has proved challenging for clinicians, as shown in chapter 4, a problem that was then addressed with the generation of evidence summaries in readily accessible formats.

Not unexpectedly, the most trenchant criticism of the direction taken at McMaster University came from Alvan Feinstein. Despite his founding-father status, when interviewed in 1991 he wielded the scourge, accusing clinical epidemiologists of being obsessed with randomized controlled trials, a condition he called "randophilia." He accused clinical epidemiologists of not recognizing the randomized controlled trial merely as an effective method for assessing whether treatment A was better than treatment B, and of assuming instead that it possessed some superior form of truth. While such criticism attached to clinical epidemiology in general, the McMaster University department came in for special attention because of its potential to do better. Says Feinstein:

My main trouble with the McMaster gang, whom I dearly love, is that they have, in my opinion, assembled under one roof more brainpower under the title of clinical epidemiology than anywhere in captivity, and I just think that they have totally blown it. All the fundamental challenges, they have evaded. Instead of taking on the challenges of developing a clinical taxonomy, they have just promulgated randomized trials. And when you couldn't do randomized trials on the big scale, you did N-of-one randomized trials. And when randomized trials couldn't give you the answer, you then did meta-analysis. I mean it just shocks me.

In the process, according to Feinstein, clinical epidemiology reinforced in clinicians a blind trust in theories and models drawn from other disciplines. The randomized controlled trial was particularly seductive, but it did not fit well with clinical practice: "The reason we are in such profound trouble today is that the bloody models don't fit what is going on clinically. Furthermore, because clinicians have not articulated what they are doing, they keep hoping that they will get an intellectual handout, either from the social scientists, the clinical epidemiologists, the statisticians, or the biomedical researchers. Clinicians will be immensely grateful for anything that will keep them from having to think about what they are doing. I would have no model whatsoever. I think that we have been destroyed intellectually by all of these models."

How else should clinical epidemiology have proceeded? Feinstein's view is that clinical epidemiology should have learned from patients, that patients should not have been fitted into "little pigeonholes." It could be argued that Feinstein's own clinimetrics does just this, reduces the human dimension to numbers, but for Feinstein the numbers are merely an input into the methodologically more difficult problems of analyzing clinical care itself. He accuses clinical epidemiology of failing to address this second stage. The focus of evidence-based medicine on the best available evidence comes in for further criticism (Feinstein and Horwitz 1997). While it is obviously good to appreciate good evidence, the problem is that only evidence seen as most scientific is then taken into account. This restricts the scope of evidence, and what is excluded is evidence that may be necessary for clinical decision making — for example, the role of psychosocial factors and support. Says Feinstein, the authoritative aura accorded to evidence selected as meeting the criteria of excellence for evidence-based medicine "may lead to major abuses that produce inappropriate guidelines or doctrinaire dogmas for clinical practice."

If Feinstein is correct that clinical epidemiology drifted away from the complexities of clinical care, then the research will fail to persuade clinicians. Thus the "change from within" envisaged by Robert Fletcher will not eventuate. The problem, as many commentators point out, is that the McMaster University researchers are not full-time clinicians. Despite these researchers' commitment to spending time in clinical practice, clinicians may see them as missing the fine nuances of clinical decision making. A particular target for criticism is the "evidence cart" promoted by David Sackett. While critics acknowledged that this system does introduce new evidence into the decision making process, some of this evidence could be wrong or inappropriate from a clinical perspective, for a particular patient. Unless doctors making the decisions have well-developed clinical skills, they will not be able to make this judgment.

Jack Hirsh, working closely with the department, has a different view. He regards clinical epidemiology as an important step forward in providing clinicians with a basic scientific training other than biomedical science. However, in practice, the translation of clinical epidemiology into direct clinical applications is no easy task. In the early days, he admits, they were too sanguine, but they learned from their mistakes: "Both Sackett and Gent learned a lot of clinical epidemiology by becoming involved with my group in performing randomized studies in the diagnosis, prevention, and treatment of venous thromboembolism, and discovering that the so-called universal truths such as sensitivity and specificity are not constant. Until we began to perform these studies in the 1970s, and then through the 1980s and 1990s, clinical epidemiology was very much a theoretical discipline. Sackett and Gent taught us how to design the studies appropriately, and how to analyze the results. In the process they learned a lot about applied epidemiology."

Hirsh cites the example of applying the results of evaluative studies of the accuracy of diagnostic tests in the field of thrombosis. The original measures of test accuracy, sensitivity, and specificity tended to be seen as constants, he says, but his clinical experience indicated that this was not so:

We thought that noninvasive testing was very sensitive and specific. Let's take impedance plethysmography for symptomatic venous thrombosis as an example. We applied it as a screening test in patients at high risk of venous thrombosis, and we made the assumption we would still have the same sensitivity and specificity in asymptomatic as symptomatic patients. It turned out that sensitivity and specificity are poor in screening, because the asymptomatic thrombi are in general much smaller than symptomatic thrombi. The sensitivity for proximal vein thrombosis is probably no better than 30 percent in asymptomatic patients, yet it is in the midnineties for symptomatic patients.

There were good physiological reasons why a test like impedance plethysmography did not pick up thrombi (blood clots in veins) in asymptomatic patients. According to Hirsh, "In order for the test to be positive, the thrombus should be obstructive and fairly large. Patients who develop symptomatic venous thrombosis have large obstructive thrombi. In contrast, high-risk patients who have been screened often have small nonobstructive thrombi, which are therefore not detected by impedance plethysmography. But many of these nonobstructive thrombi are dangerous. For example, the vast majority of patients with a major embolism (diagnosed by angiogram) have no symptoms in their legs because the thrombus is not obstructive, but approximately 70 percent have venous thrombosis if a venogram is performed."

Hirsh candidly admits, "We were kidding ourselves." There were two reasons. First, they thought they could extrapolate the observed sensitivity of impedance plethysmography when used in symptomatic patients to its sensitivity when used as a screening test. They were also wrong in accepting studies done by various groups reporting very high sensitivity for impedance plethysmography when used as a screening test. These studies were nonblinded and therefore subject to bias. Only when blinded studies were performed, in which the readers of the impedance plethysmography and venography results performed their assessment independently and without knowledge of the other result, was the poor sensitivity of impedance plethysmography brought to light (Wells et al. 1995).

The problem not recognized was that the clinical population in which a particular clinician is working is inevitably different from that on which the studies were done. Says Hirsh:

What happens initially is that you do your study on really sick people. And then you set up a diagnostic screen program, and they send all of Hamilton and southern Ontario to you. And then you begin to see patients at an early stage of their disease, and then the sensitivity of the test falls. For example, in Hamilton the thrombosis group is asked to see patients with atypical leg pain who often have not been examined by the referring physician. What we should do is to see the patients before they are tested, and not perform tests on many of them. Because of the system, we don't do this; it is inefficient. This has changed now, and patients are rated on the basis of pretest probability and then tested accordingly.

When they realized these problems, they went back and looked at patients clinically. It turned out that they had done better than they thought in predicting the probability of disease on simple clinical grounds: 85 percent of the people whom they predicted as being in a high probability group had thrombosis, and only 5 percent of those in the low probability group had thrombosis. When they combined their pretest predictions with the results of noninvasive tests, this greatly simplified the diagnostic approach. Hirsh observes, "So we have come full circle in the diagnosis of venous thrombosis. Clinical diagnosis was considered to be unreliable, but people doing the studies — including us — failed to include two important items in the clinical testing. These are the risk factors for venous thrombosis and a probability of another disease. When we add these two items to the symptoms and signs, we are much better than we thought."

Instead of seeing the resolution of a clinical question in a single randomized controlled trial, Hirsh recognizes the need for a gradual, iterative research approach. Despite the strong emphasis on clinical trials in his own book, Henrik Wulff is also concerned about the limitations of trials in everyday clinical care. First, he points out a theoretical incompatibility of trial results with the clinician's knowledge base: "If you do a controlled trial and end up with a p value, then that p value is a probability of the result of the trial, given that the null hypothesis is true. What you want to know as a clinician is the opposite probability, the probability that the null hypothesis is true, given these results. That conversion cannot be done unless you use your prior confidence in the null hypothesis. Therefore you can *never* interpret the result of a clinical epidemiology study or a randomized trial without bringing in knowledge of a different kind."

Wulff emphasizes the need for additional kinds of information when interpreting the results of clinical trials, and he agrees with Feinstein that this additional information does not come from conducting still more trials. Thus he is concerned that the capacity of trials alone to resolve the fundamental problems of clinical medicine should not be overestimated. Says Wulff, "The randomized clinical trial was thought of as the panacea of medicine: if everybody did randomized clinical trials, then all the problems would be solved. Of course, that's nonsense for a lot of reasons. It's just a tool." In particular, it was difficult to generalize the results of trials to clinical practice: "It's one thing finding out that treatment is effective with a randomized clinical trial. But then comes the problem, do we want that effect? And then, of course, it may have been the perfect RCT, but people will use the treatment for other conditions and other patients, and therefore we have the need for constant quality assurance."

While the statistical understanding of probability has been fundamental to the development of both public health and clinical epidemiology, it remains a difficult concept to understand, Wulff says:

There is also the problem of clinical epidemiology being concerned with groups. I have yet to find a clinical epidemiologist who openly acknowledges the ambiguity of the probability concept. They see in a scientific study that 90 percent of patients were cured, and then they take it for granted that there is a 90 percent chance that Mr. Brown will be cured. But that is an extremely interesting problem. What is a probability of one person being cured? Either he is cured or he is not cured. What if Mr. Brown is very old, and another study has shown that old people in general have a worse prognosis? How do you combine these probabilities? It is extremely complex, but that is what clinical medicine is all about.

Fraser Mustard is concerned that an overcommitment to the randomized controlled trial at McMaster University could lead to distortion of the clinical research agenda. Trials, he says, "can run you ragged on the trivial." The problem was that clinical epidemiology was technique driven, which placed its emphasis on the outcome of the trial itself rather than how the results of the trial articulated with the total knowledge base. Hirsh argues that the results of trials have to take account of clinical complexities in order to provide new and useful information to the clinician. Mustard adds the additional concern that trials are very expensive, and human subjects have their lives disrupted while participating in them, so trials should be designed to provide a definitive answer to a research question. This requires closer collaboration with the laboratory sciences. Trials of antiplatelet therapy, he believes, were based on a poor understanding of the pathway in thrombosis, including the Antiplatelet Trialists' Collaboration (1994). When this happens, the trials of a particular intervention proliferate rapidly but yield no clear answer.

Criticisms such as these come from within the clinical epidemiology movement and draw attention to the degree of scrutiny directed at clinical epidemiology and evidence-based medicine by the pioneers of this initiative. They acknowledge that clinical epidemiology and evidence-based medicine had an important role in developing a scientific approach to clinical care. There are, however, reservations about the adequacy of this science. These reservations are particularly acute when evaluating the adequacy of these methods for assessing disease in the community, an area specifically excluded by David Sackett. The critics reject this delimited approach and see an understanding of disease in the community as playing an indispensable role in the decision making of clinicians. Arturo Morillo's account of the role in less industrialized countries of fellows trained in clinical epidemiology echoes these concerns, and such internal concerns are amplified by others who reflect on clinical epidemiology's failings from outside.

The Problem of Disease in the Community

The strategic location of clinical epidemiology in the medical school at McMaster University may have limited the attention that could be paid to community health, and this means that the researchers have not addressed what John Evans calls the "expansionist, multivariate" presentation of disease in the community. There is, however, no denying that the practice of clinical care in community context is demanding, especially when embodied in a style of practice that explicitly acknowledges the psychological, social, and political context of illness. Two personal accounts illustrate these points.

When I interviewed him in 1991, John Stoeckle was chief of medical clinics at the Massachusetts General Hospital. He retired in 2001, after a career of nearly half a century in internal medicine. He believed that primary care had been neglected in the United States and elsewhere in favor of an emphasis on hospital medicine and acute care. This was driven by the profit motive: there are large sums of money invested in hospital medicine, and very small profits to be made in primary care. Thus the medical system had swung away from the prevention of disease and care for the chronically ill in the community, to curative interventions for the sick-in-bed. What emerged was what Stoeckle calls the "garage" view of medical care: "You can get everything tested and repaired." This discouraged clinicians from making explicit the social considerations that went into their decision making. "A great deal of what looks like fairly straight garage work is concealing a lot of social decisions," he says. "Every day at conferences, I hear social reasons coming out. There would be shrieks if I said so, but you hear them. There are social reasons for doing both tests and procedures. Occasionally I tease a colleague and make them almost admit [this]. They don't like it much, but it is there — the presence of the personal, social, and psychosocial in decision making."

The market-driven proliferation of acute care is deeply cultural, affecting both clinicians and patients. This has serious implications for the patient-doctor relationship and for any attempt to mute a predisposition to intervention. According to Stoeckle:

We are ambivalent as a profession. How much participation do you want the patients to have in decision making? We are very ambivalent. Some of us say, "OK, whatever you want you get. OK, right here." Others say, "I don't think you really need that, but if you want it, you know, I will order it for you, but I want you to know what I think, OK?" Another practitioner will say, "Listen, over my dead body! I don't believe that is important, and I am not going to do it. But I will continue to see you." The ambivalence is enormous.

Medical decisions should be mediated by what the doctor knows about the patient's social background, including social class. With the decline of primary care in the United States, clinicians were increasingly ignorant of the social circumstances of their patients. The drive for efficiency in hospitals meant that the emphasis fell on developing skills in deciding which intervention to order, rather than on taking a good patient history and getting to know the patient. This articulated well with the focus of clinical epidemiology on the technical aspects of care: when a test should be done and when an intervention is technically justifiable. Such technical evidence limited the clinician's discretion in decision making but, Stoeckle argues, this very discretion is necessary if the social context of disease is to be taken into account. This includes the patient's social class but also the general social background, as well as the patient's psychology and the way in which this mediates, for example, requests for tests:

The system locks them in. Some people called me up from downstairs in the emergency room: "Dr. Stoeckle what about Mr. Miller?" — at five o'clock in the morning. I said, "Yeah I know him. What about him?" They said, "He is down here, and he has got this chest discomfort. Do you think we should admit him to rule out MI [myocardial infarction]?" And I said, "He is one of the gypsies. You know that the gypsy clan that we have in Boston has one of the highest rates of coronary heart disease of any other group here? If you check his medical record, you will find out that his cholesterol is about 344, and he has had one MI before, down in New Jersey." The problem is the system. Staff often don't have the time to know the background of patients or to find out about it. I think that is how the system is organized. That is the reason primary care is essential. I think some- where along the line somebody ought to include patients in the system. Somebody in the system must know who they are.

The drive to be quantitatively rigorous was based on the belief that this would make clinical care "scientific," but variables to do with social net- works were never captured when assessing the outcome of a procedure. Stoeckle notes:

I was thinking the other day about a patient who came in; I was wondering how they ever could do an outcome study of this lady, who had spinal surgery. I sup- pose if you put her in an outcome study, she would come out well. She came in to see me, and she said, "I want you to write a letter for me, Dr. Stoeckle; I am not feeling good." And I said, "Why is that?" She said, "Well, you know Jimmy is down in Norfolk Prison, and Billy is in prison too, and you know my brother is up for murder." I said, "Yes, what do you want me to do?" She said, "I want you to write me a letter just so that I can be able to visit them more often, because they feel ter- rible. You know what I mean?" And I wondered how you would ever process that sort of thing as an outcome variable as to whether the surgery really did her any good? She is still in some discomfort, [but] she has things she has to do.

Stoeckle believes that the evaluation of clinical care should focus not only on how well doctors deal with the technical dimensions of care but also on how well they deal with the psychosocial dimensions. He recognizes the limits to changing medical practice. Unless the system of rewards from medical practice is changed, people will respond by curtailing what they deliver to patients.

Howard Waitzkin considers himself indebted to John Stoeckle as mentor and friend, and he credits Stoeckle for his leadership in studying and promoting community health centers. These had started as "a form of largesse," dealing with potentially problematic indigent minorities and culturally different patients (Stoeckle and Candib 1969). Waitzkin trained at Harvard Medical School, where he specialized in internal and geriatric medicine while, at the same time, completing a doctorate in sociology. As a Robert Wood Johnson Clinical Scholar, he pursued issues related to the patient-doctor relationship. The clinical part of this training period took place at a United Farmworkers' clinic. From there he entered community practice. At North Orange County Community Clinic, a clinic providing a teaching and research site for primary care medicine at the University of California, Irvine, he again became interested in the problem of evaluation, including the evaluation of coronary care units, an issue that had drawn his attention when he was a senior resident at Massachusetts General Hospital. This came about as a result of an experience with a patient who had had a heart attack, but who refused to be admitted to the hospital. Waitzkin recalls:

He realized what was going on, but he would not go to hospital, so he rested at home. It was kind of dangerous for me to be involved in this, so I started reading the literature about what the rationale was for coronary care units. Like most people, I had just accepted this dogma — you know, that's where people should be treated. So I became familiar with the British studies, the criticism, and I found them very startling, and then I started going back to the original sources by Bernie Lown and others about the rationale for coronary care units. At that point I realized that, as in so many other areas, the rationale was very dubious.

If this was so, why then did coronary care units flourish? Waitzkin's thesis was that this could be explained only in terms of the financial interests involved in developing and running coronary care units (Waitzkin 1979a). His research used Marxian social theory (Waitzkin 2000) to explain the social and political dynamics not only of medical technology but also of how doctors interpret their patients' problems in the clinical encounter (Waitzkin 1979b, 1991).

Given this background, Waitzkin feels skeptical about the proposed aim of much of the evaluation of medical care. The flawed assumption, he believes, is that the fiscal problem was caused by irrational medical practice:

A study by the National Academy of Sciences compared the financial impact of the maximum cost savings from reducing the ten most overutilized procedures by 5 to 10 percent, which was seen as the best feasible result. The total saving nationally was on the order of half a billion dollars. Whereas, if the billing bureaucracy and other administrative waste could be eliminated by a National Health Program, that would save $80 billion a year. So there is a strong ideological force that is motivating attempts to clean up the doctors' act: define standards of practice and then make them do it! The cost savings are not going to be worth a hill of beans compared to other more basic structural changes.

The necessary structural changes would require analysis of the role of the insurance industry and the pharmaceutical industry. In the United

States, for many people, the issue was actually getting access to medical care, but, Waitzkin argues, powerful financial interests opposed structural change: "Congress has not been prepared to act on this because of financial support through political action committees, which are tied to the insurance industry and banks." Such a political climate meant a lack of interest in epidemiology with a critical focus on the role of social class and racial inequality in health. "So what you have, then, is a flowering of epidemiologic work looking at noncontroversial variables in terms of the society as a whole, or a small part of the picture in clinical practice, but not looking at the whole other important set of variables that relate to the structure of society. It's very interesting, and I feel very sad that the intellectual cutting edge of the field has shifted — especially in the more recent trends within clinical epidemiology — to put the focus on a very micro level."

Waitzkin believes that the McMaster University team had a profound intellectual influence on developing methods of critically evaluating the medical literature that were readily accessible to clinicians. On the other hand, he was surprised, given the more critical attitudes to health care in Canada, that the team had buried some of the more critical intellectual questions of clinical care itself. Unable to deal directly with the effects of social structures on health, clinicians turned to technologies as a defensive measure, and the end result satisfied neither patient nor doctor. But what is the alternative? It is Waitzkin's view that medical doctors alone should not be dealing with these problems: "The need is to recognize the limits of traditional medical procedures to deal with these social structural problems, and then to develop social structures that allow other groups in the community, workplace, women's organizations, and others to help deal with problems. It doesn't take a radical restructuring of society to bring about these changes." Alternatives such as these have little chance of serious consideration when the intellectual preoccupation is with issues that do little to address the effects of social structural problems on health outcome.

Is This a Paradigm Shift?

Thus far, one set of criticisms points to the limitations of clinical epidemiology in establishing a scientific basis for clinical care. The second set of criticisms concerns its failure to address the demanding and troublesome issues raised by the social and political contexts within which patients live and within which the medical system is located. Essentially these criticisms point to a need to give evidence-based medicine a broader agenda. But it should be borne in mind that a narrow agenda may have been a critically important part of the reason clinical epidemiology was accepted in medical schools, where its institutionalization represents a substantial shift in the focus of medicine. While the charismatic leadership of the founders was important in forging a committed band of promoters, its value also lay in how its subject matter articulated with the basic science of medical education. The discipline has set clear boundaries to its enterprise, applying them primarily to the technical aspects of care. Within these limits, has a paradigm shift in scientific decision making occurred? In order to consider this issue, we must examine how succeeding paradigms of medicine have operated.

When Alvan Feinstein set up the Sydenham Society to challenge the activities of annual clinical meetings of the societies of academic internal medicine, he was mounting a protest against the dominance of laboratory medicine. Feinstein proposed instead to study empirical patterns of disease and issues of prognosis and therapy. In doing so, he invoked the work of Thomas Sydenham (1624–1689), who had led the way in systematizing the key task of the physician, clinical observation, by developing finely detailed classification of observations. What Feinstein wanted to do was rescue this past way of seeing patient care by bringing to bear new mathematical procedures that would make it compatible with scientific medicine. The reason his effort failed may well be problems of paradigm.

The shared worldview of a coherent tradition of scientific research is what Thomas Kuhn (1970) called a paradigm. In the seventeenth-century paradigm of bedside medicine, the taken-for-granted set of rules and standards for studying clinical practice emphasized taxonomic classification of signs and symptoms. In the taxonomic sciences, causality is not a primary objective. The medical understanding was that illness had to run its course, and treatment was limited to interventions like bloodletting, purging, or a change of air for restoring the equilibrium of the sick person. This view of medicine was displaced in the next centuries by scientific medicine, which saw disease as being located in the biological processes of the body and drew on science to develop disease-specific treatments. When such a shift in paradigm occurs, the assumptions of the old paradigm appear obsolete. Feinstein's move to resurrect an old paradigm may therefore have been met with blank incomprehension.

The emergence of a new scientific paradigm rests on the emergence of new facts that require new explanations, and Kuhn argues that new technologies have often generated these new facts (1970, pp. 16–17). When this happens, the new objects of study are investigated with "detail and depth that would otherwise be unimaginable" (Kuhn 1970, p. 24). In the early days of the scientific paradigm, for example, the stethoscope developed by René-Théophile-Hyacinthe Laennec in 1816 became the key technology for "seeing" into the living body. The facts generated aroused intense interest: "Through its agency, the morbid mysteries of nature, which had hitherto baffled human experience, were now to be unveiled to the crude perception of the merest tyro in the profession of medicine" (*Lancet* 1826, p. 471). The stethoscope became the emblem of the scientific doctor, despite the overall lack of treatment for the diseases diagnosed.

A new paradigm produces a new set of preoccupations, but it does not have to provide a fully detailed answer to all questions in an area. Instead, it focuses the attention of its adherents on a bounded set of phenomena that are amenable to analysis by fitting them into the relatively inflexible "boxes" that the paradigm provides. Phenomena that do not fit these boxes are simply not seen. Similarly, criticism by proponents of the old paradigm is ignored. In the early days of the stethoscope, when critics pointed out that diagnosis had little benefit for patients, the response was not to address the criticism but to invoke the new paradigm: "This is an objection that should never come from the lips of a man of science. In the pursuit of science every truth, every fact discovered, is of value" (Corrigan 1828–1829, p. 588).

In *Evidence-Based Medicine: How to Practice and Teach EBM,* we find Sackett and his colleagues' response to criticism in a section titled "What EBM Is Not": evidence-based medicine is not old hat or too difficult to practice, it does not replace individual clinical expertise but informs it, it will not be hijacked by purchasers and managers because it shines a light on quality rather than cost, and it does not see the randomized controlled trial as the gold standard, except for judging whether a particular intervention does more good than harm (1997, pp. 3–5). The criticisms are not addressed explicitly, nor are arguments mounted against criticism. Instead the book outlines reasons for evidence-based medicine: the accumulation of new evidence; the inaccessibility of this evidence to clinicians; deterioration of clinical performance over time; traditional continuing education programs that do not improve clinical performance; the capacity of evidence-based medicine, as set out in the book, to improve clinical performance (1997, p. 5). The book then offers three strategies for overcoming these problems: becoming an evidence-based-medicine practitioner, using summaries developed by others, or accepting evidence-based protocols developed by colleagues. Driving the need for this initiative is the emphasis on the proliferation of medical knowledge and the role of evidence-based medicine in solving this problem. The key technology producing the new facts is the randomized controlled trial.

This suggests that evidence-based medicine has at least these features of a new scientific paradigm for clinical care. The new way of accounting for facts is seen as superior in a self-evident way. Expertise in the scientific appraisal of the literature, and databases that extract valuable information from this literature, are certainly new. The point at issue is the extent to which evidence-based medicine is incommensurate with current practice. We need to distinguish between new ways of seeing the world and mere claims to new ways of seeing the world, even when the latter are presented with charismatic fervour.

While medical practitioners have a formal knowledge base underpinning practice, their work may also, at various times, have to be justified to the outside world. Usually this is done by referring to a simpler set of ideas that argues there is personal, social, and political value in a particular practice. This simpler set of ideas is called an ideology. The practical component, what the clinician does when faced with an individual patient, may be relatively unchanging in comparison with the various ideological ways in which this practice is legitimated in the outside world. This raises the question of whether evidence-based medicine is an ideological claim presented in evangelical terms rather than a shift in paradigm to a new form of practice. The very simplicity of the term adds to its utility as an ideology. Pierre-Charles-Alexandre Louis (1835) proposed a similar program of research in postrevolutionary France. P. K. Rangachari (1997) drew attention to this early work and asked whether evidence-based medicine was not "old French wine with a new Canadian label."

David Armstrong is a sociologist located in the Department of General Practice at King's College, London. He describes as "scientistic" the assumption that medical decisions can be based on a formula and does not accept "the dream of medicine that somehow we would have evidence and facts, that it would come down to numbers and concrete evidence." He sees clinical epidemiology not so much as a new paradigm but as a shoring up of the old paradigm: the aim is not a rejection of the core assumptions of scientific medicine but an attempt to bring clinical practice into line with the dominant paradigm. Again, experimental methods of research provide the means of claiming scientific status.

Like Waitzkin, Armstrong first qualified in medicine, then sociology.

Like many others discussed in this book, he was distressed to find that his clinical training did not prepare him adequately for clinical practice in the community. Disillusioned with practice and irritated by the hierarchical medical system, Armstrong turned to sociology instead of clinical epidemiology. His main research interest has been to analyze in meticulous detail the historical social context of medical knowledge (Armstrong 1983).

Like Feinstein, Armstrong argues that diagnostic categories are not just "nice little boxes" into which patients are filed. Like many other sociologists, he goes further, arguing that medical knowledge itself consists of fluid conceptions responsive to changes in social context (1987). While disease may derive from a biological reality, it always has a basis in social reality. Medical knowledge is socially constructed (Wright and Treacher 1982).

In 1977 Armstrong analyzed the effect of the controlled clinical trial on the balance of power between clinical experience and clinical science. He points out that the call for a more scientific approach to clinical care in the United Kingdom grew in tandem with the growth of scientific medicine. In 1928–1929 the Medical Research Council had made experimental study of the human patient a commitment. In 1931, it created the Therapeutics Trial Committee, which started testing therapies. Trials reinforced science, being "as near to a laboratory experiment as is practicable," but in the process, this undermined a traditional clinical hierarchy based on the authority of greater personal experience with patients. Not only could junior medical staff question authority but so could patients and outside regulatory agencies. In particular, he notes that the reorganization of the National Health Service in 1974 brought an emphasis on cost-effective care and increased the threat to clinical authority. According to Armstrong, one response could be the development of "humanist" medicine — described, for example, in the work of Balint (1961) — as a way of resisting "the incursion of clinical science into clinical sense" (Armstrong 1977, p. 601).

Armstrong's argument receives support from J. Bensing (2000). While Bensing accepts evidence-based medicine as a new paradigm, a doctor-centered paradigm, his concern was that it could displace the paradigm of patient-centered medicine. The problem of the latter, says Bensing, is that it is based on "fuzzy" concepts, ones difficult to reduce to measurements — "and that is what researchers need to do" (2000, p. 21). The article quotes J. P. Kassirer (1995) as arguing, "As our medical decisions become more codified, we should take care to ensure that critical therapeutic devices are not based exclusively on formal guidelines." Presumably bowing to the dominance of the doctor-centered paradigm, Bensing concludes that patient-centered medicine needed to develop its own evidence-based guidelines. It is worth noting here that the concept of patient-centered medicine invokes the biopsychosocial as a dimension of care. When George Engel introduced this approach in 1977, it too was hailed as a new medical model for clinical care and a challenge for bio-medicine. It has fared less well than evidence-based medicine. The expla-nation could well be that it articulates less well with scientific medicine. Another explanation (see chapter 7) is that the Cochrane Collaboration has successfully incorporated some aspects of a patient-centered approach into evidence-based medicine, with the focus shifting from patients to consumers.

Armstrong, like many other commentators, argues that outside regu-latory agencies could use the evidence of trials to demand increased accountability from clinicians with respect to the cost-effectiveness of therapy. There is certainly the potential to provide useful information for policy makers making decisions about the allocation of health resources. As Armstrong foresaw in 1977, this would have raised political tensions within the medical profession, in turn leading to the marginalization of clinical epidemiology within medicine. What happened instead, according to Jonathan Lomas, was that clinical epidemiology became an "animal of medicine," employed in the interests of the medical profession itself:

It is something that belongs to medicine and something that medicine has devel-oped and is using in some ways to colonize the rest of health care. That is a very dangerous development, but blame should not necessarily be laid at the door of clinical epidemiology. If the blame is to be laid anywhere, it may be at the feet of relatively thoughtful medical leaders of North America who realize that evalua-tion is the future for the health care system. As such, the tools of clinical epi-demiology are going to be central to the policy arguments that will allow indi-viduals to lever funds for their own particular programs and initiatives out of governments. Those skills and abilities are therefore extremely important for strategic and political reasons for physician organizations to obtain, and use, and become skilled at. It is happening at an accelerated pace throughout medicine, now that those skills are being acquired.

If clinical care was the soft underbelly of scientific medicine, then clin-ical epidemiology proved to be disciplinary armor against attacks. Not surprisingly, then, a major theme of the burgeoning critical literature on evidence-based medicine has been the identification of the "new para-digm" argument of evidence-based medicine as a professional ideology based on "over-hopeful assumptions that are unlikely to be fully realised" (Klein 1996, p. 85). Again, the term applied to this ideology was *scientism* (Frankford 1994), in recognition of the formative influence of the paradigm of scientific medicine. Neville Goodman (1999) attributes the authority of evidence-based medicine, and the small industry it was sustaining, to its methods. It was attractive as a means of challenging the dogma of the authoritative clinical specialist, but it was developing a powerful dogma of its own on the basis of a mirage. Since there was no evidence that "evidence" was producing better care, the claims of evidence-based medicine were ideological and the debate was being conducted on emotional and rhetorical grounds. Inspired by a lack of self-doubt, he argues, the proponents of evidence-based medicine ignored detailed, careful criticism, merely asserting the validity of their own approach.

However, if the people involved in generating knowledge from randomized controlled trials used arguments based on science to their own competitive advantage, they could, at the same time, be subjecting themselves to other economic interests. This issue concerned Fraser Mustard, who was alarmed at both the soft endpoints used for some trials and the motivation for doing trials. He recalls:

I went to a session that the Kaiser Family Foundation ran several years ago on measures of health status improvement. These are soft measurements — changes in the function of people, not mortality data — important but difficult measures and thus at risk of distortion. Since the drug industry is under pressure to do clinical trials to justify the effectiveness of a drug to get approval, this field is important to them. Some of the endpoints being promoted were disturbing because of their subjective character. Part of what was driving this was a commercial interest. Investigators were designing measurements to serve the needs of the trial culture. It became apparent that clinical epidemiology could be distorted in a way that could lead to misuse. In my view, if I were not doing what I am doing, and I was looking for something to do, I would go and study this area. I think there is a risk of significant distortion. In other words, a critical appraisal of clinical epidemiology!

In contrast, there was no immediate market value in studying the determinants of health or in developing policies to deal with these problems at a more fundamental level. These were powerful concerns in light of clinical epidemiology's role in training International Clinical Epidemiology Network (INCLEN) fellows. Kerr White came to believe that the INCLEN programs at Pennsylvania and Newcastle Universities remained broad, but that the largest program, at McMaster University, failed to broaden its perspective. "There has been some regression towards the mean there," he says; "I think that it became too narrowly focused." Fraser Mustard's view was that some of the best people trained in the INCLEN program might do what Arturo Morillo anticipated, move research out into the community. On the other hand, two forces would oppose this: the resistance of medical schools to a questioning of their authority and the role of drug companies in directing the kind of research done.

Mustard himself developed a commitment to what may in itself be a significant shift in research and policy analysis. His view was that high-quality research should be used to eliminate ineffective medical interventions, but that the freed-up resources should then be used to create the wealth necessary to sustain a healthy society. This vision was incorporated into the Canadian Institute of Advanced Research with the aim of mobilizing talented individuals to tackle complex problems without conventional institutional barriers. Says Mustard, "The barriers to the new frameworks of understanding are that, while clinical epidemiology could, as we found at McMaster, be with time incorporated into a medical school (admittedly a new one), population health is more difficult. Also the broader work on the determinants of health can threaten a profession. McKeown's work raised such a challenge. McKeown's obituary in the *Lancet* said, 'He was never knighted because he threatened his profession.' The second barrier is the caliber of people needed from different disciplines to study complex problems. The structure of universities does not make it easy to bring them together." Here Mustard refers to the work of Thomas McKeown and his challenge to medicine in 1976 in *The Role of Medicine: Dream, Mirage, or Nemesis?* (see chapter 6). Mustard's institute was intended to be an investment in talented people, even troublesome people like McKeown. It would provide a way of mobilizing human capital to focus on complex problems regardless of where they were located or what their discipline might be. "Just think of the power!" says Mustard. "Because the institute can select the area and the people, there are few boundaries in terms of what you can do, other than money and modern technologies. The institute programs have members across Canada, U.S.A., Europe, Israel, and Japan. Because we leave people in their institutions, we then create nodes in the institutions around which their work can be amplified."

The institute's funds came from private donors and from governments in Canada. It represented an interesting contrast to the Rockefeller Foundation's commitment in the early part of the century to creating separate schools of public health. They too despaired of the task of directing the attention of medical schools to the problems of community health.

The strategy of Mustard's institute, however, left researchers in place in medical schools or other institutions but provided a structure for new research, the results of which could then be disseminated back to the parent institution.

If Mustard is right, then a comprehensive shift in paradigm is unlikely to occur in one section of a medical school without the whole scientific paradigm of medicine shifting. He suggests instead disseminating new ideas by stealth, sowing the seeds of new ways of thinking wherever there might be fertile ground. In turn, given the right conditions, this could precipitate a paradigm shift in medical schools in general. In this view, it seems unlikely that evidence-based medicine has achieved anything more than a shift to align clinical care a little more closely with the dominant scientific paradigm. The promoters of the initiative have acquired substantial intellectual capital in the process. On the other hand, achieving change at all required a sustained campaign emphasizing the benefits, real and ideological, that flow from the new approach.

Given that the methods used by clinical epidemiology and evidence-based medicine are based on epidemiology, the basic science of public health, this raises the question of the relationship with the discipline of public health.

The Alternative of Public Health

There is a long history of distrust between medicine, which focuses on the individual patient, and public health, which focuses on the health of populations. It was public health that first produced methodological innovations relevant to the study of populations. Many of the innovators were themselves medically trained, but their primary commitment was to population studies. While bedside medicine was classifying symptoms, John Graunt was applying arithmetic methods to bills of mortality (1661). Graunt's contemporary William Petty raised questions about the effect of doctors and their medications on the life chances of populations. Jacques Bernoulli used a theory of probability published in 1713 to calculate life expectancy. Methods involving the calculus of probability even allowed an early demonstration of the effectiveness of smallpox vaccination in 1721 in Boston, when people vaccinated against smallpox were shown to be less susceptible to an epidemic (Shyrock 1961, p. 95). Deriving from these methods were two principles relevant to medicine in assessing its treatments: the need to control for chance and an emphasis on large numbers as providing more scientifically accurate results than studies on individuals (Oakley 2000, p. 110). Together these two principles act to reduce the risk of invalid conclusions.

In France after the French Revolution, Pierre-Charles-Alexandre Louis (1835) developed methods for evaluating medical interventions, including bloodletting. Despite the widespread use of bloodletting, he failed to find any positive effect. The work of Pierre-Simon Laplace (1749–1827) further developed theories of probability, and the first book on medical statistics, by Jules Gavarret (1840), provided new methods for dealing with problems of design. The nineteenth century saw the development of surveys and statistical studies that created control from indeterminacy and generated methods for establishing apparently immutable laws from the ever-increasing supply of information generated by states that classified, counted, and tabulated their subjects. Such methods were fostered by the new professional association devoted to "epidemiology," which was giving a clear and exact delineation of disease in the community.

Why then did a new science of clinical care not eventuate at this time? Paul Starr argues that public health had developed a very broad definition of its role, to the extent that all aspects of life relevant to health came under its definition. This was "an invitation to conflict" (1982, p. 180). Thus efforts to integrate public health and medical care were unsuccessful. One example is the decision by Yale University in 1914 to establish a multidisciplinary course for training public health officers and to locate it in its School of Medicine. C-E. A. Winslow, the first chair, was a public health scientist, not a physician. A determined public health evangelist, he identified public health as "one of the most startling and revolutionary events in the history of the human race," promoted a national health program covered by health insurance, and proposed locating preventive services, including medical services, within publicly funded health centers (1926, pp. 1077–83). Such proposals were alien to medical practice based on individual patient care.

These arguments were increasingly challenged after the discovery of germs as specific agents of disease and the development in medicine of some disease-specific treatments, with the promise of more to come. Medicine took on laboratory-based science as its fundamental basis. An exponential increase in medical research and a steady stream of therapeutic advances then made their appearance. By 1946, American doctors were occupying an exalted position in comparison with that of their colleagues a century earlier (Shyrock 1947). In the 1950s, with the development of molecular biology, the basic science of the scientific paradigm became known as biomedicine. The allure of the laboratory produced a rush to specialization in the biological sciences, and medical care practiced in the community became an unattractive option. Even less attractive was public health with epidemiology as its basic science. The ideological tables were turned. Epidemiology now seemed vague and uncertain in comparison with laboratory science.

John Paul, professor of preventive medicine at Yale University at the same time as Winslow, had a different, more pragmatic approach to the relationship between medicine and public health. Clinicians dealt with the disease of individual patients. This required training in the "hard core" of biomedical science. They also benefited from knowledge of epidemiology, so that they could start with the individual patient but then also take account of the communities and settings in which these patients lived and became ill. The term that Paul used to describe this activity was *clinical epidemiology*. In studying this "ecology of human disease," medical students would learn about the scientific possibilities for preventing as well as treating disease (1938).

With enthusiasm roused by the growth and promise of scientific medicine, these arguments were lost to view until the 1970s, when David Sackett at McMaster University saw epidemiological method as an important skill for clinicians at the new medical school. Clinical epidemiology excised the community concerns of public health but retained the methods and restricted the leadership roles to those with medical training. The clinical content was seen as an important step in wooing medical students disenchanted with public health.

Alvan Feinstein went further, becoming a vocal proponent of the view that "big E" public health epidemiology lacked methodological skills. Given the many contributory factors to health in the community, it is hardly surprising that epidemiological studies should pose complex methodological challenges and therefore come under critical scrutiny. Feinstein attacked public health epidemiology with considerable energy, targeting the scientific standards of epidemiological studies that established the menaces in daily life: coffee, alcohol, and pharmaceutical treatment of hypertension (1988). He argued that epidemiologists had gone astray in their attempt to establish the health risk posed by lifestyle factors. Epidemiologists pointed out Feinstein's own methodological errors (Savits et al. 1990) and accused him of failing to keep up with methodological developments in epidemiology and of becoming more advocate than scientist (Greenland 1991). Alfredo Morabia (2002) concludes that Feinstein was biased against disease prevention based on behavior modification.

Feinstein certainly presented a cutting critique of research addressing lifestyle risks, but criticism of his activities intensified when he turned his attention to studies that identified the risk of exposure to passive smoking. In an article fittingly titled "The Controversial Controversy of a Passionate Controversialist," Morabia (2002) argues that Feinstein became a key figure in the attempts of the tobacco industry to discredit studies that identified the risks of environmental tobacco smoke, and this is particularly important in light of what Morabia identifies as significant financial support from the tobacco industry. It is difficult to see how such issues of personal bias and institutional power could have been presented and debated within the limits of the research program proposed by Feinstein.

If clinical epidemiology was locked into a struggle for legitimacy with public health, it was largely an unequal struggle. Milton Terris, past president of the American Public Health Association, who is famous for his defense of public health, argued in 1988 that public health epidemiology provided a much better basis of training for the INCLEN program than did clinical epidemiology, but that this was overlooked for political reasons:

The Rockefeller Foundation people are selling this program, with real money to back it up, all over Asia, Africa and Latin America. They are going to divert promising people into doing drug trials. Both the Rockefeller Foundation and the Robert Wood Johnson Foundation's "clinical scholars" program avoid public health schools like the plague. I think it is an absurdity. Here we have the Third World with all its terrible problems of famine, malnutrition, infant diarrhea, malaria, and all the other infectious and noninfectious diseases, and all this money is being spent to do clinical trials. These foundations operate under a false banner. They are misusing the term epidemiology. . . . The real reason for the program is political. As I said before, clinicians in the United States and elsewhere are afraid that non-clinicians will run the health services. That is why the Robert Wood Johnson Foundation has a clinical scholars program and the Rockefeller Foundation has a clinical epidemiology program. They want clinicians to know enough epidemiology, public health, and medical care organization to step in as leaders to run the show. And some of these people, with their medical arrogance, do not hesitate to denigrate schools of public health because they are multidisciplinary. (Terris in Buck et al. 1988, p. 984)

Terris therefore saw clinical epidemiology as an occupational ideology aimed at strengthening the control of the medical profession over the health care system. The loser was public health epidemiology, which saw its methods taken over and its funding cut.

David Sackett sees the progressive encroachment of clinical epidemiology into medical training, where it displaced public health, as positive and no more than a logical extension of the greater appeal of clinical epidemiology to clinicians in training. This view is not shared by the epidemiologist John Last of Ottawa, who argues that the clinical epidemiologists made conceptual errors, the most important of which was the perception of public health and clinical care as separate, even antagonistic, enterprises. Most of the important advances in public health in the nineteenth century and the early twentieth century were made by clinician-epidemiologists like John Snow. In the present, Last argues, there is no basic antagonism between schools of public health and medical schools: "In the best schools of public health in the United States, the same people hold appointments in both places. There are so many interconnections between schools of public health and medical schools that to say that they don't speak to each other, and especially to say things like 'all the bright people are in the clinical departments, and all the ones who failed at everything in life are in the schools of public health,' it's just arrant nonsense."

Despite clinical epidemiologists' emphasis on rational thinking, Last argues, their views, especially their antagonism to both public health and to community care, are strikingly irrational. Last strongly contends that Canada must reestablish schools of public health, especially if people from other disciplines, who would feel alienated in medical schools, are to be involved in health research. Says Last, "I'm thinking particularly of people like a very thoughtful, extremely intelligent nurse who has had experience in the Canadian north and in developing countries, and I think is probably now one of the world's top people in health promotion. She had to go to Berkeley because there were no suitable programs in Canadian institutions. More important, when she tried to communicate with the people in the University of Toronto division of community health, they put her down in all kinds of devastating and gratuitously offensive ways." What is needed within clinical epidemiology, he argues, is a return to its public health roots: "What Dave Sackett and a few others do, and what it seems to me a whole generation of very able clinicians are now doing, is quantitative and rigorous analysis of clinical decision making and things of that nature. But it's not really epidemiology, because it's not genuinely population based; and some of them (there's at least one of them over at Mc) seem to reject altogether the idea of going out into the community and finding out what's really going on there."

John Last describes as "seriously misplaced" the move to close down schools of public health in the United States as a result of the survey done by John Evans (1981) for the Rockefeller Foundation. Last is concerned about the relocation of priorities in which "real epidemiology" (population based studies, mostly in community settings rather than institutional settings) gets devalued and neglected. In 1988 Last was moved to voice his criticisms publicly when he employed as residents several recent graduates from McMaster University who had wanted to do community-based studies of clinical problems and had been "rather actively discouraged" from doing so in favor of hospital-based studies. Last argues that clinical epidemiology, as defined by David Sackett, limited participation to the medically trained researcher. The narrow focus of what passed for clinical epidemiology in medicine's "disease palaces" was more properly called "clinical decision analysis." According to Last:

> The proper distinction between clinical decision analysis and epidemiology is that epidemiology is concerned with the study of disease or health-related behavior in a defined population, even if it is a population of patients rather than a community-based population with numerator and denominator in the conventional epidemiologic sense. . . . I get uncomfortable when "clinical epidemiology" applies to studies of a single patient, as in "N of one" studies. . . . I applaud the teaching of epidemiology in a clinical setting, perhaps the most significant advance in clinical teaching in my lifetime. But if this leads to the abandonment of non-clinical teaching of epidemiology and related disciplines and concepts, the next generation of physicians, and the society they have been trained to serve, will suffer. (1988, pp. 160–62).

Admittedly, the program that produced clinical epidemiology and evidence-based medicine had turned a blind eye to issues of community health. The price of incorporation in a medical school may well be the relegation of these issues to the sidelines.

Conclusion

Criticism of the McMaster University model of clinical epidemiology brought little change in its basic tenets but saw the development of a highly polished and successful proliferation of its original principles in the form of evidence-based medicine. Criticism of evidence-based medicine has been more public and has highlighted the ideological commitment of its practitioners to a form of practice that is consistent with the scientific paradigm of medicine.

While evidence-based medicine does not provide a comprehensive science of clinical care, the issue is whether it can do so in the future.

Feinstein's argument is that it cannot do so while it relies on models drawn from other disciplines instead of developing a specifically clinical analysis of its own practice. Additional and more extensive methodological development is needed. Hirsh is hopeful but does not underestimate the difficulties. More pessimistic are those practitioners committed to incorporating into their decision making the social contexts of their patients and the political context of medical care. They see the need to extend the discipline well beyond the boundaries that it set itself.

While evidence-based medicine borrowed freely from the methodological tools of public health, it has distanced itself from the social and contextual aspects of traditional public health practice and from the same contextual elements of clinical care. In the process it has distanced itself as well from the variety of research methods that public health has developed and used. The recommended extension of evidence-based medicine beyond its limits to incorporate these additional directions may be incompatible with incorporation into the medical system (see chapter 9).

CHAPTER 6

The British Intellectual Heritage

To understand the development of evidence-based medicine in Britain requires a look at the years during and following World War II. The novelist Doris Lessing, who arrived in London from Southern Rhodesia in 1949, gives an outsider's perspective on postwar Britain in her autobiography. After suffering through the war, the British, she says, were a tired people. In direct contrast with their low vitality, however, was their optimism for the future. Central to this optimism was their expectation of a new National Health Service:

A New Age was dawning, no less. Socialism was the key. . . . The National Health Service was their proudest achievement. In the thirties, before the war, an illness or an accident could drag a whole family down to disaster. The poverty had been terrible and had not been forgotten. All that was finished. No longer was there a need to dread illness and the Dole and old age. And this was just the beginning: things were going to get steadily better. Everyone seemed to share this mood. You kept meeting doctors who were setting up practices that would embody this new socialist medicine, who saw themselves as builders of a new era. They could be Communists, they could be Labour, they could be Liberals. They were all idealists. (Lessing 1998, p. 12)

These idealists included Archie Cochrane, Jerry Morris, and Richard Doll. Social medicine provided a focus for their concerns. In 1943, Oxford University had established an Institute of Social Medicine and appointed John Ryle as director and professor of social medicine. John Ryle had become disillusioned with the way in which medicine was turning a blind eye to what happened in the community:

Thirty years of my life have been spent as a student and teacher of clinical medicine. In these thirty years I have watched disease in the ward being studied more
and more thoroughly — if not always more thoughtfully — through the high
power of the microscope. Man . . . with his economic opportunity has been inad-
equately considered in this period by the clinical teacher and hospital research
worker. The medicine of the teaching schools has, as I have suggested, undergone
a gradual conversion to a highly technical exercise in bedside pathology and therapeutic method. . . . Health and sickness in the population and their possible cor-
relations with significant and measurable social or occupational influences are outside their province. (1948, p. 2)

He turned his attention to working with members of other disciplines,
including statisticians and social workers. This multidisciplinary approach
was necessary for the broad program espoused by social medicine: it covered all aspects of health care from individual medical care to any aspect
of the environment or community that affected health. Epidemiology was
central to the new approach, which included the measurement of health.
What was different about this approach was that social medicine had one
foot firmly in the medical camp.

Ryle's views were moderate in comparison with those of the group of
doctors who founded a society in celebration of Henry Sigerist in 1947.[1]
Sigerist was a medical reformer in the European liberal socialist tradition
who argued for a close relationship between medicine and human welfare
(Sigerist 1941; Brickman 1994). The Sigerist Society met over a number
of years to discuss aspects of medicine from a Marxist perspective. They
were disillusioned with the emphasis on Newtonian, mechanistic science
and chemistry in clinical practice. The threads running through their discussion concerned science and social responsibility, recognizing the
significance of class, and eliminating commercialism through group practice and salaried remuneration. They were strong supporters of a national
health service. Richard Doll addressed the group on the significance of
social conditions in the interpretation of vital statistics.[2]

The Sigerist Society did not long survive in the United Kingdom, but
social medicine continued to give coherence to a number of initiatives that
ultimately formed the basis of the British version of evidence-based medicine. The Society for Social Medicine, established in the 1950s, defined
social medicine as "epidemiology, the study of the medical and health
needs of society, the study of the provision and organisation of health services and the study of the prevention of disease." Its members were epidemiologists, community physicians, medical statisticians, sociologists,
and economists working in the field of social or community medicine.

Richard Doll, Archie Cochrane, and Tom McKeown attended the inaugural meeting of the Society; Austin Bradford Hill sent his apologies.[3]

Central to the tenets of social medicine was a commitment to centrally determined priorities and an expanded capacity to evaluate medical services (McKeown and Lowe 1974). Later Tom McKeown (1976) was to call into question the part played by *clinical* medicine in the decline of mortality in Britain in the late nineteenth and early twentieth centuries. The concerns of social medicine included the cost of medical services and the need to define a rational basis for restricting costs. The randomized controlled trial was an early candidate for the task of demonstrating that the expected benefits of some medical interventions were not being realized.

The randomized controlled trial in medicine had been used before (Armitage 1972; Chalmers 2001), but in the 1930s Austin Bradford Hill designed a randomized controlled trial for application to medical care (Bradford Hill 1937, 1962). He used comparison groups and saw randomization as a way of controlling selection bias in the allocation to these groups (Chalmers 2001). In 1946, the United Kingdom was able to afford only a small amount of streptomycin, a new drug for the treatment of tuberculosis — enough to treat fifty patients. Under these circumstances, argued Bradford Hill, anything but a randomized trial would be unethical (Armitage 1992). The trial of streptomycin treatment for tuberculosis was published in 1948 (Medical Research Council 1948), and Bradford Hill gave lucid accounts of the value of the clinical trial in 1951 *(British Medical Bulletin)* and 1952 *(New England Journal of Medicine)*. He argued that, under normal circumstances, faced with uncertainty about the effects of treatments, doctors could randomly allocate patients in a trial with a clear conscience (1963). Bradford Hill then undertook a number of proselytizing trips around the world. Archie Cochrane saw the trial design as a "very beautiful technique," the proper instrument for the systematic evaluation of the effectiveness of medical treatments (1972, p. 22). It could serve as the basis for a *rational* health service. This perception was built on a career spent in trying to exclude bias from epidemiological studies in Welsh mining communities.

One Man's Medicine: Archibald Cochrane

Archie Cochrane is in many ways Britain's equivalent to Alvan Feinstein. Both were strong individuals. As gadflies they circled the medical profession, looking for a place to sting it into greater recognition of the need for science in practice. Their commitments, however, were almost diametrically opposed. Feinstein became a clinician, Cochrane an epidemiologist. Feinstein wanted to make a good living; Cochrane had independent wealth. Feinstein wanted to convert doctors; Cochrane accused them of wishful thinking and threw his support behind the National Health Service. Feinstein had nothing of the radical vision; Cochrane was inspired by it.

Cochrane viewed his privileged background with wry humor, claiming to be "directly descended from the illegitimate progeny of a Nelsonian admiral."[4] In the introduction to Cochrane's autobiography, *One Man's Medicine,* Dick Cohen makes this telling comment about Cochrane: "My father's butler used to say that he was the only one of my friends who had the underclothes of a gentleman" (Cochrane 1989, p. xi). After leaving school, Cochrane went to Cambridge University, where he thought he might study medicine. He was, he recalls, reprimanded: "If you wish to study a trade, you must do that in your vacations. You have come here to be educated" (1989, p. 8), He studied physiology, comparative anatomy, and zoology.

Cochrane saw the early 1930s as his wasted years. His social conscience prevented him from becoming a good laboratory scientist. Instead he underwent psychoanalysis while studying medicine in Vienna and Leyden and then in London. He was appalled at the rise of fascism. During his clinical studies, the Spanish Civil War broke out, and he joined the republican cause, serving with the Spanish Medical Aid Field Ambulance Unit from 1936 to 1937. He had left University College Hospital without permission, and he recalled that, when he turned up at a ward round a year later very bronzed, with a red beard, the physician in charge said, "Ah Cochrane, back again. Had an interesting weekend?" (1979, p. 1663).

During the Spanish Civil War, Cochrane saw that the factional conflicts of the Left proved fatal to the war effort: "Overall I had a general feeling of satisfaction that I had risked my life for a cause I believed in; but I was relieved that I had not lost it in the process" (1989, p. 44). Together with his rejection of Marxism as a scientific hypothesis, this meant that he was never to join the Communist Party. Still, according to Richard Doll in his foreword to Cochrane's autobiography, Cochrane was a "man of the 1930s," with his views forged in the cataclysmic events of those years but augmented with a "fiery independence of mind" (1989, p. ix).

These qualities came to the fore during World War II, when Cochrane spent four years as a prisoner of war. He was often the only doctor in the camp, and disease was rife. In his desperate need to care for sick fellow prisoners, he kept careful, almost obsessive records of his observations of daily sick parades, plotted graphs of the proportion of the camp that was sick and wounded, and noted any factors such as diet that might be relevant. He kept meticulous notes about everything from disease presentations to the effect of sharing food parcels.[5] These formed the basis of the two papers he wrote in 1945 after returning from the war, in which he recorded his observations on tuberculosis among prisoners of war in Germany and his own experiences as a medical officer. He later concluded, "Prison life supports the Marxian theory in many ways. After three years here I have little doubt that treachery, tuberculosis and temper are closely connected with the amount of food one is getting."[6]

During his time as a prisoner of war, when he and the other prisoners were suffering from starvation edema, he instituted what was to be his "first, worst and most successful clinical trial" (1984), giving yeast extract to ten prisoners and using ten as a control group, to prove that they were suffering from a deficiency disease. Despite his doubt about both design and outcome of the trial, it was effective in obtaining both yeast and improved rations for the camp. In the camp, where he lived in intimate contact with the other prisoners, who were also his patients, there was no question that he understood their social circumstances. What held him back, and what was to constitute an enduring commitment, was not having enough information on what worked and what did not.

He was made a member of the Order of the British Empire for his services in the war, but his quest for information was not easily resolved. In 1947 he was awarded a Rockefeller fellowship in preventive medicine, and this involved a preliminary year at the London School of Hygiene and Tropical Medicine. Here he was taught statistics by Austin Bradford Hill, professor of medical statistics and epidemiology, appointed in 1945. Bradford Hill made a profound impression on Cochrane.

In the United States, Cochrane came across the 1947 study by C. C. Birkelo and colleagues demonstrating the differences between radiologists' interpretations of the same chest films. Tuberculosis represents a historical example where the uncertainties of diagnostic categorization have presented persistent difficulties (see Bowker and Star 1999). Cochrane used the vast databank of tuberculosis cases at the Henry Phipps Clinic to study the actual outcome of x-ray diagnosis for patients with tuberculosis (Cochrane et al. 1949). On his return, with his interest in medical error thoroughly aroused, Cochrane was recommended by Jerry Morris for a position in the Pneumoconiosis Research Unit of the Medical Research Council, in Cardiff, South Wales. The unit was studying the lung disease of coal miners, and Cochrane's role was to interpret coal min- ers' chest x rays taken in the field. Cochrane regarded this as an opportu- nity "hand tailored to my dreams" (1989, p. 122), since it involved a con- siderable social problem, a return to the study of tuberculosis, and the opportunity to apply epidemiological and statistical methods.

In addition to developing diagnostic criteria for the interpretation of the x rays, Cochrane was expected to participate in surveys of mining populations to establish industrial histories and exposures. At issue was the problem that it was not clear what mediated the progression of sim- ple pneumoconiosis into the seriously disabling lung disease known as progressive massive fibrosis. One theory held that it was related to con- tinued exposure to dust; according to another, tuberculosis initiated the progression. Cochrane suggested a comparison between two valleys, in one of which every effort would be made to reduce the level of infective tuberculosis. Monitoring the rate of progressive massive fibrosis would establish whether tuberculosis was involved. This was the Rhondda Fach study (Cochrane et al. 1952). Cochrane was to spend the next fifteen years doing research on this Welsh mining valley and its thirty thousand peo- ple. It required charting the x rays of the entire adult population and test- ing all schoolchildren for exposure to tuberculosis. Once established, the study rapidly expanded as the opportunity arose to use this population for further cross-sectional studies of the diseases affecting it, including lung diseases, anemia, and heart disease.

Cochrane's aim was to get such high response rates in this population that he could claim the kind of accuracy found in laboratory studies. His achievement in this respect received widespread interest. Despite a severe winter in the first year of the study, the team x-rayed 89 percent of the tar- get population, including 98 percent of miners and former miners (Cochrane 1989, p. 138). Although the Rhondda study did help some of the people claim compensation, this was not why they took part in a study that, Cochrane claimed, made the Rhondda the most medically examined community in the world.[7] In a style reminiscent of ethnographers, the research team immersed itself in the community. Fieldworkers came from the community, and one of them had advanced lung disease. There were regular meetings in which researchers reported back to the com- munity about the results of successive stages of the study.

Despite the undoubted care that Cochrane's team took to keep the com- munity onside, there are persistent questions about the tactics used to achieve the high response rates. Julian Tudor Hart, who worked in the Welsh valleys as a general practitioner, was critical of Cochrane for not setting up a more sustained system of medical care in the valley, and he attributes the high response rates to the fact that "Archie was . . . streetwise" and his "heavy artillery" hunted out recalcitrant subjects wherever they were hiding (Tudor Hart 1997, p. 36). When clinic visits declined, researchers visited people in their homes, and visited them six times before accepting a refusal. Cochrane himself would intervene near the end of a survey, when he would go out in his Daimler and bring in one or two of the people who had refused to attend, before saying to his colleague Peter Elwood, "You finish them off, I have to get back to Cardiff." In a film made of a study in the Vale of Glamorgan, a shot shows Cochrane's car bumping over an uneven road and pulling in at the survey headquarters. Child after child after child emerges from the car. They are x-rayed, and then all get back into the car. As the car drives off, a dent on its rear is clearly visible.[8]

The Rhondda Fach study (Cochrane said the word *survey* had been colonized by detergent sellers) established very firmly in Cochrane's mind the value of epidemiological studies of populations. Meticulous charting of disease patterns, based on secure diagnostic criteria, would monitor the progression of diseases over a period of time in two comparable populations, one of which could be subjected to an intervention. The researchers were interested not only in tuberculosis but also in differences in social and life experiences that were "upstream" of clinical events. The initial charting of the whole population would yield a reference population from which random samples could then be drawn for further research. The results of these studies were relevant to preventive care.

Cochrane's work on the Rhondda studies continued until just before his death. By the second follow-up in 1960, it was clear that the study would never be able to show the relationship between tuberculosis and progressive massive fibrosis. The introduction of streptomycin had reduced rates of tuberculosis in both the Rhondda and the control valley; and miners were moved out of dust hazards before their lung disease reached advanced levels (Cochrane 1989, p. 155). In 1970, the researchers were still able to contact or determine the fate of 99.8 percent of the miners and former miners. Cochrane saw it as a rare experience to be able to knock on doors that he had knocked on twenty years before. The study showed an excess mortality in miners in comparison with nonminers. The results of the thirty-year follow-up study (Atuhaire et al. 1986) disappointed Cochrane. He had, he wrote, hoped for more in his battle against progressive multiple fibrosis (1989, p. 265).

The Rhondda studies developed in Cochrane a passionate commitment to the eradication of bias in epidemiological studies, but he was also deeply disturbed by health care services in the valleys. He states:

I had long been a supporter of the NHS, passionately believing that "all effective therapy must be free" but there seemed to be too little interest in proving and promoting what was effective. In the course of our surveys I had sufficient contact with the working of hospitals and clinics and the delivery of health care generally to be dismayed by what passed for service. I was troubled by the variable and curious prescribing of general practitioners, the all too varied reasons for referring patients to hospitals, the attitudes and behaviour of the consultants they encountered there, and the variable ways that death certificates were completed. I sometimes thought of all this as my Rhondda Fach worm's eye view of the working of the NHS. It was a gloomy picture. (1989, pp. 157–58)

Having established the population health needs, Cochrane was well placed to start evaluating the adequacy of health services in addressing those needs. His attention was drawn to the study design used to demonstrate the effectiveness of streptomycin treatment of tuberculosis. He realized that the randomized controlled trial, with its random allocation of subjects to the treated and the control group, could be a telling step forward from clinical opinion and subjective observation (1989, p. 158).

In comparison with the Rhondda studies, the randomized controlled trial looks simple. In 1960 Cochrane became a professor of tuberculosis and chest diseases in the Welsh National School of Medicine in Cardiff. His aim was to continue his interest in health services research as well as promote the use of the randomized controlled trial in clinical medicine. He needed the cooperation of medical colleagues, and this proved to be a difficult task. He saw a great inertia against change in the university, and in particular, he became concerned that students from the Third World who came to take their course in tuberculosis and chest diseases were being given information that was misleading, even dangerous in the context of their own countries. He struggled to introduce epidemiology and biostatistics to the medical curriculum (1989, pp. 179–92). Above all, his proposed trials were repeatedly blocked.

One of the first trials he proposed was designed to evaluate the effectiveness of the anatomy course in training medical students by assigning students at random to training in Cardiff and Bristol, only one of which would teach anatomy. A questionnaire at the end of their training would compare what they knew. The professor of anatomy objected. Cochrane then tried unsuccessfully to persuade schools and judges to evaluate methods of punishment. He then turned his attention to screening. He found this period of his life frankly bewildering. His message, he argued, was simple: early diagnosis of disease did not necessarily prolong life. His view was that there was little evidence for introducing a cervical screening program in Britain, but that a trial program should be introduced in one area after a careful epidemiological study of the community. His views drew abuse from the public and from medical colleagues.

Cochrane again aroused antagonism when he became interested in the place where patients were treated, especially with respect to coronary care units. His colleagues in Cardiff refused permission for a trial of hospital versus home treatment after a heart attack, but the trial went ahead in Bristol (Mather et al. 1976). In the course of the Bristol trial, Cochrane took his revenge. At an early stage of the trial, there was some indication that patients treated at home were faring better than patients treated in coronary care. Cochrane recounts how, before a meeting, he showed colleagues the results but switched the trial's arms: "They were vociferous in their abuse: 'Archie,' they said, 'we always thought you were unethical. You must stop the trial at once. . . .' I let them have their say for some time and then apologised and gave them the true results, challenging them to say, as vehemently, that coronary care units should be stopped immediately. There was dead silence and I felt rather sick because they were, after all, my medical colleagues" (1989, p. 211). This story, perhaps apocryphal, illustrates Cochrane's confrontational style. He delighted in finding an unexpected answer to a significant health problem, but in contrast with Feinstein, his aim was to unsettle clinical rather than public health colleagues.

The preventive role of wine in coronary heart disease exactly fitted the bill as a readily accessible nonmedical preventive in highly palatable form. In classic epidemiological style, Cochrane started with an international comparison of mortality rates, carefully excluding confounding variables. He concluded with the "unhappy" proposition that, for some population groups, mortality rates were inversely related to the supply of health services (Cochrane et al. 1978), but that the consumption of wine was negatively correlated with mortality from heart disease (St. Leger et al. 1979). The next step would be to find supportive physiological evidence. The final test would be a trial, but Cochrane recognized that, in this case, a trial was unlikely to be practical or ethical (Doll 1997). This is exactly the kind of carefully focused research strategy that Doll and Bradford Hill had used to establish the relationship between smoking and mortality from lung cancer (Doll and Bradford Hill 1950, 1964). A randomized trial of the effects of smoking was clearly impossible. Where possible, however, a trial was valued as a decisive conclusion to a suite of studies that had started with analysis of mortality data, followed by meticulous observational studies, leading to a randomized trial of an intervention — in this case, interventions to help people stop smoking.

Cochrane's studies added fuel to his impassioned campaign against bias. Bias became his personal enemy. But he was equally opposed to prejudiced thinking by those clinicians who resisted having their interventions put to the test. In the foreword to *One Man's Medicine,* Dick Cohen (Lord Cohen of Birkenhead) recalls, "I used to enjoy watching him at meetings reacting to some overauthoritative subjective judgment from some of the Establishment; first he would bristle, then proceed to dissect his opponent's argument with the air of a plumber looking for an escape of gas which his nose assures him must exist somewhere. . . . His concentrated singlemindedness, when he was in full cry, sometimes made him forget that others too might have ideas and interests that seemed important to them" (Cochrane 1989, p. xvi).

Cochrane may have been no more than a thorn in the flesh of clinicians, except that his work then received backing from well-placed individuals in the health ministry and trusts. At the Nuffield Provincial Hospitals Trust, George Pickering, chairman of the Medical Advisory Committee, was said to be "amused by and an admirer of his radical outlook" (McLachlan 1997, p. 14). There was concern about the rising interest in screening, sparked by strong interest in the United States, but a lack of evidence of reduction in mortality. The Provincial Hospitals Trust set up a committee to look at the validation of screening procedures, to be chaired by Tom McKeown, professor of social medicine at Birmingham. It included Dick Cohen, senior medical officer at the Department of Health and Social Security, who agreed on the need for clinical evidence. The report put out by this committee, *Screening in Medical Care,* was sympathetic to the idea of undertaking trials (Nuffield Provincial Hospitals Trust 1968; Cochrane 1989, p. 209).

Cochrane recognized the value of this support. Perhaps through this influence, he was awarded the Rock Carling Fellowship, which entailed delivering an introductory lecture, followed by publication of a monograph. This was *Effectiveness and Efficiency.* In 1976 Tom McKeown's Rock Carling monograph followed: *The Role of Medicine: Dream, Mirage, or Nemesis?* Together these books had the potential to contribute to a reassessment of the resources flowing into medicine. The Black Report on inequalities in health asserted where the resources should be committed instead and made substantial reference to both books (Black et al. 1980).

Effectiveness and Efficiency transformed Cochrane from a gadfly into a charismatic seer. The argument of Cochrane's book was simple: Medical care was often ineffective; if ineffective procedures could be identified and eradicated, the savings could be better committed to the caring function.

The randomized controlled trial, as it developed in Britain, provided a key technique for demonstrating what worked and what did not work. He listed ineffective practices, including coronary care units and cervical screening. In the new scheme the pathologist would disappear as the final arbiter, to be replaced with the medical scientist, who would conduct trials to establish what really caused more good than harm. This was indeed a radical attack on the practice of scientific medicine. Newspapers focused on "the wishful thinking that guides doctors" (*Sunday Times*, 19 March 1971). Ten years later the *Times Health Supplement* (22 January 1982) recorded that the medical profession had been "reeling in fear that further chunks of its work will be shown to be ineffective or plain dangerous."

The response of colleagues to the book was varied and somewhat critical.[9] Tom McKeown wrote, "Having elevated the R.C.T. [randomized controlled trial] to the status of a religion, are you not mistaken about the identity of its high priest? With all respect to Bradford Hill, I think you overstate his contribution to the approach." Cochrane replied, "I gave Bradford Hill the write-up because I am convinced he made the randomized controlled trial respectable by selling it to the M.R.C. [Medical Research Council]. Later his book spread the idea very widely indeed. I think without him the idea would never have really penetrated into medicine." Julian Tudor Hart gave cautious encouragement: "It is a very good book and breaks important new ground. It could lead in various directions so far as social action goes: some of them very dangerous and unpleasant, others altogether good. Certainly we cannot go on as we are, and will not be allowed to anyway." E. H. Hare thought Cochrane had been too kind to psychiatry: "Attempts at RCTs — and there have been a few — are sabotaged more or less unconsciously by the psychotherapists who initially agreed to take part. But not many psychotherapists want to take part, believing that psychotherapy is like prayer and that one should not tempt the Lord Thy God."

The shock waves from Cochrane's polemic spread to the United States. Kerr White considered Cochrane to be "an icon and an iconoclast." From 1961 he and Cochrane had met regularly at the meetings of the International Epidemiological Association. Cochrane's views exactly reflected White's own views. In 1974 White was elected to the newly established Institute of Medicine, and he used this as a strategic opportunity to ensure that both the book and its ideas would get full exposure in the United States (White 1997, p. 3). Gordon McLachlan, formerly secretary of the Nuffield Provincial Hospitals Trust, was then consultant to the American Hospital Association's Research and Education Trust. He believed that *Screening in Medical Care* had already been used by policy departments in the United States "to halt a lot of costly pie-in-the-sky nonsense from the hi-tech aristocrats aching to get into the health scene, who were very much in the ascendancy in the United States, after the moon landing" (1997, p. 16). It was in the health policy field, partly as a result of White's efforts, that Cochrane's book was first noticed, rather than in academic departments of clinical epidemiology. While attributing most of the credit for the proliferation of trials to their scientific appeal, Robert Fletcher argues that *Effectiveness and Efficiency* and Cochrane's "persuasive and entertaining" lectures contributed to the proliferation of trials in American medical journals (2002, p. 1184).

In 1979, Cochrane had also called for each specialty to maintain an up-to-date list of all trials in its field of operations, to be followed by a regularly updated critical summary of these trials. In 1992, four years after his death, the U.K. Cochrane Centre was established to identify trials and to facilitate a comprehensive overview of each specialized field.

To return to the 1960s, as Cochrane walked into the international spotlight, the work in the Pneumoconiosis Research Unit was taken over by Peter Elwood, who was to assume the role of director when Cochrane retired.

The Researcher: Peter Elwood

Peter Elwood came from Belfast in Northern Ireland, where his father was permanent secretary in the Ministry of Health. All five of the younger Elwoods studied medicine. Thus Peter Elwood had a respect for the policy process, but his aim was to find a specialty where the intellectual challenge would be sustained in the long term. He ended up in general practice "with no great hopes," then went back to get a diploma in public health. This is when he got the chance to work on a study of chest disease in flax workers, flax being an important industry in Northern Ireland. The team studied 2,528 workers in flax mills in Northern Ireland; sixteen years later they achieved a 97 percent follow-up (Elwood et al. 1982). Elwood recalls:

I was the boy on the team. It was terribly dull work, terribly repetitive. But we were getting at some truth that would stand for all time. We were working towards truth; whereas in clinical practice, we never knew what we were doing, whether it was beneficial. If it was beneficial we took the credit. Dealing with samples of one — although I didn't think of it in those terms — we were just floundering. But on this study we were getting estimates of prevalence, estimates of association, and putting confidence limits on these. I thought it was beautiful! It was not certainty, but it was closer than a clinician would ever get.

Inspired to a life of research, Elwood developed an interest in iron deficiency anemia, said to be the most common disease in the community at that time. His particular interest was in the identification of the disease on the basis of a normal distribution of a quantitatively measured variate. He discovered that the cutoff value used to identify disease was flexible, and thus, he argued, the prevalence was arbitrary. He resolved to evaluate anemia in terms of symptoms, and in association with lung function and exercise levels as well as mortality. In addition he was interested in testing ways of preventing iron deficiency; and he was interested in trials. In the late 1950s he ran an ambitious randomized controlled trial, adding iron to bread and distributing this to three hundred households and looking at the effect on iron deficiency (Elwood et al. 1971).

Elwood joined Archie Cochrane in 1963, when the Rhondda studies were beginning to diversify. Cochrane recalls that when he met Elwood they did not stop talking for three days (Cochrane 1989, p. 217). Elwood says they worked together very successfully and were like-minded about epidemiology and about randomization:

We used to say that testing by randomized trials should be part of life. Archie loved two examples that I described to him. One was a plea to my wife to try different creams on half the baby's bottom, selected at random. If applied to the whole bottom, she would learn nothing! The other idea was more ambitious. During the days when the possible effects of hard and soft water was a topic of research, I told Archie that my children wanted tropical fish, so I was going to get two identical tanks and stock them with exactly the same numbers and types of fish, but one would have hard and the other soft water. Archie was taken with this, and he insisted on paying for the tanks. We were both absolutely intrigued with the evidence that collected over the next few months — the fish population in the soft water tank slowly increased, while the numbers in the hard water appeared not to change. We thought this was even more interesting than any answer relevant to heart disease — hard water is contraceptive! Alas, one of my children blew it — there was a cannibal fish in the hard water tank.

Elwood saw Cochrane as "the right man for the time." His irrepressible urge to throw out concepts and goad clinicians about bias gave Cochrane the reputation of being an enfant terrible long before *Effectiveness and Efficiency* was published. Elwood recalls: "At meetings somebody would give a paper. Archie would stand up and I would duck. He would challenge the man: 'Have you any evidence for that?' This is what gave him his impact on people, locally and elsewhere."

Elwood himself was interested in mechanisms of heart disease, including platelet aggregation and the part it played in heart attack and stroke.

Reflecting the concern of Fraser Mustard that physiological mechanisms should be considered as a way of limiting the proliferation of trials (chapter 5), he made use of extensive laboratory evidence, but it held no fascination for him. Studying the mechanisms of disease seemed too long a way to make a difference to community health. It was reproducibility that fascinated him, not precision. It was differences between populations that mattered, and in these comparisons the unit of measurement was not very important as long as measurement was consistent: "You can get over lack of precision by using larger numbers," says Elwood; "you can't ever get over lack of reproducibility." This is an important aspect of epidemiology.

Despite Cochrane's strong emphasis on randomized controlled trials, it was ironic that Cochrane himself never ran a trial. His "first, worst and most successful clinical trial" in the prisoner-of-war camp was not randomized and was published only in 1984, after Elwood asked him to talk to a seminar group about his experiences. Cochrane said it would be too painful, but Elwood persuaded him that it would help him come to terms with the experience. Elwood recalls that Cochrane nearly broke down when he gave the talk, but afterward the latter said it had helped him and he wrote up the paper.

The trials proposed by Cochrane often failed to be implemented, because of the resistance he encountered from colleagues. He felt that they resisted having their interventions put to the test by claiming that the randomization of patients to a placebo, nonintervention, group would be unethical. At one stage Cochrane discussed with Elwood a study to expose differences in the standards set by different ethics committees. There were, they believed, also differences in how the same ethics committee viewed different kinds of research. It seemed that invasive clinical studies were accepted as ethical, while population-based trials were rejected. In order to expose regional differences, the two men would submit a number of bogus research protocols to a range of ethics committees. The aim was to promote discussion and achieve some level of conformity between types of study and between ethics committees across the country. In Cardiff this proposal was ruled unethical, thus providing another wry but cutting anecdote to Cochrane's list.

The trial that brought them "seven days of fame" was the first trial of low-dose aspirin as a preventive for patients after a heart attack (Elwood et al. 1974). Elwood did the trial on a budget of a few thousand pounds. He was less concerned about the mechanisms of platelet function than about saving lives. Says Elwood, "That's what we are in the business to do!" While the reduction in all-cause mortality did not differ significantly, the total incidence of cardiovascular events did differ significantly. Cochrane and Elwood believed that judging success on the basis of the latter had not been the original intention and would therefore constitute special pleading. Only mortality data were therefore reported.

Elwood (2001) was later to report fifteen years observation of a number of platelet tests and challenge the whole concept of platelet aggregation and vascular disease, but at that time the challenge was to conduct further randomized trials (see Elwood 1997). Elwood's next trial also had results that were not statistically significant, but as in the first trial, they suggested a reduction by about 20 percent in the mortality rate of patients during the year after infarction. Their third trial of aspirin given during the acute phase of infarction gave no evidence of benefit (Elwood 1983). At this stage, Richard Doll comforted them with the reminder that their evidence was no worse than it was for "most of the other drugs in the *British Pharmacopoeia*" (Elwood 1997, p. 114).

By 1980 six trials had had similar results, and, taken together, Cochrane saw this as providing virtually conclusive proof that aspirin worked. On the other hand, a number of writers conducted subgroup analyses and claimed that aspirin would work only in males. Alarmed at the misinformation that might be coming from studies based on small, selected subgroups of subjects, Cochrane and Elwood conducted a "somewhat primitive overview" of the six trials. Given the combined total of 10,857 patients, the evidence of benefit from aspirin was clearly statistically significant. More recent overviews, with very large numbers of trials and of patients, have abundantly confirmed this early conclusion, and the use of aspirin for patients after a heart attack or stroke is now standard practice (Elwood 2001).

Results such as these confirmed for Elwood that trials were a most powerful tool for evaluating interventions. On the other hand, an overemphasis on trials at the funding stage could exclude valuable studies using other designs. According to Elwood:

I am told (but how do I know; I haven't tested it by randomized controlled trial!) that some funding bodies are beginning to say, "Randomized controlled trials go to the top of the pile; everything else to the bottom of the pile, and we'll ignore most of them." I think it is very dangerous, because there are certain things that you cannot test in a randomized controlled trial. We took part in a very large study of childhood cancer; six thousand children were admitted to this study: two thousand children with cancer, and four thousand controls. Very, very detailed information was taken on emf exposure, x rays, chemicals, radon — all imaginable things. There is no way you can test these in a randomized controlled trial. It's unthinkable! But where a trial is possible there is no adequate substitute.

Because of the dangers of chance giving a misleading answer, the move now is toward very large trials, even gargantuan trials, and some recent studies have been based upon twenty thousand to fifty thousand subjects. While this development makes it difficult for the small-time operator to conduct adequate studies, on the other hand it has to be acknowledged that small trials can be misleading. Elwood notes:

One of the things I am very interested in is chronic magnesium deficiency and the risk of a future heart attack or stroke. This has never been adequately tested in a randomized trial, though observational evidence of harm from low magnesium levels is fairly consistent. The benefit of an infusion of magnesium immediately following infarction has however been repeatedly tested. The early published evidence comes from no less than six trials. These all suggest benefit, and on this evidence many coronary care units and intensive care units started giving magnesium infusions to infarct patients immediately on admission. The six trials had, however, all been quite small, but a much larger trial (LIMIT-2), based on over two thousand patients, later confirmed benefit. Not long after this, however, the gargantuan ISIS-4 trial, based on over fifty-eight thousand patients, reported a total absence of benefit from the magnesium infusion.

A reason suggested to explain the confusion in this situation is that all the early trials, including even LIMIT-2, were small and, by chance, had had a positive outcome. Other trials in which there had been no evidence of benefit may not have been reported. This problem of selective reporting is, however, compounded by authors who, in reviewing the literature on a topic, reference only those studies that conform to their personal bias (Ravnskov 1992). The matter of the selective referencing of published studies is exactly the issue that led to establishment of the Cochrane Collaboration (see chapter 7). On the other hand, the problem of selective publication led to a number of leading journals calling for an amnesty on small trials, and a request that the details of trials that had never been published be sent to the Cochrane Centre in Oxford.

The bedrock of both Cochrane's and Elwood's work in South Wales was composed of new hypotheses about disease generated in observational epidemiological studies based upon representative population samples. Elwood, however, has a major and growing concern that large-scale epidemiology is becoming increasingly difficult:

In a prospective epidemiological study, baseline measurements are made and are related to disease outcomes ten, fifteen, or more years later. To be acceptable to a funding body, such a study has to be hung on a popular hypothesis; yet one can be sure that, by the time adequate disease incident data have [been] collected, research agendas will have moved on and that particular hypothesis will have become of little or no interest. For example, the main prospective study in

Cochrane's unit, the Caerphilly Cohort Study, was hung on hypotheses about HDL-cholesterol. These hypotheses were popular enough at that time for both funding to be gained and approval by an ethics committee. Ten years later, when enough outcome events had collected for an examination of the HDL hypothesis, the shouting was over and few were interested in HDL-cholesterol. Expecting this, we therefore built into our study a whole battery of tests on thrombosis, on platelets, on psychosocial factors, on homocysteine, and other factors that were never mentioned in the original request for funding. Furthermore, large numbers of blood samples were stored to enable the later testing of hypotheses that would arise after the study had been set up. As a result, the Caerphilly Cohort Study has made important contributions to knowledge on a wide range of issues [see Elwood et al. 1996]. Funding bodies are, however, unlikely to be impressed by reference to possible, future undefined hypotheses and possible long-term spin-offs from a study. Nor will ethics committees be likely to approve a study with undeclared aims.

Elwood therefore sees the need for large-scale, population-based prospective studies addressing diseases like heart disease, stroke, cancer, and dementia, in which a major aim is to collect a wide range of blood and other samples to be used for the testing of as-yet-undefined hypotheses. Elwood now feels he must leave this and other possible developments in epidemiology to younger research workers; but in the meantime he is ensuring that the data collected in the studies by Cochrane and himself are exploited as far as possible.

The epidemiological approach used by Cochrane and Elwood was not unusual in itself, but their commitment to giving meticulous attention to representativeness and to reproducibility of measurements — in the general population and in clinical areas — was unusual. Another colleague, Jerry Morris, also earned a reputation for his views on the contribution that this work could make to health services.

The Epidemiologist: Jerry Morris

Jerry Morris graduated with an master's degree from the University of Glasgow and completed his medical studies at University College Hospital, London. Before World War II he became interested in research into social medicine, including health services. He recalls, "It was striking how thin the research base was at that time, how thin the knowledge, how feeble the public recommendations were. It was clear that here was a major, important area of public life where the application of scientific methods could help. The application of the kind of methods which we were using, epidemiological methods, very likely could be appropriate." During this time he began his long association with the social scientist Richard Titmuss, who was working on studies of poverty and populations (Titmuss 1943). While Morris served as a clinical specialist in the Royal Army Medical Corps in the war, he and Titmuss published three papers addressing conditions selected to demonstrate the social origins of rheumatic heart disease and peptic ulcer (Morris and Titmuss, 1942, 1944a,b). Morris also had a firm grasp of the need to plan for postwar reconstruction. In 1944, as Major J. N. Morris, he published from India a handbook for discussion groups titled *Unless We Plan Now: Health* (Davey Smith 2001). These publications count as early efforts at articulating the role of health in the new welfare state. After the war, in 1948, they led to the founding of the Social Medicine Research Unit of the Medical Research Council. One focus was to be on infant mortality, another on coronary heart disease as "a major new lethal epidemic." In the unit, they would also study health services, as these would clearly relate to the treatment of chronic diseases and seriously affect people's health and well-being.

In India during the war, Morris had come across "operational research," the systematic study of the functioning of complex systems like the army, and its tasks. With others, he had debated how this could be applied to health services in peacetime. When discussing the reorganization of the health service after the war, it "struck a major chord with me." He recalls, "I proposed to the M.R.C. that one of the interests of our new unit should be 'operational research on the health service' — and they disapproved. This was the only issue of difference between us; they didn't want this. Why? Because straightaway 'you got into difficult politics': 'There's plenty for us to do. Why rock the boat and get into trouble with government?'" Unlike a charitable foundation, the Medical Research Council had national responsibility for government funding of research but set its own agenda. When Morris and Titmuss persuaded them on "scientific policy grounds" to take a new approach, the council secretary told them, Morris recalls, "I don't know what you boys are up to, but you had better get on with it."

Morris saw that epidemiology was central to providing a systematic approach to the study of disease, so he trained in public health at the London School of Hygiene and Tropical Medicine. In 1955, he wrote an article describing the "uses of epidemiology," which he expanded into a book in 1957. Morris defined epidemiology as a method of asking questions and getting answers that raise further questions. In particular it was useful for asking questions that could not be asked in clinical practice "about the health of the community and sections of it, present and past; by setting clinical problems in community perspective, describing their behaviour as group, not individual, phenomena, indicating their dimensions and distributions, and how much, and where, action is needed; by revealing problems and indicating where among populations these might best be studied" (1955, p. 401). George Davey Smith argues that this book had a wealth of prescient ideas and appealed to a broad readership. The book demonstrated that there were very large variations in practice; instead of only seeing them as a discredit to the medical profession, Morris saw them as an opportunity for research into wasted health service expenditure. For clinicians, specifically, the book provided a "fresh and new outlook on clinical problems," but it could also provide a gold mine for any postgraduate research worker "looking for a subject or cause" (Davey Smith 2001, p. 1147). In contrast to more recent trends in epidemiology texts that emphasize decontextualized methods, the book inspired an interest in the health of populations.

Included in the opportunities outlined by Morris was the use of operational research in studying the provision of services in the community. At that time, John Last was a general practitioner in Adelaide, Australia. He claims that Morris's article transformed his life. Last left Adelaide and went to London to apprentice himself to Morris with the aim of combining his medical training with "concern about the disorders and dysfunctions of industrial civilization" (Last 1994, p. 110). In helping Morris refine tables for the book, it struck him that, of the diseases existing in the community, only a small proportion ever presented in hospital practice. General practitioners were in a unique position to "complete the clinical picture" by addressing the hidden bulk of the iceberg (Last 1963).

Morris says that John Ryle was critical of the work he did with Titmuss because it paid too much attention to poverty in the causation of disease, but the studies for which Morris in fact became best known were epidemiological studies of heart disease and exercise. For forty years he analyzed and hypothesized this relationship (Morris et al. 1953; Morris 1992). He and his coworkers first compared occupations with different levels of exercise: conductors versus bus drivers in London buses; postmen versus sedentary clerical workers (Morris et al. 1953, 1966). When it transpired that the more active occupations apparently had a protective effect, the question was, what activity was needed to confer this effect? An overview of these data, as well as consideration of mechanisms of protection, led to the hypothesis that the occurrence of heart disease in middle-aged men is reduced by current, vigorous exercise. The public health implications are a greater emphasis on sustained physical activity and physical fitness.

While doing this work, Morris kept a wary eye on the rise of clinical epidemiology in Canada and the United States, where it had introduced clinicians to the use of simple but accurate methods of analysis and notions of validity and reproducibility, of specificity and sensitivity. He recognized that it might be attractive as a way of introducing a more critical approach to clinical care in Britain, especially in conservative medical schools where social medicine had failed to penetrate. In the late 1960s both Morris and Titmuss were involved in committees planning to restructure the National Health and the Social Welfare Services. At this stage, Morris could have supported the development of something akin to clinical epidemiology, but he turned instead to community medicine, a concept derived from his analysis of the uses of epidemiology in providing the basis for an efficient administration of health services in the context of the people's health (1969).

As part of the restructuring of the National Health Service in 1974, a Faculty of Community Medicine was established within the Royal Colleges of Physicians. The new specialty would subsume social medicine as well as public health, and practitioners would be trained in a variety of fields, including epidemiology and management. Archie Cochrane became its first president. Sir Austin Bradford Hill was given honorary membership (Cochrane 1989, p. 243). Central to the redefinition of what would now be a professional medical discipline was a master of science degree in social medicine focusing on theory and practice. Morris undertook its development in 1968 at the London School of Hygiene and Tropical Medicine and thus made an important contribution to both teaching and training. On the occasion of Morris's ninetieth birthday, past students attested to how the course had made them "citizens of an entirely different world": "Jerry, it seems, provided an anchor for the aspirations, and in some cases the desperation, of people looking for something to marshal their energies and commitment" (Loughlin 2001, p. 1198). What he gave them was a broad vision of health and the methodological tools for addressing the problems they saw.

At the ascent to power in 1979 of the prime minister, referred to by Morris as "that woman," the pressures on health services shifted. There was rising concern about costs, and the government looked to managers rather than community physicians for constraining cost increases (Lewis 1991, p. 33). In comparison with the situation twenty years earlier, argues Morris, costs had become a significant issue, and this opened up an opportunity for renewed interest in social factors:

The kind of money involved in health services used to be so much smaller than the money involved in major social policies, in any kind of social security improvement or any housing development. It was a different order of magnitude. You didn't say that, if you don't spend on health services, you could perhaps lick the homelessness problem. But this was no longer true, and in recent years, health services have cost so much that, in fact, you're talking of the same kind of money, the same orders of magnitude, as you're talking about in improving child benefit, or abolishing some kinds of housing shortages, or dealing with certain kinds of poverty or the plight of the chronically unemployed.

In this atmosphere, in the 1980s, Morris saw the possibility of instituting some of the more challenging applications of health services research: "This kind of thinking has become very important, paradoxically, with the forms of health service which this government was introducing. The kind of thing that the social medicine epidemiologists, who were interested in health services, had been saying for a very long time — like what are the effects of health services on the health of the population? — has suddenly been accepted by this government, at least verbally."

The problem was that epidemiologists with methodological expertise had been reluctant to turn their attention to these difficult applied social aspects. According to Morris, "It's an awful lot less difficult to study the impact of smoking on some disease than the impact of a combination of health and social services on the well-being of old ladies!" Like Feinstein, he saw the need to have good methods available for these studies, but his focus had been on the study of risk factors: exercise, smoking, fat in the diet, and so on. In comparison, studying health services was very, very difficult. In addition, research funding bodies in the United Kingdom were becoming short of funds and were increasingly reluctant to fund health services research. They were also nervous, as before, about the political implications, "because as soon as you get into health services, you get into politics." Governments themselves were primarily interested in quick returns: "They didn't care much what happens after the next election; and civil servants are similarly interested in the next few years and the next step up the ladder." This gloomy picture rubs some of the gloss off the promising support that had been given to Archie Cochrane in the 1970s.

Contrasts with Canada and the United States

Kerr White organized a conference at Chapel Hill, North Carolina, in 1952 and invited Jerry Morris as keynote speaker. White believes that this is what introduced health services research to the United States. Iain Chalmers believes that Jerry Morris was a critically important contributor to the development of health services research in the United Kingdom, but has some doubt about whether the Morris approach to health services research was applicable in the United States: "Well, they haven't got health services in America, have they? It's certainly ironic, that all of the work on health services research in the United States is in the context of this incredibly inhumane system, a system which results in a third of the bankruptcies being due to inability to pay health care bills, 14 percent of the gross domestic product being spent on health care, doctors being overpaid in the most obscene way. It's almost like fiddling while Rome burns."

This comment gives a striking illustration of the different approach to what became evidence-based medicine in the United Kingdom and the United States. In the United Kingdom, the pioneers of this movement had a strong commitment to the National Health Service and to ensuring that it delivered good service. This could be done only in collaboration with the health bureaucracy. What held pride of place in the United States was not the health service (although Kerr White viewed the health service as the most important health care institution) but the academic institutions in which new and challenging programs could be generated. From this perspective, health services research in the United Kingdom could be seen as caught up in traditional commitments with little new thinking being tolerated. And indeed, there is support for Robert Fletcher's view that British medical training was bound by tradition, so that clinical epidemiology did not take hold in Britain. Says Fletcher, "Their epidemiology came out of a concern for the population at large, not a clinical population; that's their whole history, and I think they weren't prepared to break with it. The strong suit for the United States is that, by and large, if you have a good idea, you can figure out some way to do it; people say, 'It's crazy, but if you want to, do it!' And there's money from foundations and so on. So the United States gave [clinical epidemiology] a chance, and England has not."

Clinical epidemiology certainly made little headway in the United Kingdom, but the picture is a little more complex. Public health epidemiologists themselves were not faring all that well either in the United Kingdom, except when they drew support from policy makers and trusts who shared a commitment to an effective national health service. Alvan Feinstein was the critic who found the actions of these epidemiologists least acceptable. His particular target has been Richard Doll, whose epidemiological studies he dismissed because he saw Doll as no longer knowing "which side of a patient is up." In essence, these criticisms paint the United Kingdom as being in thrall to public health epidemiology, and as we have seen, there is some substance to this view. What particularly irked Feinstein was that the term *clinical epidemiology* was used cynically — not for intellectual purpose but for fiscal reasons: it allowed medically trained researchers working in epidemiology to get an additional salary allowance, a "clinical loading." Walter Holland was one of those accused. Holland countered with the argument that clinical epidemiology, as a distinct entity, was an American aberration. In the United Kingdom the term *clinical epidemiology* reflected the original meaning attached to the term by John Paul, and it indicated the application of epidemiology to clinical practice. Walter Holland was also a keen observer of the administrative transitions that transformed community medicine into public health medicine.

British Clinical Epidemiology and Walter Holland

Walter Holland's first medical interests were physiology and clinical practice. Working on the influenza epidemic in the 1950s persuaded him that not enough was known about the source of respiratory infections. The direction he chose was to try to prevent people from getting ill rather than treating them once they had become ill. He trained in epidemiology at the London School of Hygiene and Tropical Medicine and at the School of Hygiene at Johns Hopkins University. In 1962, when he returned to the United Kingdom, it was difficult to find a term to describe his continuing clinical interests as well as his commitment to epidemiological research. There were two alternatives available: *epidemiology* and *social medicine*. Each implied a commitment to the application of statistics to the study of disease as well as a concern with the social change in order to reduce the risk of disease (Acheson 1991). Some colleagues, like Ryle and McKeown, preferred *social medicine;* others, like Cochrane, emphasized methodological rather than political commitment and called themselves *epidemiologists*. Holland sought a compromise in the name of his chair in the Department of Community Medicine, St. Thomas's Hospital Medical School, London. He recalls:

The reasons for my department and chair being called "clinical epidemiology and social medicine" were: (a) the advice that, if it had been only "social medicine," I would not have been invited to visit the United States (said half-jokingly by the Establishment at that time), and (b) the need to have the word *clinical* in the title of the department, to make it clear that we were a clinical subject and not a preclinical one. My own pay would never have been at risk, but that of individuals coming to work with me would have been, and it was considered important to set the precedent of the department being part of the clinical curriculum rather than preclinical. John Pemberton and I headed the only two departments at that time in the United Kingdom that were regarded as clinical rather than preclinical.

From Holland's perspective, *clinical epidemiology* was an unfortunate term that split epidemiologists into those who did clinical work (and were respectable) and those who were not medically trained (Holland 1983). At any rate, much of what was done under the guise of clinical epidemiology in the United States was really clinical research. Holland remarks, "They are concerned about the validity of tests. OK, that is a part of epidemiology, but it is only one very small part of it. They are studying the validity of diagnosis and decisions and things like this. That isn't really epidemiology. Epidemiology is concerned with defined populations. OK, if you take a definition of a defined population of patients in a hospital — that is fine, but what does it mean? How do you generalize from that?"

In Canada and the United States, the problems that lead to the rise of clinical epidemiology surfaced, Holland argues, because of the lack of expertise in public health epidemiology: "In the 1950s and 1960s, U.K. epidemiology was considered far ahead of American, and it was recognized as such. That was largely because we had changed more rapidly from concern with infectious disease to concern with chronic disease. There were the major studies by Bradford Hill and Doll on cancer of the lung, by Jerry Morris and others on vascular disease, and so on. The Americans were still paramount in infectious disease. The Framingham study, in spite of the amount of publicity that it has had, is not, by modern standards, a very good study."

This backlog was part of the explanation for the explosion of interest in clinical epidemiology. In Holland's view, epidemiology in its various guises in Canada and the United States was concerned with "little fiddly bits of statistical technique, rather than being concerned with health, with the major problems." What clinical epidemiologists had done was to stake out the area of large, randomized clinical trials as their particular field of interest, but "we have never thought that was our prime purpose." Nor does he think this notion of evidence-based medicine has much to offer. It has advocates, some with "great charisma," and it makes a contribution to providing medical practice with a more rational basis, but medical practice "still depends on careful, thorough collection, analysis and dissemination. And its interpretation is still subject to personal or political idiosyncrasies, as in the past!" (2001–2002, p. 3).

It should be added that, in the face of such criticism, Sackett is unrepentant. Clinical epidemiology, he argues, succeeded in areas where public health epidemiology had failed (2002). It was a better way to teach medical students: it persuaded them of the relevance of clinical epidemiology as a basic science for clinicians. Departments of clinical epidemiology not only were growing in size and number but also were producing better research into clinical practice.

Conclusion

In comparison with the United States, the United Kingdom has a much more fluid relationship between clinical medicine and public health. While public health may have a tenuous hold on the imaginations of some, or even most clinicians, they operate in a National Health Service that constrains their opportunities for private clinical practice. The founders of social medicine were medical doctors who threw their weight behind the National Health Service, producing evidence about health services that strengthened this arm of government. They employed a range of study designs, of which Cochrane saw the randomized controlled trial as the most promising for evaluating health services.

By the time Cochrane wrote his book, he had been sorely provoked by the rejection of his ideas. It could be argued that he strayed well into the field of polemic, and that his agenda then found support with leading members of the health bureaucracy. He was well supported by the parallel activities of the epidemiologist Jerry Morris and benefited from the influence Morris exerted through both his research and his activities on government committees.

Kerr White is widely credited with having imported the British version of health services research into the United States. While Cochrane's ideas had some effect in the United States, the Cochrane Collaboration constituted the primary form in which they were to proliferate in Canada and the United States.

Notes

1. Wellcome Library for the History and Understanding of Medicine, SA/SIG Sigerist Society.

2. Wellcome Library for the History and Understanding of Medicine, SA/SIG Sigerist Society, Folder A17.

3. Wellcome Library for the History and Understanding of Medicine, SA/SSM C.36, Folder A1.

4. South Wales Echo, 28/4/1984, p. 13.

5. Cochrane Library of University of Wales College of Medicine, Llandough Hospital, Wales, ALC/2/1.

6. Cochrane Library of University of Wales College of Medicine, Llandough Hospital, Wales, ALC/2/3, Spanish Civil War and World War Two, typescript draft attributed to Cochrane.

7. Cochrane Library of University of Wales College of Medicine, Llandough Hospital, Wales, ALC/8/2, Film research in the Rhondda, produced by Newport College of Art, n.d.

8. Cochrane Library of University of Wales College of Medicine, Llandough Hospital, Wales, ALC/8/2, Vale of Glamorgan x-ray survey, 1955, the Medical Research Council, Llandough Hospital.

9. Cochrane Library of University of Wales College of Medicine, Llandough Hospital, Wales, ALC/5/1/2. Personal letters to Cochrane after the publication of his book.

CHAPTER 7

The Cochrane Collaboration

The strategic epidemiological approach used by the epidemiologists Archie Cochrane, Jerry Morris, and Richard Doll can be compared with a pyramid whose base is a broad range of studies of mortality and morbidity data. The hypotheses from these studies lead to a smaller number of more carefully focused, and demanding, field studies. These, in turn, together with evidence from physiological studies, can lead to a specific hypothesis to be tested in a randomized controlled trial, where possible and appropriate. This trial forms the apex of the pyramid, providing secure scientific knowledge on which to base policy decisions.

In 1979, Archie Cochrane reviewed the use of the randomized controlled trial and proposed that each medical specialty should identify all the trials done in its field and then prepare up-to-date, critical summaries of the relevant ones, so that practitioners would have easy access to information on effective care. With the rapid growth in the number of trials in the 1980s (see Chalmers 1988), this raised the possibility of a different pyramid, one whose base is a large number of randomized controlled trials and whose apex is a scientific overview of the trials. When it was recognized that there could be sources of bias in the overview because of publication bias (the tendency for preferential publication of studies with a positive outcome), the resolution lay in including in the overview not only trials with a positive result but also those with a negative result and those that had never been published. Central to these efforts was the methodological contribution of Thomas (Tom) Chalmers. A contemporary and sparring partner of Alvan Feinstein, he was located at Harvard

University in Boston. While Chalmers's work was well recognized in the United States and Canada, it was Feinstein who provided the key input to the development of clinical epidemiology in Canada and the United States. Chalmers, however, made a critically important contribution to the development of the Cochrane Collaboration.

The Meta-analyst: Tom Chalmers

Tom Chalmers was the third Thomas Clark Chalmers, M.D. His father was financially ruined during the Great Depression, giving Tom a first-hand view of the effects of deprivation on a community. Tom recalls:

My father was a family doctor in a nouveau riche community, a suburb of Forest Hills, New York, outside of the city. The people there had made all their money in the 1920s on the stock market; then they all became destitute. We had a big house, and at one time we had five or six patients living in the attic. Their chief complaint was starvation — and they had been bank presidents and business owners. Finally the mortgage company also took our house, and they had to kick them all out. The house stayed empty for two years, and all these people went on the streets. The mortgage company established the fact that if you don't pay your mortgage you lose your house.

Faced with this experience, Tom Chalmers decided to follow his conscience even if that meant taking on his father's rather precarious profession. After graduation he practiced primary care but soon realized that he was constantly making mistakes. He knew about trials as "a very important tool for finding out whether small increments are worthwhile" and decided that trials could help him make better decisions when treating patients. What followed was what he saw as three further careers, which he summarizes as follows:

And I got an opportunity in the middle of my practice to go to Japan and to study the treatment of hepatitis in a randomized control trial with bed rest and diet [see Chalmers et al. 1955]. It convinced me that that was the way to go. I quit practice and became a full-time chief of medicine so I could do clinical trials. After thirteen years I went to Washington because I felt, at the Veterans Administration, I could do control clinical trials in a lot more hospitals. President Johnson was going to make the VA hospitals into perfect examples of what socialized medicine would do. Nixon axed all that, so I went to the NIH [National Institutes of Health] for a while, and then decided the only way to get doctors to do more clinical trials was to get them young. So I accepted a job as head of a medical center and dean of the school in Mount Sinai in New York.

Chalmers had found through personal experience that biostatistics was central to clinical trial research. His saw his efforts to introduce this training in the medical school as unsuccessful. He had obtained a commitment from the trustees to create a Department of Biostatistics, based on the argument that biostatistics was more important to medical students than biochemistry. Chalmers recalls, "It didn't go over very well with the rest of the faculty. In fact it went over so badly that when I left in 1983 they proceeded to dismantle the department. Apparently anybody can do biostatistics." Although he was able to have some positive effect on medical training, he was concerned about taking on an administrative role: "I had gathered an impression that every dean and hospital president that I had ever met was incompetent, and they were incompetent because, when they became an administrator, they stopped doing their clinical work and stopped doing research. I was determined that I would continue doing research, but I found you can't do research and go to committee meetings all day; and you can't see patients if you are chairman of a committee."

When he tried to keep abreast of research, he found that he could not remember the contents of articles soon after reading them. This led him to start extracting data from papers, combining it, and publishing the results (Chalmers et al. 1977). His conclusions allowed him to argue with faculty members about the best way of doing things instead of just accepting "what the loudest and most effusive person said." He was in his office one day in 1982 when he received a telephone call to say that he had won the research medal of the Evaluation of Research Society. "I said, 'What for?' They said, 'For your meta-analyses.' And I said, 'What are they?' And that is how I learned what I was doing. Apparently I had been doing meta-analyses for years and hadn't known it."

Chalmers gave up his administrative role in 1983 to concentrate on this fifth career, meta-analysis. Simply put, he saw meta-analysis as using statistics to combine the results of multiple different trials addressing the same problem. In the case of trials with samples too small to show a statistically significant result, meta-analysis could produce an answer. He argued that meta-analysis was generally a much better alternative than spending research funding on ever bigger trials with the purpose of resolving the uncertainties in existing, smaller trials. He supported the rule that no one should be allowed to start a randomized control trial without first completing a meta-analysis: "Because it is when you do the meta-analysis that you discover what has to be in the trial." His contribution therefore spans methodological papers on both trials (Chalmers 1981) and meta-analysis (Chalmers et al. 1987), as well as reviews of therapeutic interventions (for example, Chalmers 1988).

Chalmers believed strongly that medical information should be based on cumulative meta-analysis, where a combined effect is calculated after the addition of each new trial to assess when a new treatment becomes significantly effective. In this way clinical recommendations could be synchronized with accumulating evidence. The case that particularly impressed Iain Chalmers of the Cochrane Collaboration was the meta-analysis of treatments of myocardial infarction (see Hunt 1999 for a personal account by the researchers involved). Joseph Lau and colleagues (1992) conducted a progressive meta-analysis of trials of treatments for myocardial infarction in the order in which they were published. Their meta-analysis showed that intravenous streptokinase used as thrombolytic therapy for acute infarction showed a consistent, statistically significant reduction in total mortality by 1973. The recommendations of clinical experts lagged behind (Antman et al. 1992). Without cumulative meta-analysis, argue Lau and Chalmers (1995), there could be delays in treating patients with effective drugs and delays in abandoning potentially harmful ones.

Keenly aware of the amount of time it took to identify the trials done in an area, Tom Chalmers argued that most clinicians would not have the time to take on this ongoing task, nor would they have the skills to do the meta-analyses. He became convinced that "someone in government" should set up a unit that would find all the randomized trials in a field, combine them, update them when new trials came out, and then find some software to disseminate the results. As he puts it, "Everybody has been advocating that this happen, but nobody will pick up the bill, the tab."

When interviewed in 1991, Tom Chalmers was located in the Department of Health Policy and Management at Harvard University. He strongly supported the role of schools of public health, but his vision was of a school of public health with integrated departments that concentrated on treating people, preventing disease, and generating health policy. These views placed him much closer to the British model than either Sackett or Feinstein were. He had also established a close relationship with Iain Chalmers, whom he described as "one of my best friends, cousins two hundred years removed."

The Collaborator: Iain Chalmers

Iain Chalmers was also developing an interest in meta-analysis, which he sees as a statistical technique that combines estimates from similar trials addressing the same intervention with the purpose of deriving a more statistically precise overall result, reducing the uncertainty that can result from considering studies one at a time. Sometimes clinical authorities could underestimate the benefits of treatment, as meta-analyses showed in the case of treating breast cancer with tamoxifen and polychemotherapy. But in the case of the routine hospitalization of women with twin pregnancies, meta-analysis showed that there was unlikely to be an important benefit (Chalmers et al. 1993; Crowther 1991). In the United Kingdom, argues Doll (1994), Richard Peto and Iain Chalmers pioneered the use of meta-analysis, but Iain Chalmers preferred the term *systematic review* to cover meta-analysis as well as other processes for the scientific synthesis of studies. According to Chalmers:

> They are techniques to reduce bias of various kinds. If you want to reduce the impact of publication bias, then you look behind bushes and under stones for every trial that might be relevant, every study that might be relevant — qualitative or quantitative — to your question. . . . Systematic approaches are required to address bias, but that raises the question: what system? As in any scientific endeavor, people are required to describe what it is they set out to do, what methods and materials they used to do it, how they made sense of the data they collected in terms of their analysis, and then what they concluded: what did it all mean?

In this process, he and others built the Cochrane Collaboration, named after Archie Cochrane. Vast in its international reach, the Cochrane Collaboration depended heavily on the capacity of Iain Chalmers to direct the burgeoning functions of the organization.

Iain Chalmers trained at the Middlesex Hospital Medical School (now combined with University College, London), the closest medical school to Harley Street. There were no courses in public health, and he did not learn about epidemiology or the randomized controlled trial until six years after qualifying. Says Chalmers, "I had managed to be let loose on the public as a medical graduate without having any conscious recognition of these terms and what they implied. That is a pretty damning comment on me and on the education system to which I was exposed." He believes that people who wanted to retain their hold on the curriculum actively blocked the introduction of a public health course:

> The nearest thing that I had to something really enlightening was a wonderful three-month psychiatry course where the professor had recruited psychiatrists with very different views on the world. It was clear that no one could speak with any certainty about what was the truth, and that was very liberating. In other places we were told there were certainties, and you had to regurgitate these certainties in exams if you wanted to pass. It was really not an education. We were

like parrots that had been admitted to this institution: "We have got to teach them to speak what they did ought to speak!"

During his training, he liked to go on "bumming" holidays, and he decided to visit the Middle East. A fellow student originally from Beth-lehem introduced him to his family, who were then in Jordan. Meeting them inspired Chalmers to read a book called *The Arabs* by Edward Atiyah, a Palestinian historian. Chalmers recalls:

It was absolutely shattering to realize what we had done to them. Appalling. Like everyone else at the time, I was a default Zionist: poor little beleaguered Israel sur-rounded by a hundred thousand saber-brandishing Arabs. What on earth could one do but say, "Give them their own plot of land," even if it belonged to some-body else? It has not been like that at all, and some of the people I admire most are the Israeli revisionist historians who are now writing about what actually did happen, in the light of papers that have now become available. I felt ashamed. I remain very angry but utterly impotent in the face of continuing disgraceful things happening there with the connivance of the great powers.

After graduating, Chalmers went to work in Gaza as "a rather pathetic gesture," but it turned into an intensive learning experience. Like the local clinicians, he had available to him only the rituals of Western medicine. These proved to be inadequate. Says Chalmers:

In the 1960s when I went to medical school, there was enormous worry about penicillin-resistant bacteria. People who were taught therapeutics at that time really had it rammed home to them that you should never give anyone an anti-biotic unless you were absolutely certain they had a bacterial infection. When I worked in a Palestinian refugee camp for two years, and children with the early signs of measles came to me, I said, "Well I know that bacterial superinfection can occur." But supplies of antibiotics were very limited in the camps I was working in; they were usually supplied at the beginning of every month, and by the third week we were usually out of them. And I had been taught that you shouldn't give antibiotics before there are clear signs of bacterial infection. I used to tell the par-ents to come back if they were worried about the child so that I could listen again to the chest or look again in the ears or for neck stiffness. Children died in the intervening period because measles can absolutely race through malnourished children. They can be overwhelmed by bacterial superinfection very fast. It was an extremely sobering experience, as you can imagine.

The intensity of this experience persuaded Chalmers not only of the uncertainty of clinical practice but of the real dangers that this posed to patients. On his return to the United Kingdom in 1971, he decided to train in obstetrics and went to a hospital position in obstetrics in Cardiff. Here were new sources of uncertainty. He was disturbed by the realization that, when he was woken at three in the morning to attend to a woman in labor, he had to take account of who the woman's obstetrician was. Various obstetricians had firmly held views on treatment, and their views were inconsistent, but it was not clear to him that these firmly held views made any difference. As a result, starting in 1973, he did two studies comparing the caseload of one obstetrician — about five thousand women over five years — with the five thousand women who were the responsibility of another, who had very different views. One was a radical interventionist, the other far more conservative. Chalmers and his colleagues could not detect any differences (1976a). He then tried to allow for the fact that the two obstetricians in the study had somewhat different patients referred to them because of their clinical interests; but even a comparison of fifteen hundred women who were as alike as possible did not show a difference (Chalmers et al. 1976b). A third study analyzed secular trends and was unable to detect any decline in perinatal mortality in Cardiff over a time when there had been increased intervention rates, including Cesarean sections, instrumental delivery, and the start of ultrasound screening (Chalmers et al. 1976).

It was during these studies that Chalmers was alerted to the difficulties involved in dealing with bias. He was left with the insecure feeling that he really could not tell if he had managed to exclude all the biases in the studies. What added to his building skepticism was disclosure of the disastrous harm caused by some pediatric interventions, including children left blind following oxygen administration after delivery.

Soon after its publication, a colleague gave him Archie Cochrane's newly published book to read, and he felt as if he were "being given a compass in the jungle." Randomization would provide a powerful method of excluding bias in studies on the effect of medical interventions. Chalmers states:

And that's what is so special about randomization. You are controlling for things you have not measured. For example, the fact that you have not measured neuroticism, on some scale invented by some psychologist, between two comparison groups does not matter. If it does matter, then you stratify by it and see if there is any effect within that stratum.

I went off and did Jerry Morris's course in social medicine, and that was terrific. It was the best year of formal education I've had, his course at the London School of Hygiene and Tropical Medicine — in spite of the fact that they hardly mentioned randomized trials. I can forgive them that because it really was an incredibly exciting year. What was exciting was that, for the first time in any part of the education that I've had, we were encouraged to challenge our teachers. And that was an amazingly liberating and wonderful thing!

He met Archie Cochrane during that time. In 1974, inspired by Cochrane, he started collecting reports of randomized controlled trials in obstetrics and neonatal pediatrics and campaigning for a register of these more reliable studies. In 1976 he wrote to a psychologist colleague, Martin Richards, outlining a plan for the combined analysis of trials that were sufficiently similar. In 1979, Chalmers published his first systematic review and meta-analysis of trials of fetal monitoring during labor. Archie Cochrane tried unsuccessfully to raise funds to support a systematic search for and analysis of the trials that Chalmers had begun to identify. The Maternal and Child Health Unit of the World Health Organization gave a small grant for hand searching sixty journals.

Chalmers's earlier work challenging obstetric practice had drawn the attention of the Royal College of Obstetricians and Gynaecologists and the British Paediatric Association. Alec Turnbull, professor of obstetrics and gynecology at Oxford University, had previously collaborated on Chalmers's Cardiff studies (Chalmers et al. 1976a) and much impressed Chalmers when he admitted publicly that he had been promoting induction of labor without reliable evidence of benefit of its widespread use. Simultaneously, there was pressure to establish a national perinatal epidemiology unit to house the epidemiological surveys that had been conducted in 1946, 1958, and 1970. Chalmers believes that political pressure for such a unit also flowed from a campaign run by the Spastics Society, focusing attention on an unacceptably high rate of handicapped children being born and attributing this to lack of support for maternity and neonatal health services. The National Perinatal Epidemiology Unit was funded, and Iain Chalmers was appointed to be its first director. He was still in Cardiff at the time, but he asked for the unit to be located in Oxford, where he had support from Alec Turnbull and Anne Anderson, a reproductive physiologist.

Chalmers recognized that changing medical practice was difficult, but his trust lay in evidence to help clinicians mount a challenge to harmful practices. He says, "Once you start to get trials which show, for example, that fifty years of radical mastectomies have not been justified, then you can start to see what a powerful weapon such evidence is for those who wish to challenge authority. In principle, that's what scientists should be doing the whole time; but it's sometimes difficult when you are involved in a priestly profession like medicine." This means that strong evidence is important but not in itself sufficient to ensure change: "I am under no illusions, however, that carefully validated evidence about the effects of care are likely ever to become the major influence on patterns of practice. There are simply too many other vested interests impinging on decisions made within health care systems. Nevertheless, I continue to hope that good evidence about the effects of interventions of one kind or another may become more influential" (Chalmers 1991, p. 137).

All the same, evidence was an important ingredient for change, and Chalmers committed the unit to gathering this evidence. From 1978 onward, properly designed trials in the perinatal field were collected, classified, and entered onto a register. He was helped in this task by Murray Enkin of McMaster University.

The Obstetrician: Murray Enkin

At the time of the founding of McMaster University, Murray Enkin was an obstetrician in Hamilton, Canada. McMaster University had the aim of setting up contacts with local practitioners, and Enkin was invited onto the faculty of the Department of Obstetrics and Gynaecology. He saw this as a tribute to his large private practice, to which the university wanted access, rather than to his academic interests. At that stage, he had not heard about the Department of Clinical Epidemiology and Biostatistics.

Enkin was a strong proponent of natural childbirth, and for this reason he was invited to a meeting titled "Maternity Care in Ferment: Conflicting Issues," held in New York in 1978 to mark the sixtieth anniversary of the Maternity Center Association. There he heard Iain Chalmers speak about a new edited book, *Benefits and Hazards of the New Obstetrics* (Chard and Richards 1977). Enkin stayed up all night reading the book, including the chapter by Chalmers. He concluded that Chalmers was "the guy who's got the answers" to the problems of obstetric practice. He was particularly interested in the science, because "science is the best kind of rhetoric that you can get." In addition, he saw that Chalmers had charisma and wrote a brilliant analysis. Enkin took a year off and went to work with Chalmers at the fledgling National Perinatal Epidemiology Unit in Oxford.

When Enkin arrived in Oxford, it soon became clear that he needed to be trained in epidemiology, so he did a course at the London School of Hygiene and Tropical Medicine. In hindsight, he believes the McMaster University course would have suited his needs better. At first his attention was focused on building up the register of trials. On the basis of the growing register, Chalmers suggested a series of monographs in which the evidence in the whole perinatal area would be collected. Their first book was to focus on antenatal care, the second on elective delivery.

Effectiveness and Satisfaction in Antenatal Care (Enkin and Chalmers 1982) provided an appreciation and critique of antenatal care. The book emphasizes the importance of the randomized controlled trial in controlling for bias. Two chapters came from social scientists working at the unit. Ann Oakley covers the historical origins of antenatal care and Jo Garcia concentrates on qualitative studies to demonstrate women's somewhat negative views of antenatal care. The authors are international: Judith Lumley and Jill Astbury from Australia provide an analysis of advice to pregnant women to refrain from harmful activities. While one authoritative prohibition was shown to be without foundation (sexual activity), another with compelling evidence of harm (cigarette smoking) concerns an addiction, and the advice may be impossible for patients to follow; in still other cases the evidence was inconclusive.

A chapter by Adrian Grant, a clinical epidemiologist at the unit, and Patrick Mohide, a professor of obstetrics and gynecology at McMaster University, draws on clinical epidemiology to analyze the use of screening and diagnostic tests in antenatal care. They argue that screening tests should not be introduced without evidence — from an admittedly laborious task of assessment — that the prerequisites of a screening program had been met. These are that the condition should be an important one, the test should be acceptable and cost-effective, early diagnosis should lead to effective management, and resources for the program should be available. Their chapter is unusual in that it contains a systematic review of four then-recent trials of fetal heart-rate monitoring during pregnancy. Two trials had been published, but Grant and Mohide also obtained the details of two unpublished trials from the researchers themselves. On the combined evidence of published and unpublished studies, they conclude that there was no evidence of benefit. The final chapter, by Enkin and Chalmers, cautions against the bias that arises in clinical practice when an obstetrician extrapolates experience with a limited number of patients. It also warns of the bias inherent in observational studies, but it concludes with an acknowledgment of "a curious mixture of science and magic involved in antenatal care" (Enkin and Chalmers 1982, p. 286).

Effective Care in Pregnancy and Childbirth

The proposed second book on elective delivery did not eventuate, but the database of trials was becoming impressive and had gone electronic when the World Health Organization provided funds for a microcomputer. Chalmers, Murray Enkin, and Eleanor Enkin identified and classified over three thousand reports of trials from 250 journals. Chalmers and colleagues (1986) listed a growing number of author-collaborators and set out the four components of the database: a register of published trials, a register of unpublished trials, a register of ongoing and planned trials, and overviews or meta-analyses. They surveyed forty-two thousand obstetricians and pediatricians in eighteen countries, obtaining data on 395 unpublished trials, and concluded that prospective registration of trials was the only way to tackle the problem of publication bias (Hetherington et al. 1989). They recruited reviewers and developed a process for preparing reviews and summaries of their relevance; after being edited, reviews were entered onto the database. As new evidence accrued, reviews were updated or amended.

In parallel an edited book was prepared to cover the whole field of pregnancy and childbirth. Chalmers suggested that Murray Enkin should participate in this book too, commuting between Oxford and Hamilton, but that they should be joined by Marc Keirse, professor of obstetrics at Leyden in the Netherlands. Keirse had experience in tertiary obstetric care. The book, *Effective Care in Pregnancy and Childbirth*, consists of two massive volumes, one on pregnancy and one on childbirth (Chalmers et al. 1989). There is a paperback summary, *A Guide to Effective Care in Pregnancy and Childbirth* (Enkin et al. 1989), which was prepared so that women could have inexpensive access to the findings of the research. The database was published as the *Oxford Database of Perinatal Trials* (Chalmers 1988).

Contributors to the book were asked to review an area of practice with which they were familiar. The reviewing process had to be scientific, open, and accountable. As set out in chapters 1 and 2 of the book, the focus was to be on randomized controlled trials because of their capacity to abolish selection bias in comparative studies. The trials had to be formally assessed as having met an adequate methodological standard, and published as well as unpublished studies had to be considered. Contributors were given access to the *Oxford Database of Perinatal Trials,* and the database was expanded to include any further trials authors wanted to use (later it was estimated that half the chapters were based on the database; Chalmers et al. 1993). Next the editors wanted formal quantitative syntheses of the results of similar trials. Statistical methods were proposed for the unbiased combination of information from different trials, and a standard format was required for tabulating results. Graphs offered an accessible way of presenting material, and the graph that represents point estimates and confidence intervals for each of the trials in a study later became part of the logo for the Cochrane Collaboration. Lastly, contributors were asked to address implications for practice and future research.

The ninety-eight international contributors to *Effective Care in Pregnancy and Childbirth* provided eighty-nine chapters. There is a marked shift in this book in comparison with the earlier one. Several of the papers are repeated from the 1982 book, but are updated to include systematic reviews of numbers of trials not available in 1982. While Ann Oakley and Jo Garcia had moved to the new format and acquired coauthors, a number of chapters still did not use systematic reviews of the statistical kind: Marc Keirse and Murray Enkin contributed to a number of chapters setting out the nature and location of obstetric practice. Miranda Mugford and Michael Drummond wrote a chapter on the role of economics in evaluation of care, Sheila Kitzinger addressed the social context of childbirth, and Madeleine Shearer analyzed maternity patients' movements. Jonathan Lomas and Murray Enkin contributed a chapter on variation in operative delivery rates, in which they considered nonmedical determinants of practice, both in patients and in the profession.

The major part of the book is a dazzling display of what we can learn about interventions in pregnancy and childbirth from systematic reviews of trial evidence. There is an elegant chapter in which Peter Goldstein, Henry Sacks, and Tom Chalmers demonstrate that prescribing hormones for the maintenance of pregnancy is fraught with risk in the absence of proper evaluation. They show that the tragic consequences of prescribing diethylstilbestrol for this purpose could have been avoided by a large, well-designed randomized controlled trial or by a systematic review of properly controlled trials conducted before 1955. The book ends with explicit recommendations for practice, including lists of interventions that work, others that are questionable, and still others that should be discontinued.

Later, the first Cochrane Centre brochure emphasized how useful the book had been to policy makers. The House of Commons Health Committee said that the book had "profoundly influenced our deliberations," and the Department of Health sent a complimentary copy to each District Health Authority, where it helped to inform the purchasing of maternity services. There was "informal evidence" that individual clinicians found the book useful even if some aspects of well-established professional practice had been shown to be without benefit. Iain Chalmers was particularly gratified that women found the book useful. He says:

For me the most heartening thing was that women have reacted to it positively. It is a tremendous alibi to have if women find it useful, in all sorts of ways, some of which I had not even conceptualized. There is an analysis in there making it quite clear that we do not know whether reducing salt in the diet has any impact on blood pressure in pregnancy. I heard the anecdote that one woman had said to her doctor, who was trying to get her to reduce salt, "Forget it, there is no good evidence. I like salt on my food and I am not going to reduce it until there is good evidence." So women were using it to negotiate their care. Some obstetricians resisted and called us an obstetric Baader-Meinhof gang.

The implications for policy makers were self-evident. In 1990, the Milbank Memorial Fund cooperated with other agencies and the editors to convene a meeting to discuss ways of increasing the influence of this work. With this meeting, *Effective Care in Pregnancy and Childbirth* crossed the Atlantic. In a 1993 issue of the *Milbank Quarterly,* Chalmers, Enkin, and Keirse (1993) provided a detailed description of the processes involved in the project. In the same issue was Jonathan Lomas's analysis, "Retailing Research" (see chapter 9 of the present volume).

McMaster University was aware of this new development, and Brian Haynes fully appreciated the achievement of Chalmers. Says Haynes, "He has the ultimate example of what all medicine should be doing in sorting out the trials that have been done. It's hardwired to the evidence, so a practitioner can just look up in what looks like an ordinary textbook what to do." Haynes notes that Chalmers had achieved this in a narrow area, perinatal medicine, and even then "a monumental amount of work" was required to keep it up to date. Murray Enkin was less enthusiastic, as he gradually become aware that the collection of facts in a database was not useful in and of itself. His interest remained in the collecting of facts in a book so that these facts could be humanized: "Facts without feelings are useless, feelings without facts are dangerous," he says. His concerns about the new directions of the database in the Cochrane Collaboration came to a head when David Sackett came to Oxford in 1994. Enkin notes:

I think that sometimes too much attention is paid to the facts, to the data, to the randomized trials. I consider these as means to an end, to be used when they provide useful answers, to be ignored when they give wrong answers. I don't mean that sarcastically. Let me give an example. All the trials of nutritional supplementation of impoverished, malnourished women showed no benefit. Are we to assume that we should not feed these hungry women? That is a pretty extreme example, but there are other trials where I just don't believe the results. That does not mean that trials are not valuable; it's not a question of dropping trials.

Chalmers confirms that the database had become a primary interest. By 1992 he felt that "I had basically shot my bolt in the perinatal field." The question was whether this approach could be extended to other fields.

The Cochrane Collaboration

The publication of *Effective Care in Pregnancy and Childbirth* coincided with the inauguration of the National Health Service Research and Development Programme. The director, Michael Peckham, was an oncologist. In an article outlining the aims of the new program, Peckham (1991) referred with approval to the National Perinatal Epidemiology Unit's work. Chalmers was a member of the Central Research and Development Committee of the National Health Service Research and Development Programme and suggested the idea of the Cochrane Collaboration to Peckham. Says Chalmers, "I wrote on a single piece of paper a proposal, which I handed to Michael." Peckham asked for a full proposal and presented it to the committee. It was funded despite robust opposition that Chalmers parodies as follows: "People did not see this as proper research. It's far too applied. It is fine to have a little bit of applied research, but this is really quite unreasonable. I mean, what will happen to the reputation of researchers if we allow that to happen?"

In 1992, funding was provided for a small group based in Oxford, independent of the university and part of the National Health Service, called the Cochrane Centre. Cochrane's name was used as a personal tribute but also in reference to his work on effectiveness. Bearing in mind the contribution made by the authors of the 1989 book, Chalmers knew it had to be an international collaboration. The Cochrane Collaboration was launched in 1993 in Oxford, at what was to be the first of the annual Cochrane Colloquia.

Growing rapidly, what developed was a replication of the work on the *Oxford Database of Perinatal Trials* in a growing number of other fields. There are now forty-nine international review groups, each with a coordinating editor supported by an editorial team. The review groups were formed in response to the interests of a group of people who wanted to conduct systematic reviews around this interest. They had to commit themselves to the Collaboration's ten key principles: collaboration, building on the enthusiasm of individuals, avoiding duplication, minimizing bias, keeping up-to-date, striving for relevance, promoting access, ensuring quality, continuity, and enabling wide participation. Reviews are updated and posted on the Web, as well as being supplied on compact disk as *The Cochrane Library,* which contains a database of systematic reviews as well as a controlled trials register. It is in the review groups that the main work of the Collaboration gets done. This is voluntary work, in the sense that researchers negotiate with their institutions to devote discretionary time for research on conducting reviews.

These teams of researchers are supported by methods groups that refine the methodology of research synthesis. They meet face-to-face at the annual Cochrane Colloquium. An elected steering group of fourteen members is supported by a small secretariat, currently located in Oxford. There are fourteen Cochrane Centres, which have national or regional responsibilities for supporting and coordinating Cochrane initiatives. Brian Haynes established the Canadian Cochrane Centre at McMaster University. Peter Tugwell in Ottawa coordinates the Cochrane Musculo-skeletal Group.

It is this large international conglomerate that is seen as contributing to evidence-based medicine. The term *evidence-based medicine* was coined to describe the McMaster University aims, and Iain Chalmers believes that this is appropriate for those who are clinicians, and he is not. When Chalmers was knighted in 2001, the draft citation for his knighthood included "for services to evidence-based health care," and he asked for "evidence-based" to be deleted. He wants to distance himself because of its use as a pejorative, to describe clinical care that is provided by automatons. On the other hand, he is inclined to support evidence-based choice by consumers. For better or worse, the term is firmly attached to the activities of both McMaster University and the Cochrane Collaboration.

Given the broad scope of the new direction, it was necessary to be explicit about what was required of reviewers in terms of the processes to be used. The following checklist comes from the book *Systematic Reviews* (Chalmers and Altman 1995):

· Is the question clearly focused?
· Is the search for relevant articles thorough?
· Are the inclusion criteria appropriate?
· Is the validity of included studies adequately assessed?
· Is missing information obtained from investigators?
· How sensitive are results of the review to changes in the way the review is done?
· Do the conclusions of the review flow from the evidence reviewed?
· Are recommendations linked to the strength of the evidence?
· Are judgments about preferences (values) explicit?
· If there is "no evidence of effect," is caution taken not to interpret this as "evidence of no effect"?
· Are subgroup analyses interpreted cautiously?

This list was prepared by Andrew Oxman at the Norwegian Direct-orate for Health and Social Affairs, Oslo, Norway, who is formerly of McMaster University. He played a key role in systematizing the field, but he also illustrates the overlapping activities of the Cochrane Collaboration and McMaster University.

Andrew Oxman and International Connections

Andy Oxman grew up in Denver and was an antiwar activist during the Vietnam War. He and his friends wanted to know more about how to change the world. At the same time, they recognized that everyday skills would still be needed "after the revolution." This recognition led to his interest in community-oriented primary care and his decision to go into medicine and become "a sort of Julian Tudor Hart working in a rural area." At medical school in Michigan, he married a Norwegian medical student and accompanied her back to Norway. In 1982 he went as a gen-eral practitioner to a very small town in Norway above the polar circle. In this isolated community he would read articles in medical journals giv-ing advice that put him at odds with the other doctors in the area. After two years he decided that he needed better skills in understanding the needs of communities, and that he also needed a better foundation for clinical decisions. He applied to the master's program at McMaster University on the basis of a brochure describing the program and became a resident in community medicine.

Oxman's thesis, on the use of systematic reviews, was inspired by *Summing Up: The Science of Reviewing Research* (Light and Pillemer 1984). In the thesis, he developed his checklist to measure the quality of review articles, and measured the checklist's reliability and validity. With Gordon Guyatt he produced guidelines for reading literature reviews (Oxman and Guyatt 1988), and he contributed to the users' guides to the medical lit-erature series in *Journal of the American Medical Association,* including an article on how to use an overview (Oxman et al. 1994). After completing his thesis, he taught a course on systematic reviews on the master's pro-gram, one of the first in the world. Oxman recalls, "In line with the sort of teaching that is done in that program, the expectation was that, to get into the course, you needed a question, to get out of it you needed a pub-lishable review. Many of these reviews were subsequently published. It was a very good way of summing up what people had learned earlier in the program because, to do a review, you had to apply a lot of the prin-ciples of clinical epidemiology. People found it very challenging."

In his first year of teaching a graduate seminar, Oxman taught Iain Chalmers and Murray Enkin as students. At this stage they were finishing the Oxford database and the book by the same name, and Iain Chalmers himself recorded that he found the people in the McMaster department a "pretty daunting lot. I was dead scared most of the time." It was daunting for Oxman too to meet up with people who had completed large numbers of reviews. Oxman discussed with Chalmers the developments at Oxford. In 1993, he went as a visiting fellow to the U.K. Cochrane Centre to prepare the first edition of the Cochrane handbook and its guidelines for doing reviews. He then returned to Hamilton, where he was involved in organizing the second colloquium, in 1994. Oxman then returned to Norway, to the National Institute of Public Health in Oslo. His job description as a senior researcher included a 50-percent time commitment to the Cochrane Collaboration.

Oxman argues that the United Kingdom has a two-hundred-year-old tradition of epidemiological debate over method. This history generated the necessary intellectual and financial resources for the support of evidence-based medicine. Public health in the United Kingdom had a strong focus on the effectiveness and efficiency of medical care, something largely outside the scope of public health in the United States and Canada. Because of this history, evidence-based medicine was embraced by public health physicians and referred to as "evidence-based health care" to emphasize its relevance to decision making about health care policies for populations as well as clinical care for individuals. Reforms in the National Health Service may have been aimed at cost constraints, but if they were, the Research and Development Programme created opportunities that were realized by Chalmers for the support of the Cochrane Collaboration. The benefits were mutual. A strong emphasis on effectiveness has remained in the Research and Development Programme.

Despite these local origins, the Cochrane Collaboration drew support from a broad range of people prepared to volunteer their services because it represents an ethos that appeals to them. Says Oxman:

I think the Cochrane Collaboration is a unique and fascinating organization for a few reasons. It combines idealism with a strong commitment to rigorous science. It is idealistic but critical and questioning. It is an unusual organization in terms of the degree of collaboration. I think part of the drive that has brought people into it is an antiauthoritarian attitude, where evidence is seen as a way of leveling the playing field and making decisions fair, based on something other than who has got power and who shouts the loudest. There are a lot of people who have come from various experiences — like Iain in Palestine and my antiwar experiences — and have come into this as angry young men and women. Even if they now have gray hair, they have still hung onto a bit of that anger and have a concern with equity and social justice. A lot of people came into the pregnancy and childbirth group after the experience of working in other countries. I don't think that it is just a coincidence that people like Gord Guyatt work in the Medical Reform Group. That compares with the people in the U.K. who were involved in the Society for Social Medicine.

Activities in evidence-based medicine at McMaster University require collaboration too, but it is a more limited collaboration between the admittedly large number of members of a research team. The voluntary ethos does not have to be as strong as in the Cochrane Collaboration, and that leaves them with more of the ethos of an academic department. Ultimately Oxman was more at home in an organization without this academic ethos.

The primary emphasis at McMaster University is on incorporating evidence from trials into clinical practice rather than on the generation of reviews. Iain Chalmers has had a robust debate with Brian Haynes and colleagues about this issue. Chalmers thinks this is a potentially misleading way of making evidence available to end users: "My argument with them is that, if you are a clinician and you look at this paper, your first question is, 'Are there any other trials and what do they say? Am I looking at an outlier? It was published in the *Lancet:* is that because it had a striking result?'" Instead of individual trials, Chalmers argues, clinicians need systematic reviews of trials, because they provide more reliable evidence for practice: "When people want to know what the bottom line is, a review is a much better guide — provided that the quality of the review is sound. This is what the Collaboration endeavors to provide." The same reviews are then also useful for a number of other users, including policy makers and consumers. In more recent times, Chalmers believes, the emphasis changed, focusing greater attention on reviews. The McMaster hierarchy of evidence is now headed by randomized trials done with individual patients (N of one trials), followed by meta-analysis of randomized controlled trials with no heterogeneity.

Both Oxman and Chalmers believe that the most substantial connection between the two initiatives was forged when David Sackett went to Oxford University. The university medical school had become concerned about a lack of achievement and energy in public health. Chalmers suggested to the university that one of the problems was a lack of leadership in the field. They should set up an institute to build on their strengths, doing well-designed field trials of new interventions being produced in molecular biology (building on the work done at Oxford by Richard Peto) and conducting systematic reviews to set the work in context (building on the work of the Cochrane Collaboration). Chalmers suggested that one of the few people who could head it would be David Sackett. Sackett had spent a sabbatical in Oxford and had impressed them, and he had agreed to be the first chair of the Collaboration. In 1994 Muir Gray, director of research and development for the Oxford region of the National Health Service, and David Weatherall, Regius Professor of Medicine, created a chair in clinical epidemiology for Sackett and invited him to create the world's first Centre for Evidence-Based Medicine. Sackett was encouraged to find that "the most senior of medical schools" was accepting a program to bring clinical epidemiology/evidence-based medicine to the bedside in addition to applying it to the purchasing and providing of health services.

Sackett was well supported in these efforts by large numbers of people who had undergone training at McMaster University or attended the workshops run by Gordon Guyatt and others. Oxman says that Sackett "barnstormed" the United Kingdom and Europe. Iain Chalmers adds:

Dave set off explosions all over the place. As you know, he is a larger-than-life North American. He is a wonderful teacher but uses a style that is uncomfortable for some people in this country. Quite early on, he realized that he would be asked to speak a lot, and indeed, he was asked to speak all over Europe and further afield, about this thing called evidence-based medicine. So he got a video film made of one of his talks so that they could watch his talk. Well! There were clinicians in Oxford who saw that as egoism at its most extreme. As a consequence he made some real enemies here, but he also made some very good friends and he converted many young people. He was only here for five years, but his mark on Europe as a whole is indelible. He is a very charismatic teacher.

Sackett himself recorded that he gave more than a hundred lectures in 1998 (Sackett 2000). It was here that he participated in an international collaboration with coauthors from New York, Oxford, and Hamilton to produce the first edition of *Evidence-Based Medicine. How to Practice and Teach EBM* (1997). When leaving Oxford to return to Canada, Sackett announced a proposal for the redemption of experts like himself: compulsory retirement: he would never again "lecture, write or referee anything to do with evidence-based clinical practice" (Sackett 2000, p. 1283). He was going to turn his attention to randomized trials. What he did not do was use his experience to turn a more critical eye on the monument to evidence-based medicine that he helped to design and construct. The prophet left the field without recanting, leaving the disciples to carry a message unsullied by doubt.

Issues in the Cochrane Colloquium

The Cochrane Collaboration is a decentralized organization depending on the generosity of volunteers. When Iain Chalmers was asked in 2001 whether it also depended on the presence of Iain Chalmers, he replied:

> Oh, no, that is one of the nice things. I came off the steering group of the Collaboration four years ago, so I have had no part of the development of the Collaboration since then, except in the U.K. Cochrane Centre. There are wonderful people who are involved in helping it go forward. The point is that it has made itself essential to many departments of health. The NHS *needs* the Cochrane Collaboration. Now that it has proved itself as a result of a lot of volunteer effort, hopefully people who are going to need a bit of help to do a review are more likely to find it from those who have become dependent on the output of the Collaboration.

The ethos of generosity is central to the Collaboration, and this has worked well in Europe and Canada, but less so in the United States, where people have a different approach, often expecting payment for their efforts.

In arguing for the importance of the Cochrane Collaboration, Chalmers draws attention to the role of evidence in the prevention of suffering. The pregnancy and childbirth project had gained attention because the evidence it produced "had the potential to make a really important impact on the suffering of babies and their parents." And the systematic review of antenatal corticosteroids showed that not only did the intervention prevent morbidity and mortality in premature babies, it also reduced the cost of neonatal services. It is not only effective in reducing the suffering of babies but it also reduces the cost of their care. The interests of health policy makers therefore parallel the interests of consumers. In Andy Oxman's view, it is also the case that a combination of idealism with science leads to an emphasis on consumers: "The reason we are doing this is not to benefit ourselves or to benefit doctors, but to benefit the end users. I think that that is a logical connection." Because of his positive experience with consumer groups in the pregnancy and childbirth field after the publication of *Effective Care in Pregnancy and*

Childbirth, Chalmers sees consumer groups as playing a central role in the Collaboration. Oxman points out, however, that the interests of policy makers and consumers do not always coincide. When new forms of effective care add to costs, policy makers have conflicting interests in containing costs or providing effective care.

The Consumer Network in the Cochrane Collaboration has the role of facilitating the flow of information to and from consumers. Consumer participation is encouraged in identifying priorities and in the actual process of reviewing. There is also a Cochrane Consumers and Communication Review Group, which undertakes its own reviews of interventions that affect consumers' interactions with health care professionals, services, and researchers. Their particular focus is on information provision and communication. One expected focus for review is consumer participation in health care planning, policy, and research. A review addresses the involvement of consumers in research and agenda-setting in the National Health Service (Oliver 2001). Here too there is an emphasis on challenging authority: "In today's world it is not appropriate to assume that consumers of health care services are ignorant, or that they desire an autocratic and paternal service" (Wale 2001, p. 10). While the Cochrane Collaboration has a solid commitment to involving consumers, *The Cochrane Library* has been aimed at reading and comprehension levels comparable to those of people who would read, for example, the *British Medical Journal.*

There is a tendency in consumer groups to appreciate qualitative research as more accessible. Oxman argues that systematic reviews of qualitative studies are clearly outside the remit of the Cochrane Collaboration, as are a range of other epidemiological studies: "If we take on every new challenge that is put to us, we will never cope with what we have taken on already — which is big enough, almost overwhelming." He does see a role for qualitative researchers in analyzing how systematic reviews are conducted. These reviews involve classification and categorization of trials, and qualitative researchers are skilled in methods of making these processes more rigorous. While qualitative methods have been registered as a possible methods group for some time, he does not see the same incentive for qualitative researchers to participate in the activities of the Collaboration.

It is difficult to assess the effect of an initiative such as the Cochrane Collaboration. Certainly a wealth of material has been produced. In 2001, Mike Clarke and Peter Langhorne (deputy chair and chair of the Cochrane Collaboration Steering Group) reported that there were six thousand people in sixty countries contributing to the collaboration, the Cochrane controlled-trials register had more than thirty thousand entries, and there were one thousand completed reviews. Editors of journals were requiring editorials to refer to relevant Cochrane reviews, and funding bodies were increasingly requiring systematic reviews as part of the justi-fication for a new study. The focus of the Cochrane Collaboration was on the mammoth task of producing this information. An unpublished inter-nal paper (Holmes et al. 2001) demonstrates that evidence from Cochrane reviews has been regularly cited in national and international guidelines. Iain Chalmers, however, urges caution: "If the Cochrane Collaboration moves away from giving information to trying to tell people what to do, then it is doomed; it will put backs up all over the place. Policy decisions are made on the basis of many inputs, and Cochrane reviews can never provide more than one input."

Central to the organization is an emphasis on self-reflective analysis. This involves reassessment of challenges (Oxman 2001), as well as improved methods of implementation of the evidence in health care (Oxman and Flottorp 2001). One continuing source of concern is whether clinicians are finding *The Cochrane Library* to be of immediate benefit in comparison with some of its derivative products, including guidelines. This concern is shared by two reviewers in the very difficult field of psychiatry.

Clinical Researchers: Carol Joughin and Morris Zwi

Morris Zwi is a consultant child psychiatrist at the Child and Family Consultation Centre at the Richmond Royal Hospital. Zwi is an enthu-siastic clinician who uses a systems approach involving not just the child but also the family and his own colleagues in decision-making roles. He was skeptical about the claims to science of medicine and psychiatry, and he was drawn into evidence-based medicine by suspicion. He was con-cerned that the government and clinicians with strong beliefs in their par-ticular favored modes of treatment would misuse the so-called evidence, which he believed was often based on unsound methodology. Zwi recalls:

It was the time of the Tory government, and there was more and more emphasis on quality of services. The direction we were being pushed into was to justify what we were doing with outcome measures for everything. I decided that this was the kind of thing that was going to be rammed down our throats. In child and ado-lescent mental health, I knew that there was not much good-quality research, and

I worried that there was going to be a coup by people who believed only in cognitive behavior therapy. If you do behavior therapy on someone who is depressed, you can conduct a depression inventory before and after treatment and measure the change. I don't have a problem with doing that; I just think that that is not all that we should be doing. It would restrict the way people worked and thought. In systemic therapy we have inbuilt criticism and self-reflection in terms of having colleagues who observe and offer views for open discussion. It helps us keep on track. This acknowledges the complexity of interactions between individuals, be they colleagues or families. These are complex interventions; they are very difficult to measure.

So I wanted to understand what these changes were about. What tends to happen is that you get bullies who claim to be experts in an area, and they come and crush anything in their path. Unless you have something that you can use to stop them, like information, they ride straight over you. I could either apply some of these principles to the way that I worked and to the way that our team worked, so that we could survive, or I would know enough to construct a legitimate argument against its use.

I am very pleased that I went down that path, because that is exactly what did happen. Not in the extreme way that I anticipated, but it has been very useful to have skills in this area. It has been very useful to understand methods and statistics so that I can challenge some of the so-called experts when they are pushing a particular point of view. I have done that from time to time, just asking questions at the end of a talk at a conference or a professional forum where people have been throwing their weight around.

Zwi went to a workshop in 1997 in Oxford at the Centre for Evidence-Based Mental Health. David Sackett contributed. Zwi discovered that the focus was very much on epidemiology and on skills in asking and answering questions, as well as on critical appraisal of the literature. He had been alerted to the importance of epidemiology during his medical training in South Africa (see chapter 8) and was interested in getting more involved in the area. It was during this workshop that he was told about the work being done by Carol Joughin.

Joughin is a researcher who has also worked as a clinician and manager in a wide range of health service settings. She was introduced to the ideas of evidence-based practice through her master's degree program in health management at City University, London. In 1997, she was appointed to the FOCUS project at the Royal College of Psychiatrists' Research Unit. The aim of the project, funded by the Gatsby Charitable Foundation, was to promote effective practice in child mental health services. Joughin's approach has been to keep at an accessible level everything that is produced by the project, so that practitioners find it easy to read. She says, "There are enough people doing highbrow work in this area, and there are not enough people making it accessible to practicing clinicians and people who are really struggling with very complex work. I have worked in virtually every area of the health services, and children's mental health is the most complicated area I have ever worked in."

Joughin knew she faced a difficult task. At this time, clinical governance had not yet become an issue. She saw chief executives of health care organizations as having responsibility for running the equivalent of a large company. They were usually not medically trained, but they had to deal with a powerful medical hierarchy. It was very difficult to question what the profession was doing, and there was little incentive to do so. With more recent changes, these executives became accountable for clinical quality as well as financial management. As is evident from Zwi's experience, this brought substantial change in the approach to evidence-based practice but, initially, little of it was positive.

When Joughin started the project, she found there was insufficient evidence in children's mental health services to take on either of the then currently popular trends of developing evidence-based guidelines or doing multicenter clinical audit. Instead she decided to focus on supporting clinicians in making evidence-based decisions. Most clinicians in the child mental health field did not know what evidence-based practice was, were unaware of the Cochrane Collaboration, and, if they did know of it, were immediately put off of doing systematic reviews by the time commitment. With few practitioners interested in this approach, her first step was to "hook them in."

One of the early initiatives for the project was to produce a book on evidence, and this resulted in the volume *Finding the Evidence,* now in its second edition (Scott et al. 2001). Joughin and coauthors asked psychiatrists to address an area of practice and produce a short list of references of systematic reviews or meta-analyses, reviews, classic papers, cutting-edge papers, and books. These were the vehicle for providing additional information about appropriate Cochrane Review groups and Websites, as well as the methods of conducting searches. Joughin says, "In everything we did, we tried to combine an element of teaching about the basics of evidence-based practice with the things that we know people want to learn about." The next step was to identify one issue of high concern to clinical practice in this field: attention deficit hyperactivity disorder (ADHD). Although there was a very large literature on this disorder, and there were more clinical studies on the use of stimulants in its management than on any other child mental health problem, psychiatrists still felt uncertain about its management.

Following the standard search protocol for a systematic review,

Joughin started with a literature search, looking for trials with more than sixty patients. She found only a few with samples over thirty; there were frequent serious problems with lack of information on research processes and large dropout rates. She was "quite shattered" by the low quality of the research. Senior clinicians helped with the evaluation of these studies, but some of them were not trained in critical appraisal techniques. In addition, this is a particularly complex area in which the social and family contexts of the child have an intimate relationship with the problems experienced. It became obvious that the Sackett and Straus notion of an evidence cart for clinicians to consult was impossible: the evidence was simply not there and, even if it had been, the skills of clinicians were not adequate to the task of critically analyzing the material "on the run" and then applying the evidence to practice.

At this stage she realized she would have to take an active role in critically appraising the material. Then Morris Zwi telephoned, saying he was interested in evidence-based practice. She immediately went to meet him. They decided to collaborate and acquire the necessary methodological skills. These were accessible in a one-week course in the Systematic Reviews Training Unit at the Institute of Child Health, London. This unit was set up by the National Health Service Research and Development Programme in 1996 with the aim of training health professionals in making systematic reviews of research in order to support evidence-based practice and policy in the health service. The unit has close links to the Cochrane Collaboration and the National Health Service Centre for Reviews and Dissemination

While this training was invaluable, Joughin decided neither to do a systematic review nor to produce guidelines. Instead she and Zwi collaborated in producing *Focus on the Use of Stimulants in Children with Attention Deficit Hyperactivity Disorder* (1999), which they describe as an evidence-based briefing, a guide to promote debate around questions that clinicians see as important. The book starts with a simple and disarming description of evidence-based practice, and this style is maintained throughout. The focus is on fourteen clinical questions, and for each of these there is an outline of the background, a critical analysis of key references, and a listing of further important papers. This material serves as the vehicle for methodological discussion: it provides clear details on search strategies and critical appraisal tools, including meta-analyses and systematic reviews. The authors conclude that there was little evidence on which to judge the long-term effects of treatment with stimulants for ADHD. Although the book was not intended for parents, many parents found it useful. It was produced by the Royal College of Psychiatrists and was very well received. Major systematic reviews in the area were in progress at the time, and a second edition of the book was planned to include this updated material.

This experience persuaded Zwi to enroll in a diploma program at the Systematic Reviews Training Unit. He now combines his clinical practice with teaching evidence-based practice. Joughin continues to teach and work in the area. Her primary concern now is with the dissemination of knowledge. She is concerned that the practical limitations on practitioners may be underestimated. She argues that searching the literature is difficult, and some clinicians still do not have computers on their desks, nor do they have the time to conduct searches. Searching on-line she considers "a nightmare," and she much prefers a CD-ROM. The biggest problem, however, is that "the average person who provides the majority of care to the majority of patients does not have time to read a huge amount." While sophisticated formats are useful for clinicians motivated to read journals and reports, at the other extreme much simpler methods are needed. She is experimenting with disseminating evidence in accessible "coffee-table books" or on giveaway mouse pads with summary diagrams and contact addresses.

Joughin and Zwi have used the Cochrane Collaboration as a primary source of material. The methodological material that they promote is drawn from either McMaster University or Cochrane Collaboration texts. They have used training courses on systematic reviews when needed. What they produced was a practical product that translates the concerns of the Cochrane Collaboration into those of immediate concern to clinicians.

Initially Morris Zwi's suspicions were allayed. While policy changes may place unwelcome limitations on good clinical practice, evidence-based arguments can be used by both sides of a debate — if the skills are there. But the balance of power is unequal. When the National Institute for Clinical Excellence produced a guidance document for the treatment of ADHD, it supported the use of the controversial drug methylphenidate. The Royal College of Psychiatrists endorsed the guidance, noting that they supported what most child and adolescent psychiatrists saw as good practice.[1]

This decision on treatment of ADHD illustrates one of the problems of meeting what are pressing needs of policy makers for guidance on financing health care. The state is properly focused on constraining financial expenditure on pharmaceutical drugs. Evidence of effectiveness is essential if they are to identify and constrain expenditures on drugs that are less effective, or more expensive but with the same effect as another drug. These decisions cannot always wait until the evidence is unequivocal, and this can produce impatience with the time taken to conduct a good review and then produce evidence-based guidelines. The risk is that, in meeting time objectives, policy makers may sacrifice quality. The Cochrane Collaboration does not see the production of guidelines as an appropriate activity for itself because of local differences in the policy contexts of different countries.

Conclusion

Iain Chalmers points out that he has been a contract researcher, without tenure, throughout his time in this field. The people who do the reviews for the Cochrane Collaboration mostly do this work without payment. The Collaboration has functioned on the generosity and commitment of a large number of international researchers. It has stimulated interest in critically appraising and producing good evidence for clinical care decisions about interventions. Such care and precision in assessing outcome tends to have a conservative effect on practice, summed up by Iain Chalmers as follows: "I am undoubtedly a snail when it comes to innovation in medicine. I am skeptical of claims. Being nice to people does not need to be researched: it's something worth cultivating. But there are other ways in which you can interfere in people's lives and really mess them up; with the best of intentions, you can really mess them up. That is probably why I witter on about the need to take bias seriously."

The effects of an organization such as this are seen not only in the Websites and publications but also in how it affects what people think about health and illness. While consumers have participated in setting priorities in the Collaboration and participated in reviews of issues of clear importance to consumers, it is not clear that the effect has yet been felt by the average consumer of health care. Potentially, self-help organizations and consumer activist groups (familiar to researchers in the pregnancy and childbirth area) are the main beneficiaries.

Similarly it is not yet clear to what extent there has been a change in clinical practice. Let us return to Henrik Wulff's argument (chapter 3) about the need to combine the dominant technical interest with the practical interest in communicating with people and the emancipatory interest in freeing people from domination. The example of child psychiatry shows that the technical material produced by the Cochrane Collaboration still needs an interpreter before it is communicated to practitioners in the field. This interpreter does not have to be medically trained. For those with the commitment, the material is available, and training is accessible to help anyone who wants to take on the task of translation. Practitioners who become proficient in the field as a result of having the processes of evidence-based medicine explained to them may even find that arguments based on evidence are useful in defending territory from potential medical tyrants or political entrepreneurs. Thus emancipation is a real possibility.

There is little doubt that the Cochrane Collaboration has produced material in an aggregated form that has been useful to policy makers. Following Archie Cochrane's agenda, this should lead to cost savings, and these savings could then be diverted to improving neglected aspects of care. In contrast to Cochrane's agenda, the Cochrane Collaboration does not explicitly support the diversion of funds to more deserving but neglected areas of care. The effect, however, is the same when it challenges areas of policy by drawing attention to the inadequate evidence base in the area. Such advice is not necessarily welcomed by policy makers. Central to this organization has been its relationship with the British government. Like INCLEN, however, the Cochrane Collaboration has centers in other countries. The question, then, is the extent to which the evidence produced in highly industrialized countries is relevant and appropriate for less industrialized countries. In particular, what will the situation be if a Cochrane Centre finds itself radically at odds with a government over an issue of evidence?

Notes

1. S. Mayer, Ritalin gets the nod of approval in the UK, *The Scientist* (November 9, 2000), www.biomedcentral.com.news, accessed on April 11, 2003.

CHAPTER 8

The Cochrane Collaboration
in South Africa

In the United Kingdom, the interests of the state were coherent with the
establishment of the Cochrane Collaboration. In *Uses of Epidemiology* Jerry
Morris says, "Myself I have an old-fashioned faith in saturating the services with *facts*" (Davey Smith 2001, p. 1149). The Cochrane Collaboration
has produced a constant stream of these facts. The United Kingdom had
a government that, to some extent, welcomed the facts. This raises the
question of how a Cochrane Centre would fare in a country where the
facts being produced were unwelcome, and where, to use Sackett's
phrase, clinical authorities "resisted the egalitarianism inherent in clinical
epidemiology" (2002, p. 1163). There was also the question of the voluntary nature of the Cochrane activities. In a less industrialized country, people working in the Cochrane Centre would require significant sponsor-
ship from government and nongovernment institutions.

South Africa provides an interesting recent example of a country
undergoing substantial political change, including change in the delivery
of health care. After the election of the African National Congress government in 1994, a medical system that had primarily served the white
population was being restructured to meet the needs of the whole population. Moreover, this change was occurring in the context of an almost
overwhelming problem associated with the emergence of the AIDS epidemic. Not only could the political changes in the country not be ignored
by the proponents of evidence-based medicine, but, as a boon to the
researcher, the debate on the role of evidence in setting up a new system
of health care was readily accessible. The Cochrane Collaboration's

Colloquium in Cape Town in 2000, which I attended, presented an opportunity for analyzing exactly such a situation. It also allowed me to draw on my personal views of South Africa, my country of birth.

A Personal Account

When I traveled to South Africa in 2000, it was my second visit to the country after the fall of white majority rule and the election of the government headed by Nelson Mandela. Before the colloquium, I visited my sister who lives in the foothills of the Drakensberg in Kwa Zulu-Natal. She is inclined to be New Age and delights in finding spiritually satisfying graveyards in which she would feel at peace if she were to be buried there. As we drove past some of the graveyards on her short list, she pointed to rows of new white crosses. There was always a funeral in progress. All the local graveyards would soon be full. This is the face of AIDS in this rural area. The euphoria I felt after the election of the Mandela government rapidly faded.

On a farm farther into the mountains, there is a pottery, Ardmore Ceramic Art, established by Fee Halsted-Berning. Drawing on the local tradition of making unbaked pots, she trained local, largely uneducated farmworkers in modern ceramic techniques. The work they produce is inspired by their own traditions, and the pottery achieved an international reputation for its strong designs and powerful mythic images. Bonnie Ntshalintshali, who enjoyed a growing international reputation, was one of the most successful of the young potters. I visited the pottery in 1995, when the country was still celebrating its first democratic election. Fee Halsted-Berning sounded a word of warning. She was desperately worried about the spread of AIDS. The men on the farm would probably not use condoms, and the only solution seemed to be for the women potters to remain celibate. But they were also celebrating with Bonnie Ntshalintshali, who was in love and about to get married. With luck, at least Bonnie would be safe.

It was reassuring at that time to know that there was a pugnacious health minister in the new African National Congress government. Nkosazana Zuma was a member of the African National Congress liberation movement, and had been medically trained in South Africa and Britain. Despite her commitment and excellent credentials, her attempts at implementing AIDS prevention programs soon brought her into disrepute. Zuma was accused of squandering R14.2 million on *Sarafina II,* an AIDS awareness play—and bypassing the normal competitive tendering process (*Weekly Mail and Guardian*, March 7, 1997). She met these criticisms by referring to the racist attitudes of critics (*Weekly Mail and Guardian*, March 22, 1996). In 1997, with 2.4 million South Africans said to be HIV positive, it was reported that only about half the R65 million AIDS budget had been spent (*Weekly Mail and Guardian*, May 2, 1997). Condom distribution programs were dogged by failure. Forty million condoms that had been distributed were found to be faulty, but a secret recall netted fewer than 5 million (*Dispatch Online*, May 17, 1999). Television advertisements for condoms were relegated to a post–10 P.M. time slot (*Weekly Mail and Guardian*, July 18, 1997). With the HIV tally steadily rising, critics described the AIDS awareness program as incoherent and the education campaign as imperceptible and unintelligible (*Weekly Mail and Guardian*, October 16, 1998). Programs were being implemented in a scattershot manner (*Weekly Mail and Guardian*, March 22, 1996). These problems were compounded by the announcement that antiretroviral treatment (AZT and Nevirapine) for the 25 percent of pregnant women who were HIV positive was too costly. Zuma threw her support behind a locally produced product, Virodene. The government's support for the development of Virodene was described as corrupt by Costa Gazi, national health secretary of the opposition Pan Africanist Congress (Gazi 2000), and the product itself was described as paint stripper and a "witches' brew" (Trengove-Jones 2000).

In mid-1999 Zuma was replaced by Manto Tshabalala-Msimang, who had also left South Africa to join the liberation movement and had earned a medical degree from the First Leningrad Medical Institution. At the time of Tshabalala-Msimang's appointment, the AIDS Directorate was still not spending 40 percent of its budget. During National Condom Week, her department distributed a shipment of condoms that had been stapled to information cards. In 2000, Gazi called for manslaughter charges against the former minister of health (*Weekly Mail and Guardian*, February 4, 2000). With a growing infection rate, the Health Department seemed paralyzed and ineffective. It is in this context of repeated failure that President Thabo Mbeki started talking to researchers who denied the relationship between HIV and AIDS.

Such confusion did not bode well for any prevention program. When I visited the Ardmore pottery in 2000, Bonnie Ntshalintshali had died of AIDS at the age of thirty-two, leaving a young child. Throughout her illness, she had been described as suffering from a cold. She was the fourth of the Ardmore potters to die, and her work joined the display in the pottery's Gallery of the Dead. The number of dead has grown ever since. They leave behind them a number of children, some of whom are no doubt HIV positive. They have not been tested. Since the men's rejection of condom usage had clearly not been overcome, I asked one of the new young women potters if it would help if I sent from Australia a load of the most exotic and artistic condoms I could find: with colors, stripes, knobs, and flavors. She smiled and looked away. My sister's glance silenced me. Later she explained that it had become unacceptable for a white woman to advocate condom usage. It would be interpreted as a racist attack on black men's sexuality.

What seemed to be a rather extreme version of events was borne out when newspapers reported the death of Parks Mankahlana at the age of thirty-six. He was presidential spokesman for Mbeki, and Nelson Mandela before him — the public face of the government's denial that HIV causes AIDS, and the person who argued that HIV-positive pregnant women should not be treated because there would be no one to care for their children. Mankahlana himself had recently married, and he too had left behind a young child. There was widespread speculation that he had died of AIDS, and questions were raised about whether he had used antiretroviral drugs (Dowling 2000). The government countered by defending the privacy of the family and implied that such questioning was inspired by racism. In July 2000, Mbeki's doubt about a causal relationship between HIV and AIDS made headline news at an international AIDS conference held in Durban, not far from the rural area where the Ardmore pottery was establishing its Gallery of the Dead.

While traveling to the 2000 meeting of the Cochrane Collaboration, I saw clear signs of the failure of the AIDS policy. Airport toilets had dispensers for digestive tablets and tampons but not condoms. There were none of the warning signs about travel and safe sex to which I had become accustomed in Australia. On the night of my arrival in Cape Town, I listened to a radio program about the response of rural youth to AIDS. The young men interviewed roundly rejected safe sex messages. Their preference, they said, was for "skin on skin." What did they think about the risk? They did not believe there was a risk, but interpreted these theories as an assault on the credibility of Mbeki by the opposition in the coming local government elections. As committed African National Congress supporters, they did not intend to pay any attention to opposition propaganda.

Here then was a political situation in which well-trained and committed policy makers were caught in a deadly dilemma. The evidence pointed one way, political realities constituted an exactly opposing force.

And yet evidence could not be rejected out of hand. The issue was to give legitimacy to the rejection of evidence. In 2000, Mbeki convened the Presidential AIDS Advisory Panel, which was intended to represent diversity of expertise. The panel included people holding the view that HIV had no causal link to AIDS. Lampooned in the press as flat-earthers, they suggested that AIDS is an artifact of the system of data collection. Concluding that AIDS is not sexually transmitted, and that a major cause of death was the use of toxic anti-HIV drugs, this portion of the panel recommended a suspension of all HIV testing until it was proved to be relevant to Africa — but they supported good general public health measures. Panelists supporting the causal link between HIV and AIDS called for extensive HIV and AIDS surveillance programs and a focus on risk factors such as the behavior of youth. They recommended safe sex education and the promotion of condom usage. The process of trying to reach consensus produced results described by an anonymous member of the panel as "chaotic and terribly misleading" (All the president's scientists 2000). The final report ducked the issue on the grounds that favoring one view was contrary to the spirit in which the panel was convened. The minister lamented the failure of panelists supporting the causal link between HIV and AIDS to engage in the Internet debate about the issues.

At the Cochrane Collaboration meeting, the plenary papers by leading South African health bureaucrats focused on antiretroviral treatment of HIV, with never a mention of the preventive role of condom use. Clearly, evidence was a two-edged sword in the context of an increasingly defensive policy response to HIV-AIDS. It is exactly in a time of crisis such as this that access to reliable evidence should come into its own. Timely and effective evaluation of the cost-effectiveness of every program could have delivered a sound foundation for policy and a strong defense against charges of mismanagement. South Africa needed evidence-based medicine and evidence-based health policy. Faced with a flagrant disregard for scientific fact, however, I wondered why there was a South African Cochrane Centre at all. How had it come into being, and how had it become so well established that it could conduct an international conference a few years later?

As it turned out, the health bureaucracy in the new government provided the necessary support. The two ministers of health had been caught in a dilemma over AIDS, yet respect for evidence remained. But evidence was of most value to the people who had to implement the programs devised in haste among the higher echelons of government. Their responsibility was to health care in the longer term rather than to recurrent political crises. In addition, as this chapter argues, these approaches were sustained by a longer tradition of political struggle over health. This provided strong community support for democratic change in health, but perhaps more important, it provided a base of critical analysis and an emphasis on the need for evidence of health change. In addition, as has been a repeated theme in this account, the right people were there to take on the task.

The Political Tradition in Medicine

South Africa had a long political struggle to reach its first democratic elections, in 1994. A focus on the health of the public has been one aspect of this struggle. This tradition gives South Africa a base of critical analysis that has proved to be useful in the introduction of evidence-based medicine into the country.

There have always been health reformers in South African medicine, and they generated a well-respected critical approach to health care. Just as commonly, they ran afoul of the authorities. Some stayed on, fighting the odds. Others left the country. Included in the latter group was Kerr White's epidemiologist colleague John Cassell. Zena Stein and Mervyn Susser had distinguished careers as epidemiologists in the United States, where they moved in 1965. Inequality, repression, and social justice have, collectively, been a thread running through much of their work. As Stein put it in a 2003 interview, "The scene in which we grew up was two separate societies — poor blacks, and middle class and wealthy whites. So, it was a good situation to learn and think, if you had a social conscience of any kind" (Wilcox 2003, p. 498). Stein's career in community care started in Alexandra, a township outside Johannesburg in the 1950s, and this left her with a firm commitment to spending time in the community. This fitted well with the approach recommended by Jerry Morris in *Uses of Epidemiology,* an approach that allowed her to combine an activist approach with that of the scientist. She went on to become a pioneer in promoting safe sex for women, and it was in recognition of this work — as well as the work she and Mervyn Susser have done at the Africa Centre for Population and Reproductive Research in Kwa Zulu-Natal — that she was invited to serve on the Presidential AIDS Advisory Panel.

Over generations, these researchers built up a tradition of critical analysis of health care and its relationship to political structures. My focus is on the medical schools in the 1970s. This was the time when the need for a better evidence base for medicine became apparent worldwide; South

Africa was no exception. As in other countries, the momentum came from students who started questioning the authoritative views of clinical teachers. The difference here was that some of these students had turned to medicine as a way of addressing the gross injustices in the country. They had become further politicized by working on voluntary projects in the community. They built schools and started small health projects as exercises in "conscientizing" the community. Not surprisingly, in their medical training they were at odds with the more traditional teachers.

THE GENTLE RADICAL: MORRIS ZWI

In 1977, Morris Zwi started his medical training at the University of the Witwatersrand. At first he was idealistic about what medicine could achieve in South Africa, but he hated his medical training and cringed at the arrogance of some lecturers. Zwi recalls:

> Especially in the clinical years, it was still very much based on the British system, teaching with authority by undermining your sense of competence — which is the worst possible thing to do. I remember being asked, at a bedside with the patient there as well as nine other students, to give ten different causes of jaundice. I sort of managed to get three or four, and the consultant just blasted me: "You don't do enough reading; how do you expect to be a doctor if you don't spend time in the library?" Meantime I was spending more time in the library than anyone else because I wasn't going to lectures. It was that kind of thing, scaring you into doing reading, and then coming back the next day to show that you could reproduce their way of thinking.

Medical students at this university, most of them white, many from privileged backgrounds, did their clinical training in Soweto at Baragwanath Hospital and other hospitals serving the black population around Johannesburg. There they gained rich clinical experience. For those with a live political interest, it alerted them to what was going on in the black community and to the lack of good health services. It also generated in them a critical attitude to some of their clinical teaching. Zwi notes, "The worst example of what makes a bad doctor was a surgeon who was teaching us how to do a rectal examination. Basically he got five people to do a rectal examination on one patient. This was at Coronation Hospital. This patient had no say in the matter. It was absolutely appalling." There were also shining exceptions, brilliant clinicians and inspirational teachers who spoke kindly to patients and who asked permission before examining patients.

Zwi suggests that only about ten out of the two hundred medical students in his year were politically active. They developed considerable skill at challenging their teachers. Says Zwi:

We would say, "That is fine, teaching us about treating TB, but what are you doing about the housing conditions of people?" After all, they taught us that socioeconomic conditions like overcrowding cause the spread of TB. Overcrowding occurred because people were not free to move and live where they wanted; they had to live in ghettos. "As a doctor you have that responsibility, because you know that the health system here is as distorted as it is because of the apartheid system. So what are you doing about that?" They used to feel very uncomfortable teaching our group. Which was great!

This group of students was clearly quite different from David Sackett's cohort. They did not need clinical epidemiology and clinical evidence to challenge clinical authority. Instead they drew on the self-evident political injustice they saw in the wards and the community. In their community focus, their approach more closely resembled that of Kerr White. The methodological tools they needed to nail down their convictions came initially from public health. Les Irwig gave the public health lectures, scheduled as in David Sackett's time late in the afternoon. According to Zwi, "Epidemiology consisted of five sessions in the whole of fourth year, and that was it. They were usually late in the afternoon, and most people did not go. He wasn't inspiring, quite dour. But what I remember about it was his casting doubt on published work and saying, 'You've got to know how to unpick these things.' He just taught us some very basic things about critical appraisal and research methodology."

Zwi joined a group of students who initiated direct action in community health. Over a numbers of years, groups of students set up community health clinics in isolated and deprived rural areas. They did this in collaboration with community workers, who were highly politicized and organized as a result of the experience of forced resettlement. In these community settings, the students provided services and trained lay health workers. At that time, police were arresting people who presented at accident and emergency departments with shotgun wounds or bullet wounds. The assumption was that they had been involved in political unrest. As a result, wounded people could not get proper treatment. After negotiating with political leaders for entry into areas where there was unrest, the students helped treat people who had suffered the effects of teargas, gunshots, or police beatings. This evolved into a service to train local residents in emergency first aid.

Another initiative was a journal called *Critical Health*. It was intended to stimulate debate about and critique of the political economy of health in South Africa. The journal published the health statistics that the government was suppressing and argued for a socialist health program. The title contained the term *critical* in recognition of the dire state of health for most South Africans, but also because ongoing critique was required. The editors intended to put forward an alternative program for change at a time when change seemed unlikely. The government banned a number of issues.

These students ran afoul of the state. Most commonly they found it difficult to get into residency programs, and the police harassed them. What broke their effort was compulsory army training — and this meant active service either on the country's borders or in the black townships. Medical training delayed this call up, but postgraduate study did not count. When they finished their medical courses, they left the country. Morris Zwi became a child psychiatrist with an interest in evidence-based practice (see chapter 7).

Clinical Activist: Merrick Zwarenstein

Merrick Zwarenstein was part of this same group of medical students. He stopped going to lectures in his second year and spent his time in the library. The burning question he wanted answered was how he could know whether the community work they were doing made a difference. Ward rounds did not leave space for such questions, but, for him too, the person who provided the most insight was Les Irwig in his epidemiology lectures. Irwig taught them to ask simple questions: How do I know I am making a difference? What difference am I trying to make? How might I measure that difference? If I measure that difference, could it be explained only by my intervention? Could I find a control group? Could there be other sources of bias? Providing the answers to such questions is the core aim of clinical epidemiology, so Irwig invited David Sackett to talk at the medical school. The staff was skeptical, but the students were enthralled. These experiences changed the way Zwarenstein thought about his work. He went on to apply these methods in various community projects in South Africa.

Irwig emigrated to Australia, where he is now head of the Department of Public Health and Community Medicine, Sydney University. Zwarenstein used a fake London address to escape army service and remained in

South Africa. By this stage, in the late 1980s, it was clear that political change was coming in South Africa. Medical schools in South Africa had proved resistant to change on the grounds of social injustice; they were to prove equally resistant to the ideas of clinical epidemiology and evidence-based medicine. Echoing McMaster University's concern with changing the medical paradigm, Zwarenstein reflects on this resistance: "It's like village life. You can't be too far away from the mainstream if you are in a small village. The village does not like it. And I think that South Africa is basically a series of small villages, and if people are too different — even if it is not political — I think this is a system that does not find it easy to accept them."

With so many of the more radical members of his medical cohort effectively in exile, it was difficult to build up the necessary momentum for challenging the paradigm in the medical schools. Zwarenstein turned instead to research in the Medical Research Council in Cape Town. His research has focused on the diseases of poor communities: diarrhea (Harrison and Zwarenstein 1993) and tuberculosis (Zwarenstein et al. 1998). He has argued for the delivery of primary health care through a district health system (Zwarenstein et al. 1993) — one that employs village health workers (Kuhn and Zwarenstein 1990), thereby establishing a role for lay health workers (Zwarenstein et al. 2000). In 2001, he was involved in a collaborative project with Louis Niessen from the Institute for Medical Technology Assessment, Erasmus University, Rotterdam. They argue that World Health Organization guidelines for developing countries need to be strengthened by more extensive use of evidence from Cochrane reviews, but they note a lack of Cochrane reviews addressing conditions encountered in developing countries. If the standard of evidence required for guidelines for developing countries is lower than that required for developed countries, they say, then there is a real risk that these guidelines will promote out-of-date, second-rate care.

An important issue is that guidelines focusing on single diseases do not fit with the complex presentations and scarce resources in health care settings in developing countries. Zwarenstein and Niessen are enthusiastic about applying a World Health Organization approach, which is based on the integration of a set of guidelines into a single program. In diseases of childhood, for example, they have replaced a series of complex guidelines, one for each separate childhood disease, with an integrated package. Evidence-based guidelines are retained, but presentations are clustered and recommendations are integrated rather than being available in an amorphous pool. The aim is to enable the health service provider, who often acts alone in an isolated setting, to be more responsive to the overall care of the sick child.

Zwarenstein and Niessen are conducting randomized trials of interventions to promote practices based on these guidelines across seven developing countries. Zwarenstein and colleagues in Cape Town and the Free State are conducting the South African intervention. It is based on an adaptation of the guidelines designed to respond to the expressed needs of frontline practitioners and to the barriers to good care, identified in earlier research. According to Zwarenstein, the question is whether their intervention works in an "ordinary run-of-the-mill primary care clinic in the back of beyond." Their aim is to change the skill of practitioners, the health of patients, and the health of the community. It is essentially a top-down approach. Their primary concern is not with the community but with the delivery of good health services. Says Zwarenstein:

Forget the communities. This is not public health; it is clinical care. It is about people who show up at the door. Currently, they are getting a really bad deal. They get really bad care if they are attending private sector services, and they pay much too much for it. Patients are telling us what it is that they want. They are saying, "I feel grim and I want to be fixed." And that's what we are trying to do. Care is not delivered in a community; care is delivered in a disorganized system of clinics. Some of the best of providers have a feel for the community determinants of what they see. Some of the very, very best of them may be political activists about those determinants, but the idea that there is an unbroken continuum between public health and primary care is really too idealistic, everywhere in the world.

Niessen adds that, worldwide, 95 percent of the health budget is devoted to direct clinical care, and it follows that this is where research should be focused. This is not minor quibbling about the proper focus of academic research. Zwarenstein points out that effective clinical care for both tuberculosis and sexually transmitted disease could have minimized two of South Africa's worst public health problems:

What is the real problem that we need to address if we want to improve TB in the community? It is the fact that the quality of care is so poor that only six out of ten patients who present with the disease go on to complete treatment and effect cure. If you can't fix that, and that's the only thing you really need to fix, you can't fix TB. If you can get rates up to 90–95 percent then you are probably reducing the pool of infective cases, and this will have a *major* public health impact. There is the idea that what clinicians do is not public health. Well, for most of the important diseases, it absolutely is public health.

My real anger with the South African AIDS program is not that they delayed Nevirapine, although I think that's scandalous. In 1986 and 1987 it was becoming clear that the problem with HIV which resulted in its massive spread in Africa was untreated sexually transmitted and ulcerative disorders: gonorrhea, syphilis, and others. We knew in 1986 and 1987, even then, that if you dealt with it so that no one had a sexually transmitted disease for more than an hour after their first clinical visit, we would have an epidemic peaking at 3 percent rather than 35 percent of the population. We knew that then. *Nothing* has been done yet on that problem. So there is this really weird situation where policy makers who believe in public health do not believe in the improvement in the quality of clinical care, and the result is a major public health disaster.

From his base in the Medical Research Council, Zwarenstein feels he has the evidence for improving what primary care practitioners actually do "under laughably difficult conditions." This involves more than the top-down diffusion of evidence; he and his colleagues have learned to work with the practitioners involved in a cooperative way: "We are increasingly convinced that we have a handle on how you approach them, how you teach them, how you work with them in the field."

Both Niessen and Zwarenstein make use of the evidence from Cochrane reviews, but they do not see themselves as "Cochrane people." Their focus is not on generating reviews, but on the research that comes before the reviews and then feeds into reviews. Their other focus is on the research that follows reviews and addresses how the results of reviews can best be implemented in health care settings. In 1994, with the change in government, there was a clear opportunity to influence the formulation of health policy through good evidence of effectiveness of care. Zwarenstein decided that the Cochrane Collaboration was "potentially the most effective vehicle, the best organized" for these purposes. He notes:

I was *au fait* with clinical epidemiology; we had had several contacts with INCLEN. Useless, no possibility of getting it going here. It didn't seem possible to insert it into the clinical curriculum — nobody was interested in clinical epidemiology, nobody was taking it up, none of the departments was interested in it. One department at Pretoria was interested, and Les Irwig and I had tried working with them on a grant. We didn't get the grant, but the experience of working with a medical school was so unhappy that it just seemed to me that relying on the organized medical schools was going to be as unhelpful then as it had been in the pre–1994 era. There has been continued resistance from the top, and people who get to the top are people who fit a model of clinical excellence that does not accommodate evidence.

If Zwarenstein were limited to a national forum only, this would have presented a depressing scenario. This was no longer the case, however, as the Cochrane Collaboration was ensuring that people with similar concerns would know about each other. During a visit to the United Kingdom in 1994–1995, Zwarenstein, Iain Chalmers, Les Irwig, and Jimmy Volmink met and discussed the idea of establishing a Cochrane Centre in Cape Town. Jimmy Volmink too had been working in the Medical Research Council and was extremely well placed to take on the task of setting up the new center.

Home Town Hero: Jimmy Volmink

Jimmy Volmink is a local man, born in Athlone on the Cape flats outside Cape Town, an area zoned for "coloured," or mixed race, people under the apartheid regime. In 1975, he won a special dispensation, renewed annually, to go to the University of Cape Town, where he studied science and then medicine. He entered a world of white privilege feeling intimidated, socially and intellectually: "I felt I was from a different world," he says. "I had never even seen a Bunsen burner; I'd only seen it in pictures!"

He had as many questions as the white students from the University of the Witwatersrand did, but he felt constrained by circumstance:

Because I was at UCT [University of Cape Town] by special permission of government, there was a limit to what I could do in terms of questioning authority. It would be regarded as stepping out of line, so I did not have the freedom to do that. Yet, when I was in fourth year and I did community medicine, I think the temptation to say something was just overwhelming. I got into serious trouble with the then professor of community health for daring to contradict him. He was making a case repeatedly that people get TB in this country because they are genetically predisposed to it, and that social factors had very little to do with this. And I just could not live with myself any longer, sitting there with my mouth closed. I started challenging him openly. That was the only subject in my entire medical career that I failed. He failed me! I really believe he victimized me. I was made to repeat the exam.

From this experience Volmink realized that he enjoyed thinking independently, but that he had to do it in the world outside the medical schools. After graduating, he worked as the only doctor in a small mission hospital in Swaziland. There he saw diseases like cholera, typhoid, and malaria, which he had learned about but never seen. He returned to Cape Town to do pediatrics but concluded that his personality was still not suited to the hierarchical structure of a hospital, and that he needed to work in the community. He decided to enter primary care as a general practitioner. In order to do this, he had to leave the public sector and enter private practice. This went against his principles. Volmink recalls, "I thought, well, just because you are in the private system, that doesn't mean that you have to serve rich people. There is an alternative. So I applied, again, for special permission to set up a practice in the most underserved area in Cape Town, which was Khayelitsha. I was informed that I could not do that, because I am classified coloured and this was an African area. I could not rent a building; I could not buy a building; I could not practice there. I was devastated."

He was allowed to set up practice in the neighboring township of Mitchell's Plain, another disadvantaged area. During his ten years of practice there, he became increasingly interested in how the social context of patients influenced both how they presented in the clinic and their recovery. He recognized the political origins of many of their problems but did not see himself as a political activist. However, he had become skeptical about what doctors were doing and achieving, so he decided to do research on his own practice population. As a start he decided to document the issues making people ill and to test interventions that might improve their health. To do this, he needed postgraduate training in epidemiology. When he applied to the only training course in the country at Stellenbosch University, they turned him down on the grounds of color. Frustrated, he picked up the newspaper and noticed an advertisement for a Harvard/South Africa Fellowship. Harvard University was coming under increasing pressure from antiapartheid groups to disinvest and distance itself from any company invested in South Africa. One of its responses was to set up a scholarship allowing a small number of black students to study for a year at Harvard University. Volmink applied; the fine distinctions of color practiced internally in South Africa did not apply, and he went to Harvard University to get a master of public health degree, specializing in epidemiology.

When Volmink returned to South Africa, he split his time between his clinical practice and a research position at the Medical Research Council. There he set up a national research network of general practitioners that had a surveillance function. They drew attention to conditions seen in primary care rather than hospitals, focusing on anything from infectious diseases like measles to domestic violence in families. Then he was awarded a Nuffield Medical Research Fellowship to Oxford University for doctoral studies. His intention was to learn good research skills while conducting an epidemiological study of cardiovascular disease. But then he met Iain Chalmers. Volmink recalls:

I was cycling past the Cochrane Centre with my two-year-old son on the bars. I was going really slowly, and who should come by but Iain Chalmers. I didn't know it was Iain Chalmers. He started chatting to me — which I thought was rather strange. In England! We spent a little bit of time talking, just in general, and he was very welcoming. He didn't know me from a bar of soap, but he welcomed me to Oxford and said, "Anytime you want to come and visit and have a cup of coffee, feel free to do so." His friendliness and openness blew me away, so I thought I had to get to know this guy a little bit more. That was my big mistake! I went into the Cochrane Centre one day, and I came out two or three hours later completely brainwashed, completely taken up with this idea that we can actually do quite a lot to get the evidence straight, so that we can start making informed decisions in health care based on what interventions work and what doesn't work. This meeting with Iain Chalmers proved to be a life-changing experience for me.

While studying for his doctorate, Volmink started going to the Cochrane Centre to learn how to do systematic reviews and meta-analyses.

Volmink was at this point a rare asset, as Iain Chalmers must have recognized immediately. Volmink was highly trained for somebody with such strong links to the community, and he came from what was, in effect, a developing country. A Cochrane Centre in South Africa could help redress an imbalance in the Cochrane database. Volmink himself had noted that there was a problem with the database:

If you looked at the Cochrane database, the Cochrane reviews were largely addressing questions that were being asked by people in developed countries. And one could understand it: that is where the organization started, and one of its principles is that the initiative is driven by the interests of individuals. It is something that you make a lifelong commitment to; it has to be something that really grabs you. The only way to redress the imbalance in *The Cochrane Library* was to get more people involved from the developing world.

While many South Africans live in poverty, South Africa shares with more industrialized countries a relatively well-developed health infrastructure. At this stage there were good resources for health care. There was a potential pool of skilled researchers to support the center. People like Justus Hofmeyr had worked on the perinatal database, and both Merrick Zwarenstein at the Medical Research Council (MRC) and Les Irwig from Australia guaranteed their support.

The idea of the Cochrane Centre was welcome in South Africa too. By this time it had its first democratic government with a clear commitment to ensuring a shift in the power base of bureaucratic organizations like the Departments of Health and the Medical Research Council. Volmink, Chalmers, Irwig, and Zwarenstein (styling themselves a "gang of four") visited Pretoria, Johannesburg, and Cape Town to discuss the possibility of setting up a Cochrane Centre in South Africa (Zwarenstein et al. 1995). The idea was enthusiastically embraced by the MRC, including William Malegapuru Makgoba, who took over as chair of the MRC board in January 1999. Shortly afterward, he accused Mbeki of being "medically and scientifically naive" with respect to the AIDS debate (*Weekly Mail and Guardian,* March 17, 2000). The center was established in Cape Town and shares the MRC premises.

Nandipha Solomon was employed by Makgoba to manage the MRC's corporate affairs and stakeholder function. She clearly articulates the problem that the MRC faced: They had a commitment to move from doing "blue sky" research to addressing research priorities determined by the burden of disease in the country. While accepting that medical research could do little about the major source of ill health, poverty, they had to justify the money given to medical research. Investment in medical research had to be shown to be more worthwhile than "putting roofs over the heads of homeless people." According to Solomon, "Sixty percent of our funding comes from the taxpayers through the government, so in essence, our bosses are the people on the street. We've got to show that whatever we do in our science is being done in such a way that it impacts on the people's health. We've got to justify our existence. We can't just be the organization that exists behind four walls and accumulates journals that sit in an archive somewhere."

She too invokes the notion of a paradigm shift. In this case it is not one involving a shift to scientific practice, but one involving the idea of scientists becoming responsive to the community. Says Solomon:

> It is a mind shift. It is moving away from saying, "I'm the scientist and I've got the expertise and you don't really know what you are talking about," to saying, "I am the scientist, and yes, I do have expertise, and yes, I have studied" — but then listening to the other person say, "I respect you for that, but you can also hear my point of view. Maybe I don't have your qualifications and experience, but I do have the experience of being in the community. That disease or problem you are trying to deal with affects me. So, hey, let's work together here, because at the end of the day, I'm paying taxes, and I pay you so that you can assist me."

Solomon describes herself as very passionate about this approach. Hard evidence about the good things science is achieving makes it easier for her to get a dialogue going in the community, so she is a keen supporter of the Cochrane Centre.

Those who promoted the idea of setting up a Cochrane Centre were gratified to find that Nkosazana Zuma, who was then national minister of health, had encouraged the MRC to support the unit. She was clear on the need for the center. The MRC responded by funding almost all the center's operating costs, a most generous move.

The South African Cochrane Centre started conducting its own research into important local issues in community care, including a systematic review of strategies to promote compliance with treatment for tuberculosis (Volmink and Garner 1997; Volmink et al. 2000). The center ran workshops to train people in using systematic reviews, and these have proved highly successful, prompting a growing demand from practitioners and policy makers in local government. The center has also started collaborating with individuals and other academic centers in Africa to set up an African network for doing and using Cochrane reviews. Jimmy Volmink is in some doubt about how effective they have been in their third major effort, that of providing evidence for national health policy making.

In 1999, the South African Cochrane Centre was commissioned by the minister of health, Manto Tshabalala-Msimang, to produce a report on mother-to-child transmission of HIV, especially the effect of antiretroviral agents. The report found evidence that treatment was both effective and safe. It was submitted but ignored, and all further attempts at communication failed. Volmink, Patrice Matchaba, and Zwarenstein conclude, "It seems that scientific evidence is not yet a powerful force in government decision making in South Africa. It appears to be eclipsed by political agendas and entrenched prior views that give undue weight to unsubstantiated opinion" (2001, p. 173). Volmink and colleagues believe that action in these areas is still possible: "We have given her [Tshabalala-Msimang] the kind of information that she can act upon even if taking these actions is going to be very difficult politically." Less kind was the conclusion by Makgoba (2000) that the government was in a state of denial over the AIDS epidemic, and that this explains why it turned to pseudoscience for answers.

Given what Volmink and colleagues described as the "high-level politicization" of the topic of HIV (2001, p. 173), Volmink's most difficult assignment was serving on President Mbeki's AIDS advisory panel, where he had to engage with people whose understanding of evidence about the AIDS epidemic in South Africa seemed to overlap his own very little. As Volmink puts it, "Ooh, that was an interesting experience — just the kinds of people who were on that panel. Some of them appeared to be from Mars in terms of their understanding of what was happening." One of the topics on which the panel was asked to advise was antiretroviral therapy.

Volmink's appointment to the panel was an acknowledgment of the center's importance as well as an opportunity to talk about the importance of having solid evidence as the basis for decision making. However, after that experience in particular, he is under no illusions about the role of evidence in determining policy directions: "I think when evidence supports what policy makers have already decided they want to do, then they snap it up just like that [snaps fingers]. That's very clear; that's been the pattern. But I guess that's the same everywhere else. When the evidence is going against what they would like to do, or what they don't have resources to do, then it becomes a little more difficult. Then they bring in all sorts of other inputs that would compete with this."

Competing demands for funding can be weighed in a rational manner, but if policy makers are interested in a course of action that goes against the evidence, a common tactic is to bring in experts who make contradicting but authoritative announcements based on very little evidence, and this then justifies government inaction. At first Volmink found this response discouraging, but then he realized that a lack of response from top policy makers is a common problem in all countries: "Policymakers cannot predict or control the evidence they receive, and may have to ignore it if it goes counter to the other social and political factors that determine policy. The challenge, however, is to find a way for researchers and policymakers in South Africa to maintain dialogue over such health care issues. Appreciation on the part of researchers for the constraints under which policymakers operate would help to promote such dialogue. Policymakers, on the other hand, would assist by discussing their concerns with researchers more openly" (Volmink et al. 2001).

With patience, the Cochrane Centre could still contribute. Partly in response, the staff has now started working with local health bureaucrats, whom they are asking to identify questions important to them so that the center can conduct reviews on the topic. Another group enthusiastic about their reviews is made up of the managed care organizations, but Volmink has some doubt about how useful the evidence is for this group. He remarks,

They certainly flock to our workshops, and they've also been making some noises about commissioning reviews in the future, but we'll see what happens there. The trouble with people such as managed care organizations is that they are interested in cost cutting. Now, sometimes the evidence helps you to do that, but it doesn't always go in that direction. And I think that is something they need to learn. It's not about cost cutting; it's about doing the right thing in terms of choosing interventions that have been shown to be effective — and then ideally choosing interventions that are both effective and cost-effective.

A clear understanding that the Cochrane Centre is not allied with cost-cutting initiatives is reassuring to the clinicians who must be persuaded of the relevance to practice of evaluative sciences. The center has to set up direct contact with clinicians. Ideally, it could contribute to medical training and instill a respect for evidence at an early stage, when students are open to critical approaches. Unfortunately the medical schools have continued to resist this, and the Cochrane Centre staff does not contribute to medical training. Volmink believes that this is because the medical hierarchy fears they will undermine traditional medical authority. On one occasion when he was given access to sixth-year students at the University of Cape Town, students were enthusiastic. He was not invited back. The center did, however, contribute to postgraduate training in public health.

Health Bureaucrat: Leana Olivier

Without Leana Olivier, the Cochrane Centre might well lack its present community focus. She serves on the center's advisory board and articulates a strategic approach to the integration of Cochrane Centre functions into comprehensive primary health care services. Olivier is a nurse by training who became aware of the challenges of providing holistic care for patients. In the 1980s, she went to work in community services at a local health authority. She then transferred to the Department of Health, Western Cape Province. After the major restructuring of the department in 1994, she was appointed as provincial deputy director of the subdirectorate of maternal, child, and women's health, which includes adolescent health, school services, and human genetics. Her area of responsibility is the whole of the Western Cape Province, its four regions and twenty-five districts. She appears to be undaunted by the scope of these responsibilities.

Olivier argues that the approach of the Cochrane Collaboration was clearly useful at the level of the senior health bureaucracy, where clinical experts understood that it offered them evidence on the multitude of health problems that they face, and which present a constant challenge to their expertise. These range from epidemics of cholera, tuberculosis, and the ever present threat of AIDS, to relatively commonplace problems like an epidemic of parasitic skin infections. The more difficult task for the Cochrane Centre was to engage health care providers in the field and engage communities in the work of the center. While staffs in hospitals and urban clinics face a demanding task, those in the far-off rural areas, where care is provided only by mobile clinic vans, experience the greatest need.

The Cochrane Centre, Olivier argues, would have failed if it had merely developed guidelines and used them to tell health care workers what they should be doing in these primary care settings. "In our history in South Africa," says Olivier, "we have had *enough* of that. If you take that type of approach, you are just going to scare people off. So you *have* to tread very lightly with the message 'How can we support you to do your job better?'" Central to this approach is the validation of the expertise of people working in the field. Like Nandipha Solomon, Olivier had a clear appreciation of the need for dialogue: The way to approach providers in the community, she states, is to say, "You have got the expertise, so let's put our expertise together and *then* we are going to tackle this challenge. *We* are going to do it!"

In the health departments, they worked against a background where health care workers associated research with the statistics they had to collect and submit to a head office or district office. Olivier remarks, "There was no ownership of what they did. There was not a culture of doing research and getting involved in research. So, if you come to them and say, 'We will summarize whatever you need and give it to you in a way that will be helpful, interesting, or whatever,' they are not interested. There is still no ownership. So we must actually prepare the way, wait, and take the right opportunity to get the message across."

The people whom she saw as being ready for participation were the new district managers who needed immediate information and who could see the Cochrane Centre as a source of information for formulating policy, planning services, and responding to crises. In this task it helps to have available to them people who are respected by the community. This is where Jimmy Volmink's background is invaluable, as are Olivier's own roots in the community. George Swingler, a pediatrician working with the center, also has credibility, but he has earned it through working with the community, where, says Olivier, he is "very much respected and loved because he is a wonderful and knowledgeable person." Like Solomon, Olivier emphasizes that change must start with going out into a community and starting a dialogue: "They need to go out, and will say, 'How can we assist you to build capacity and help you to deal with health care problems? What about, for example, acute respiratory infections? And, by the way, you are saying that you've got a problem in the Western Cape with skin conditions that you don't know how to treat. Do you know that the Cochrane Centre can help with this? Dr. So-and-so or

Nurse So-and-so' (in the audience), 'How about working with us in this project?' That gets people involved, that type of phased-in approach."

Central to her vision of the function of the Cochrane Centre is the belief that topics for systematic reviews must come from the community, but that all levels of the health system have to be involved, particularly policy makers who do not have the time or expertise to generate the evidence they need for decision making. Olivier says, "Ask the people! Work according to the needs of the community, but remember that health care providers are part of the community they are serving. If you don't work according to these principles, you've had it. Because you need these people. Why are you doing systematic reviews? To ensure that better health care is provided. And who must ensure that that happens? Surely the policy makers and health managers. So, if you don't get them on board at all levels of health care, you've had it. It will just be another academic exercise."

Essentially this scheme rests on trust at all levels of the system, and this is difficult to achieve. The strength of the situation in Cape Town is that there is a devoted team of researchers, practitioners, and policy makers with a common commitment to better care. "We've all got this commitment to make things better," says Olivier. "We want to make it better. You find that kind of philosophy or vision or mission in the people now working in the services in the Department of Health and related institutions like the Medical Research Council and the Cochrane Centre. We feel we owe it to the community at large, we owe it to our families, and lastly, we owe it to ourselves to make the situation better and to use whatever we can to get there."

Administrator with Commitment: Bernadette Bredekamp

Remarkably, the commitment expressed by Leana Olivier characterizes all the people working for the Cochrane Centre. The administrator Bernadette Bredekamp sees her work at the center as one of the ways she can help with the "mammoth task" confronting the health system. During an outbreak of cholera early in 2001, it became clear to her that there was a serious lack of resources for dealing with health problems. Without clean water, people were going back to stagnant pools. When children became ill, they did not get help at hospitals where there were too few resources and insufficient staff to treat them: "It's one vicious cycle after another," she says. "Sometimes I feel just so helpless!'

Bredekamp's family is fortunate in having private medical insurance, but a recent experience of a friend brought home to her the reality that good health care was not accessible for most people:

My friend had a baby two years ago and could not afford to go to a private hospital. She went to the local day hospital. On giving birth she was kept for observation for six hours and then discharged. She was lying there, freezing cold, and she was saying that the sheets still had blood spatters on them. The framework of the bed just wasn't clean at all. She asked for a blanket, and they said, "Sorry, we don't have any. You have got to bring your own." That just made me so angry. That is just such a simple, bare necessity that you would expect from a hospital. Those are the conditions that people are faced with every single day.

As a consumer, Bredekamp places a high value on information about health, but first, she says, people want the very basics: a clean bed and a blanket. This echoes Merrick Zwarenstein's view on priorities in the health services. As a taxpayer, Bredekamp wants to know that the resources are well used. She values the workshops that she helps organize for the center, because they promote an approach that will ensure that funds are spent in an effective way. The first step is a wide understanding about the role of evidence in the health care system. The second is political action. Evidence about the lack of resources and about the best use of resources may not have an immediate effect, but "with evidence, you can at least knock on the minister's door."

In a system sadly lacking in public resources, Bredekamp recognizes the value of individual initiative. Since she is aware of the terrible consequences of a lack of information about condoms in the school system, this is one of the issues she has taken on personally. Says Bredekamp:

We need to inform the children; it is our responsibility. We are tasked with this. Where better to start than within your own family? It is essential that they know, and I constantly say to the young people in my family, "If you need to speak to someone, if you feel awkward speaking to your mum, speak to me." They need to know! They need to know about teenage pregnancies, they need to know about sexually transmitted diseases; and the only way they are going to find out is if people take the time to inform them. I know it is very little, but I am very passionate about it, and I try to help wherever I can.

With people like these, how could the center not succeed?

Conclusion

In many ways the South African Cochrane Centre in Cape Town was born into a uniquely supportive social and political environment. There was a well-established tradition of critical thinking to draw on. It was initiated at a time of political change, when there was a need to generate new visions for a better health care system. On the other hand, the political process was more intent on subverting than displaying evidence, and the medical schools were obstructive. Support came from research institutions, from individuals at a number of levels in the health system, from the local bureaucracy, and from researchers. Providing the glue for this mix is the passionate commitment to community health held by the people involved in the center and by those in supportive roles. They maintain this commitment both as a requirement of their employment and as members of the community. Here is the ideal situation for setting in place a group responsible for generating evidence that contributes to the activities of policy makers, practitioners, and consumers.

Ideally, this group fulfills many of the rather utopian visions of the researchers who preceded them. Members of this group are conducting trials into health services that would delight Archie Cochrane, and their meta-analyses would win Tom Chalmers's approval. In many ways they represent exactly the qualities that inspired Kerr White to write about the ecology of medical care. It is perhaps a sign of the times that they were unaware of Alvan Feinstein's work, but it is unlikely that they would, under pressure, conduct studies of sufficient mathematical refinement to satisfy the Feinstein program. The more pragmatic McMaster University approach, and the clear purpose of the Cochrane Collaboration, is much more amenable to their needs.

Their ideals have yet to be realized, and the challenges are considerable. In a country that lacks trained people with strong ties to the community, retaining staff is a constant problem. In 2001, Jimmy Volmink, Patrice Matchaba, and Merrick Zwarenstein coauthored the chapter "Reducing Mother-to-Child Transmission of HIV Infection in South Africa" in *Informing Judgment: Case Studies of Health Policy and Research in Six Countries*. Matchaba, a qualified obstetrician and gynecologist, saw the effects of HIV in his practice in Kwa Zulu-Natal and joined the South African Cochrane Centre in 1998. He left to become director of Novartis South Africa, a pharmaceutical company. The problem of struggling against almost overwhelming odds in the public health system is recognized as a strong incentive for emigration. Jimmy Volmink left in 2001 to become director of research and analysis at the Global Health Council in Washington, D.C. Merrick Zwarenstein left for Canada soon afterward.

In January 2002, Volmink returned to Cape Town as Glaxo-Wellcome Professor and Chair of Primary Health Care at the University of Cape

Town. His responsibilities include developing community-oriented, problem-based learning and promoting an evidence-based approach to health care.

The biggest challenge, however, remains to develop the capacity to tread a careful line through the political realities of a health system. There seems to be little point in providing evidence only to legitimize decisions taken on political grounds if evidence that contradicts these decisions is ignored.

CHAPTER 9

Achievements and Limitations

Clinical epidemiology defined the basic assumptions, and set in place the methods, for a new academic medical discipline; it then generated the idea of evidence-based medicine to describe how its research could be applied in clinical practice. Both clinical epidemiology and evidence-based medicine inculcated skepticism about therapeutic claims based on subjective clinical opinion, except when these were supported by good evidence. In the Cochrane Collaboration, international groups of researchers checked evidence from systematic reviews for errors, and evidence-based medicine evolved into an international collaborative enterprise. The effect of the Cochrane Collaboration has been "characterized as equal in importance to the human genome project" (Sackett 2002, p. 1165, quoting Naylor 1995, who wrote that it had this "potential"). The Cochrane Collaboration has been described as a gift from Britain to the world, with the potential to change health care internationally (Smith and Chalmers 2001).

This is an appropriate time to acknowledge the achievements of the field, but also to point to its limitations. In chapter 5, the criticism directed at clinical epidemiology focused on its narrow vision: it did not represent a comprehensive science of clinical care, it ignored disease in the community context, and, thus, failed to address some of the pressing concerns of clinicians. From 1995 onward, another series of criticisms appeared, and many of these were directed at evidence-based medicine, especially that promoted by the Cochrane Collaboration. These criticisms are the focus of this chapter.

Achievements

The work of the Cochrane Collaboration depends on volunteers who respond to the idea that they are involved in something worthwhile, that they are part of a social movement. The Collaboration has the political aim of collective liberation from the traditional medical system: volunteers, perhaps feeling slightly oppressed in clinical and other settings, are able to counter traditional clinical authority using the evidence that they and others have produced. Having destabilized traditional authority by pointing out the uncertainty of its conclusions, the Cochrane Collaboration has found increased certainty in the superiority of evidence produced collectively and sustained by high and transparent standards of rigor. Activities are systematized and constrained by articles of faith set out by a charismatic leadership. The annual colloquia are designed to function as a showcase for open democratic debate involving clinicians, consumers, policy makers, and anyone else interested in contributing.

Commitment to the principles of the Cochrane Collaboration has turned on its head many of the incentives of academic research. Instead of focusing on their own academic careers and the time-limited requirements of most research funding, researchers who join the Cochrane Collaboration voluntarily donate their time to work collaboratively in a task that draws no financial support except what might be provided by local funding sources. They also make a commitment to continue updating the results of their review, taking account of new trials and developments. Together these constitute a considerable commitment of time and effort.

A key factor in the way that evidence-based medicine operates has been the rise of information and communications technologies. Computer technology played a key role in the coming-of-age of evidence-based medicine, starting from the early years of clinical epidemiology, when Charles Goldsmith at McMaster University fed cards into a large computer kept in an air conditioned room. Computer programs provided a centrally important simplification of the effort required to collect data, generate analyses, and maintain databases. The result has been a rapid growth in the literature reporting trials of interventions, reviews of such trials, and electronic dissemination of this information.

The Cochrane Collaboration requires a global organizational network. Communications technologies have linked researchers in different countries into international teams working together on specified problems with the aim of synthesizing what is known. The advantage to this is that researchers from a variety of settings can contribute their skills, bringing to the task their local knowledge. This is useful in searching for unpublished material or for monitoring ongoing research so that these can be taken into account in reviews. The refereeing process is facilitated by sending documents for review electronically to any country in the world. The results of this activity are published electronically for ease of access.

A note of caution here: A burgeoning literature is a feature of every contemporary academic discipline, not just medicine. Electronic access to any number of journals is available long before they arrive in the mail, and practitioners in many fields face the problem of keeping up-to-date with research findings. But it was in medicine that the evidence-based movement arose and where it has flourished. A major source of uncertainty for clinicians has long been doubt about how well-informed they are about the literature (Fox 1979). Evidence-based medicine amplified this problem by emphasizing the need to be fully informed about that evidence specific to clinical practice. At the same time, it provided the solution: accessible summary evidence with scientific authenticity.

The ease with which this good clinical information is communicated has to count as a fine achievement. The problem is that achievement is mirrored by a difficulty: ease of access to good evidence raises the expectation that clinicians will act on the new information. At the very least, no clinician should be able to claim ignorance of the literature as justification for failing to prescribe the best available interventions. Evidence-based medicine has certainly produced changes in how health care practice is understood, but the issue is whether evidence has entered seamlessly into clinical care and transformed how it is practiced. If this has not yet happened, can we look forward to it in the future? It is in addressing these problems of implementation that evidence-based medicine faces its biggest challenge.

The Problem of Implementation

While evidence-based medicine does not constitute a comprehensive science of clinical care (see chapter 5), it has been an important initiative in providing additional scientific evidence for clinical decision making. But what is the real extent of its achievements? Perhaps the claims made on behalf of evidence-based medicine have been a trifle extravagant and have set too high a standard for success. A revolutionary paradigm shift has not occurred, but it would be gratifying at least to see good evidence that clinicians readily incorporate evidence from evidence-based medicine into their decision making, and that this has resulted in health benefits for patients.

Unfortunately it seems that clinicians have not responded as expected. Despite a number of implementation strategies that have been subjected to assessment in randomized controlled trials, clinicians appear resistant to change, and clinical practice does not seem to have changed to a marked degree (Haines and Donald 2002). It is tempting to see still further proliferation of computer technology as the solution. Internationally there are certainly many clinicians without adequate access to these technologies, but the answer is likely to be more complex.

The problem of moving from evidence to practice is not new. This problem has dogged the movement from its early stages, attracting the interest of the Milbank Memorial Fund after the publication of *Effective Care in Pregnancy and Childbirth* (Chalmers et al. 1989). The fund was concerned to ensure that research on the effectiveness of medical procedures influenced clinicians, policy makers, and consumers (Cleary and Fox 1993). In 1993, a special issue of the *Milbank Quarterly* was devoted to this issue. Here Jonathan Lomas set out a program for ensuring the dissemination of good evidence. It remains relevant.

Lomas, at this time, was still at McMaster University. The number of clinical trials was growing, but these were having little effect on clinical practice. McMaster University itself was doing some of the research, with Brian Haines showing that peer-reviewed publications had only a loose connection to what happened in clinical practice (Haynes 1990). A paper in the special edition of the *Milbank Quarterly* by Lomas, J. E. Sisk, and B. Stocking (1993) argued that practitioners still used textbooks as their primary source of information, despite the evidence in the textbook *Clinical Epidemiology: A Basic Science for Clinical Medicine* (Sackett et al. 1991) that much of this information was outdated or wrong. Concerns about cost containment and quality assurance had triggered interest in changing physician behavior, and there was interest in summarizing this evidence in practice guidelines, but these were not effective in bringing about change.

Lomas (1993b) proposed a program for change based on the assumption that there was a need for a cultural bridge between researchers and practitioners. There were three models for bridging this gap. Researchers traditionally communicated with practitioners by means of passive diffusion, an uncoordinated process in which information was assumed to flow from researcher to practitioner through the literature by a process resembling osmosis. This model respects the autonomy of the professional practitioner. The problem was that information did not readily diffuse to practitioners, a proportion of whom did not read research studies, preferred summaries, and practiced in a way that deviated from the directions implied by research.

The second model differs from passive diffusion by accentuating active dissemination, with an emphasis on good quality evidence in a synthesized and accessible form. *Effective Care in Pregnancy and Childbirth* (Chalmers et al. 1989) provided one such example, with skilled intermediaries able to relay research information to practitioners. Active dissemination would rest on intervention in the information marketplace by "retailers": "organizations and *ad hoc* groups that are ideally credible to both producers and consumers and are able to accurately synthesize and disseminate the research information, and its implications for clinical practice" (Lomas 1993b, p. 442).

The third model of dissemination takes a direction beyond the relaying of information, in however accessible a form, through coordinated implementation. It involves careful assessment of what drives the potential consumers' behavior. A variety of groups would employ a variety of ways to persuade clinicians of the need for change. The groups involved could be patients, administrators, policy makers, and professional organizations. In the further development of this model, Lomas saw the answer to the problem of putting research into practice.

Lomas's analogy of retailing an academic product to its practitioner-consumers allows us to examine where evidence-based medicine has succeeded and where new gains may still be made. I deal with each of the models in turn.

Passive Diffusion

Three assumptions underpin the passive diffusion model: "that practitioners actively seek out research information, that they can select and appraise the information appropriately, and that they make research-driven probabilistic patient care decisions" (Lomas 1993b, p. 440). These assumptions fit well with the aims of *Clinical Epidemiology: A Basic Science for Clinical Medicine*: "Just as your ability to achieve accurate diagnosis and efficacious therapy determines your clinical effectiveness today, it is your skills in self-assessment and in tracking down and assessing biomedical knowledge (most of which resides in the journals) that will more and more determine your clinical effectiveness tomorrow" (Sackett et al. 1985, p. 246). Clinicians were seen as suffering from a knowledge deficit, and the McMaster University textbook produced a well-polished product for addressing the deficit, training the scientific practitioner to gather information from the literature and apply it in practice. The assumption was that, rationally, changes in practice would follow.

In these early years, clinical epidemiology faced a real problem with establishing its share of the medical marketplace (to continue with Lomas's retailing analogy), and there were constraints on the strategies it could employ. It was marketing a new product, and the problems involved in gaining a market share were considerable. Before it could even enter the market, it had to persuade medical wholesalers that the product was worthwhile. This was a difficult task. The assumption of the scientific paradigm is that objective science effects change, progress is inevitable, and researchers only have to publish new evidence for it to replace the old. Indeed, consideration of the social context within which dissemination occurs might well be seen as introducing a bias into a scientific study. Clinical epidemiology gained entry to the market by asserting the objective scientific basis of its activities.

Active Diffusion

Once admitted as a medical discipline, clinical epidemiology turned to active dissemination, using enhanced marketing strategies to sell its product to practitioner-consumers through persuasive, charismatic, inspirational salespeople. When practice did not change and criticism mounted, the shift was not to a different product (which is what critics like Feinstein were recommending). Indeed, changing the product would have jeopardized the tenuous hold that clinical epidemiology had in the medical marketplace. Instead, the clinical epidemiologists polished their product more highly and marketed it under an attractive new label, evidence-based medicine. Evidence-based medicine was explicitly promoted in workshops and in an extensive literature as the best response to everyday problems encountered in clinical care: insufficient time, limited search skills, and limited access to burgeoning evidence.

When some of the practitioner-consumers of evidence-based medicine found the product inaccessible, the product itself did not change, but there were changes in design to better suit the needs of clinical consumers.

While the passive diffusion model left practitioners to sort the wheat from the chaff, in the active dissemination model the evidence is presorted, formatted and highlighted, and promoted by credible intermediaries. The problem of accessibility was resolved by producing prepackaged, condensed versions of the product. The textbooks made a determined effort to improve presentation. *Evidence-Based Medicine: How to Practice and Teach EBM* (Sackett et al. 1997) was revised; the second edition included a CD-ROM carrying clinical examples, and there was a Website to update the evidence. *Users' Guides to the Medical Literature: A Manual for Evidence-Based Clinical Practice* (Guyatt and Rennie 2002) also has a problem-based CD-ROM, and the rather hefty book comes accompanied by a condensed pocket version.

These initiatives in undertaking active dissemination should not be a cause for criticism, although some critics responded negatively to the "proselytizing zeal of EBM proponents" (Charlton and Miles 1998, p. 373). An editorial in the *Lancet* (1995, p. 785) sums the problem up as follows: "The voice of evidence-based medicine has grown over the past 25 years from a subversive whisper to a strident insistence that it is improper to practice medicine of any other kind. Revolutionaries notoriously exaggerate their claims; nonetheless, demands to have evidence-based medicine hallowed as the new orthodoxy have sometimes lacked finesse and balance, and risked antagonising doctors who would otherwise have taken many of its principles to heart." The problem then is the perception of exaggeration and evangelism, rather than the narrow focus on one grand product and delivery of that product in shimmering style. The problems intensify when the expected revolutionary changes to clinical practice do not eventuate. Perhaps then a different product? The problem is that the product is relatively inflexible, being designed around scientific principles that define the limits of adaptation. If diversification is difficult, this puts the emphasis on polishing the product further and improving marketing strategies to compensate for an apparent lack of appeal.

The Cochrane Collaboration introduced an additional strategy. It trained volunteers in the process of systematic review by defining processes for conducting a review, and putting these into practice in review groups. The Collaboration thus developed an additional market response by involving its consumers (both medical consumers and patient organizations) in the actual generation of its product. In retailing terms this may be the equivalent of a franchising operation, engendering fierce loyalty in owner-operators, who are also the ultimate consumers of the product. The Cochrane Collaboration's approach to involving patient-consumers finds an echo in the initiative by Brian Haynes to develop patient information systems in consulting rooms.

In parallel with these efforts, a range of organizations had a role in retailing the evidence in the form of guidelines. Clinical guidelines are formal statements about specific aspects of clinical practice with the aim of assisting those who make decisions about what is appropriate health care. Ideally a panel of specialists in a field assesses the rational implications of evidence for practice in a country or region, with allowances made for local circumstances. While capturing the evidence from systematic reviews, guidelines take a broader focus on the overall management of a condition (Grimshaw and Eccles 2001).

McMaster University and the Cochrane Collaboration have provided evidence of the effectiveness of interventions, and this presents a starting point for consensus development in the process of generating guidelines. Neither group has focused on direct dissemination of evidence through guidelines; indeed, the Collaboration actively distances itself from this activity. The more usual process is for intermediaries like health professional or administrative organizations to take on the task. The guideline movement has grown in parallel with evidence-based medicine and could reasonably be expected to reinforce a respect for evidence-based decision-making.

There are, however, a number of problems. Guidelines may not filter through to clinical practice any more effectively than does the raw evidence or its synthesized form. This is complicated by the problem that guidelines can be produced by a variety of organizations; the results can be contradictory, causing confusion or even controversy (Stuart et al. 2002). The development of guidelines is still another step in the process of research synthesis, and there are not yet sufficiently rigorous methods for generating guidelines, especially when the evidence is sparse and expert opinion has to be taken into account. Guidelines are expected to be contextual, so it is not surprising that they often failed to describe formal processes for combining evidence and expert opinion (Shaneyfelt et al. 1999). Thus the generation of practice guidelines is still beset by trials and tribulations, but the imprimatur of a professional organization makes them more acceptable (Cook and Giacomini 1999). In 1993, Lomas had concluded that evidence provided in this accessible format was a necessary, but not a sufficient, condition for change. Stephen Harrison added a later note of caution: From the perspective of health policy analysis, it is "extraordinarily naïve" to think that any set of bureaucratic rules would be self-implementing (1998, p. 22).

The production of guidelines has not been without risk for the organizations involved. Conceptually, guidelines are a strategy to enhance the quality of health services, and this generates an overlap with health services research. Jerry Morris notes that "as soon as you get into health services, you get into politics," and this has certainly been true in the United States, where the generation of guidelines was undertaken by the Agency for Health Care Policy and Research, established in 1989 as the successor to the National Center for Health Services Research. The agency struggled under budgetary constraints, and one of the problems faced by the agency in defending its budget was its clinical guidelines program. The guidelines were seen as "weak and not user-friendly" and unlikely to change clinical practice, but they had also made "committed enemies" of the medical specialists whose practices were under question (Gray et al. 2003, pp. 295–97).

If guidelines are a dubious form of retailing evidence, how else might evidence be retailed? One long-term, direct strategy has been to familiarize students with the advantages of evidence-based practice at an early stage of their training, but this requires that those not trained in this way be converted. The International Clinical Epidemiology Network disseminated clinical epidemiology to selected faculty members from less developed countries with the aim of having them disseminate the message further upon returning home. An important educational component of change has been the intensive workshops conducted by McMaster University team, attended by an international audience, which provided intensive, hands-on introduction to the intricacies of the method, taught by senior members of the team in their inimitable style. This is peer education in its most polished form.

A more gradual approach is that of Carol Joughin with the FOCUS project at the Royal College of Psychiatrists' Research Unit in the United Kingdom. She argues that change requires a slow process of engaging the profession in the actual generation of knowledge synthesis. Given the complexities of decision making in mental health, and the absence of good trial evidence for conditions that are troublesome in practice — conditions like attention deficit hyperactivity disorder — this change must occur before guidelines are even attempted. Joughin's project prepares clinicians to make evidence-based decisions by developing their skills in finding evidence and then focusing on an evidence-generating project concerning a topic of keen interest to them in their clinical practices. Thus any professional organization must take account of the knowledge base of its discipline, and skilled interpreters of the evidence may then be needed to familiarize clinician-consumers with the function and benefits of evidence.

What has been described so far are the first two models of dissemination: passive and active, which, Lomas argues, are based on the assumption that knowledge changes behavior (and, indeed, we know this happens in cases where a new form of knowledge provides a breakthrough treatment for a previously intractable problem). It could be argued that the intensity of the activities described above are more properly classified under the third model, which goes beyond mere provision of information, in however accessible a form, to employ dissemination through coordinated implementation.

Coordinated Implementation

In clinical practice, new knowledge is usually accommodated amid other competing influences on practitioner behavior — and many of these influences are social, political, and economic. Successful implementation therefore involves careful assessment of what drives the potential practitioner-consumers' behavior. The third model uses multiple routes of influence in the practitioner's environment to bring to bear a variety of influences on decision making. Potential candidates include groups with specific tools of persuasion, including patients and patient organizations (through public pressure), health administrators (through regulation), public policy makers or private insurers (through economic incentives), and clinical policy makers in professional institutions and in peer groups (through education and peer approval). In this way clinical accountability rides in tandem with economic accountability.

McMaster University has concentrated on a refined model of peer education, although many of the people attending their courses are health policy makers or come from health insurance agencies. Gordon Guyatt has turned to the media for further public dissemination of the policy implications of evidence. The Cochrane Collaboration has turned to a range of additional avenues for bringing about change. Evidence can be disseminated more effectively if it finds consumers at a variety of levels of the health system, perhaps particularly at the level of the health bureaucracy that has influence over funding. The example of the South African Cochrane Centre demonstrates this multilevel activity and shows that support for its activities rested on a long process of change. Ideas diffuse gradually, promoting a climate for change. When political change came in South Africa, support for the Cochrane Centre was, in some ways, opposed to the interests of policy makers at the ministerial level. Support came in a diffuse form from different levels of government, ranging from the higher echelons (where support needs to be strong) to grassroots community workers (where the products may need to be promoted by a person with local credibility). Without such support, the center could not have been established and could not function. Ideally, in a sustained process of change, people in various roles become committed consumers or retailers of the product they helped produce.

Based on this analysis, the more recent manifestations of evidence-based medicine appear to constitute tentative steps toward dissemination of evidence through coordinated activity. Enhanced marketing of evidence by health administrators, policy makers, and consumers depends on how these groups see their role in the dissemination process. The issue, finally, is whether these additional activities benefit those who ultimately make clinical decisions: the clinicians.

Relationship with Policy Makers

Drawing on the analysis of Archie Cochrane, D. W. Light (1991) argues that the first step in setting up an efficient health service is to establish which services are worth providing and which should be discontinued, given the health needs of a population. The next step is to provide only those services that most effectively deal with the health problems. Here Light applies what he calls the Cochrane test for a well-functioning health system:

1. Consider anything that works.
2. Make effective treatments available to all.
3. Minimize ill-timed interventions.
4. Treat patients in the most cost-effective place.
5. Prevent only what is preventable.
6. Diagnose only if treatable.

In 1991, Light saw the National Health Service in the United Kingdom as scoring well only on item 2 (making treatment available) and 6 (diagnosing only treatable disorders). There was clearly a long way to go. Evidence-based medicine was well placed to provide the evidence base that would be needed to implement this vision for a more effective health service.

Both Light and Cochrane before him saw the problem of overuse and inefficiency in health services as originating in the practices of doctors who persist in using "costly, ill timed, or ineffective practices" (Light 1991, p. 1253). While there may, as Howard Waitzkin argues (see chapter 5), be more fundamental systemic reasons for inefficient practice, it seems reasonable to hold doctors accountable by means of outcomes research, protocols, and medical audit. Certainly this should be easier to achieve in a centrally administered health system. Unfortunately there is little indication that evidence, however carefully collected and synthesized, will ever be the determining influence on practice. In the view of Iain Chalmers, "vested interests" stand in the way of both changes in practice and the generation of evidence-based policy (1991, p. 137). Prominent among these are the interests of clinicians that are potentially in conflict with the interests of health administrators.

The Cochrane Collaboration does not see a relationship with health administrators and policy makers as a cause for concern. It does not take a prescriptive stance: if the government and its health bureaucrats are using the same evidence as clinicians and consumers, then the issue for the producers of evidence is not how evidence is used but only that it be scientifically irreproachable. Their commitment is to provide the same information to any group interested in evidence, be they clinicians, consumers, or policy makers. How this evidence is then interpreted has to depend on local contexts, including the resources available for health care and the priorities for policy.

Given the financial commitment that made the original Cochrane Centre possible, and given the financial support of national Cochrane centers by some governments, the expectation was that policy makers would indeed make use of the information generated. The Cochrane Collaboration monitors the extent to which systematic reviews are put to use in national clinical practice guidelines (Holmes et al. 2001). Chris Silagy and colleagues (2001) argue that the use of systematic reviews in guidelines was a measure of "payback" for funding committed to research synthesis, and they show that national smoking cessation guidelines commonly drew on Cochrane reviews, but that this was most extensive in the United Kingdom.

In practice, the relationship with policy makers has been a complex one. In the view of Iain Chalmers, the Cochrane Collaboration has been willing to respond to policy concerns, but policy makers have been unwilling to nominate their priorities in terms of the questions that the policy makers would like to see addressed. One possibility here is that the Cochrane Collaboration is seen as being integrally connected with clinical care, and governments are wary of intervening in clinical practice as this can meet with as much resistance as success. An alternative is for the state to generate its own evidence and guidelines.

In the United Kingdom, the National Institute for Clinical Excellence is a government body established, in 1999, to produce guidance for the National Health Service on treatment and care, including technology appraisals, clinical guidelines, and the assessment of interventional procedures for safety and effectiveness. With a government center taking over policy-directed evaluation, effectively this means that the Cochrane Collaboration receives financial support free of overt political commitments. This has decided advantages in an organization where researchers are encouraged to nominate (with suitable justification) their own issues for analysis, and where there is an expectation that the nature of the evidence produced will be independent of the policy processes operating in specific countries.

If health administrators in the United Kingdom have not consumed evidence to the extent that might have been expected, why has there been state support for evidence-based medicine? Rudolf Klein (1983) analyzed the politics of the British National Health Service. Klein and colleagues argue that the National Health Service in the 1960s to mid-1970 was dominated by an ideology of efficiency: "the idea that policy should be directed towards squeezing the greatest possible output of health care — that elusive concept — out of an inevitably limited input of resources" (1996, p. 64). Members of the medical profession saw the answer in increased funding and were locked into a political struggle with successive governments reluctant to target new financial sources. Policy makers feared an ever increasing health budget, particularly troublesome in a time of financial constraint. Finally, the political system was moving to a format favoring small government and participatory democracy. Rationing was the answer, and what was needed was a formula for a fair division of resources. Evidence-based medicine provided a rational means of meeting new demands not by increasing funding but by diverting resources from less effective interventions to those promising a better "health gain" (Klein et al. 1996, p. 53). Purchases of health services on the grounds of effectiveness were finally formally incorporated into managerial decision making in 1993 (Harrison 1998). Was it a problem that there was little evidence for the effectiveness of much of routine clinical care?

Not if the use of evidence was largely ideological. In fact, argues Klein and colleagues, the lack of evidence was part of the attraction: "For if demonstrable effectiveness, based on scientific evidence, is to be the only criterion for purchasing, if the onus of proof is to be on doctors to show that their interventions improve outcomes, then most of the existing services provided by the NHS would fail the test and could be scrapped. No wonder ministers and managers embraced the new faith with enthusiasm. For it appeared to offer them the prospect of less pain, less responsibility for taking difficult decisions and a legitimate way of curbing what were often perceived to be the idiosyncratic and extravagant practices of doctors" (1996, p. 104).

This was not quite what Cochrane had in mind in terms of the diversion of funds to the caring function of medicine. Controversy surrounding the National Institute for Clinical Excellence (NICE) gives some indication of the depth of feeling surrounding the issue of the relationship between evidence and rationing. Julian Tudor Hart sees NICE as being involved in "a disgraceful retreat" and warns, "We all use the term rationing when what we really mean is that the scope of the NHS should be reduced" (2001, p. 490). An editorial in the *British Medical Journal* describes NICE as "an instrument for rationing" that "corrupts the concept of evidence-based medicine" (Smith 2000, pp. 1363–64), and Lipman sees the health bureaucracy claiming "extra legitimacy by invoking the mantra of evidence-based medicine" (2001, p. 489). A review of NICE recommended that the institute adopt more rigorous processes, and it noted "concerns that NICE has become the scapegoat for controversial rationing decisions" (Burke 2002, p. 2120). The government was "hiding behind the 'figleaf' of NICE" (Gulland 2002, p. 406), but there was a real risk that NICE guidelines would lead to increases in expenditures without matching increase in health improvements and increased inequities in the availability of services (Gafni and Birch 2003).

In the United States, the Agency for Health Care Policy and Research in the U.S. Department of Health and Human Services has to operate in the context of a complex system of public and private organizations that offer health services, pay for these services, or administer them. It too came under pressure. The appeal of health services research had been that it would generate systematic evidence for policy making. Of particular concern were issues of quality and cost raised by evidence of practice variations and inappropriate use of procedures (Gray 1992), but there were more important issues at play. According to Bradford Gray, the legislation that established the agency signaled the trend toward managed care, with decisions moving "from judgment to standards, from expert to science, from the individual physician to objective criteria agreed upon by expert panels" (1992, p. 64). Clinical guidelines were central to this program. Reducing ineffective practice would help to reduce those health care costs that were troublesome for "administrators of private health plans or sickness funds and of public insurance programs, employers, insurers, and patients" (Lohr et al. 1998, p. 14).

Gray and coauthors (2003) outlined the problems faced by the Agency for Health Care Policy and Research. The word *policy* in the title had unfortunate repercussions. In 1994, with both the House of Representatives and the Senate under control of the Republicans, it was taken to imply a partisan link to the health care reform plans of President Clinton that had been defeated in 1993–1994. The expectation of Congress had been that the agency would both change clinical practice and save costs. This had not been realized, and the agency stood accused of wastefulness, with the guidelines program seen as "unwarranted interference with the practice of medicine."

It is clear that the path from evidence to policy is not linear, and that evidence may have no more effect on policy than it does on clinical practice. We must approach the idea of "evidence-based policy" with caution, warns Nick Black (2001). Policy makers have to deal with the full complexity of any problem, accommodating social, economic, strategic, and a variety of other influences. Researchers traditionally rely on emphasizing the strength of their evidence — as in the passive diffusion model. But evidence-based policy can become a reality only if there is improved communication between researchers and policy makers to generate a more complex model in which researchers get a better understanding of the policy process, and if policy makers are more involved in planning and conducting research.

When the Agency for Health Care Policy and Research was recast as the Agency for Healthcare Research and Quality in 1999, the changes instituted took account of this more complex approach to the generation of evidence-based policy. As outlined by Gray and colleagues (2003), the reference to policy in the title was dropped to distance the agency from the health policies of particular governments. The new agency was seen as serving three consumers. The first were "people making clinical decisions," and these included patients, families, and clinicians. Then there were the purchasers and providers making managerial decisions. Finally there were those making policy decisions at all levels of government. Instead of engaging directly in guideline development, the agency provided funding for a series of twelve external evidence-based practice centers to conduct systematic reviews of the evidence on topics nominated for their relevance to factors like disease prevalence, significance to health programs, and cost, as well as the availability of scientific data. This evidence could be used directly by health plans and payers, and by public and private organizations to develop practice guidelines.

Arguably, the agency, which derived from the broad interests of health services research, now functions as a considerable sponsor for evidence-based medicine, drawing on the skills of evidence-based medicine practitioners across Canada and the United States, including many of McMaster University's evidence-based-medicine researchers. The National Guidelines Clearinghouse, an Internet-based resource sponsored by the agency, provides ready access worldwide to detailed information on practice guidelines. In this structure, evidence is strategically located in a collaborative approach involving the agency with organizations that take responsibility for health care decision making in its various forms, including the American Medical Association and the American Association of Health Plans.

Lomas's third model requires that clinicians be persuaded of the need for change by groups including administrators, policy makers, and professional organizations. Irrespective of the health system, this path to reform seems to be a thorny one, and so the alternative of turning to patients and patient organizations for help becomes more attractive. Patients are increasingly recognized as being involved in the decisions regarding their care, but the interests of patients have also been at the center of many political struggles over health care. As Ann Daniel notes, "In politically contested arenas, patients are rather like icons held high above the battles over who decides, who controls and who gets what" (1995, p. 58). Instead of merely invoking the interests of patients, the Cochrane Collaboration has taken the additional step of actively involving consumers in its organization.

The Role of Consumers

The authors of *Effective Care in Pregnancy and Childbirth* were sympathetic to the interests of patients and interested in working with consumer groups. Murray Enkin had had a long commitment to working with women as patients and consumers in his obstetric practice. In the perinatal arena, Iain Chalmers had found it essential to work cooperatively with consumers who had concerns about how women were being treated during pregnancy and childbirth. Women's health lobby groups had been a powerful force in drawing attention to inadequacies in the maternity services. The advisory committee of the National Perinatal Epidemiology Unit, under the directorship of Chalmers, included representatives of women using maternity services. He also worked closely with Ann Oakley, a sociologist who had conducted qualitative studies of women's experience of childbirth (Oakley 1980). His aim was to focus on questions that women saw as significant, rather than have issues of concern defined by drug companies, equipment manufacturers, or the medical profession itself.

From this we could argue that, if there is a bias in consumer views, the experience of the childbirth arena suggests that it would be in the direction of questioning medical authority, a central tenet of the evidence-based-medicine movement. The commitment to involving consumers in the Cochrane Collaboration led to two out of twelve positions on the Cochrane Collaboration Steering Group being reserved for consumer representatives. There is a Consumer Network, which provides training and runs a Website. Consumers are given financial support for attending meetings.

These initiatives owe much to the representations of Hilda Bastian, who was appointed to the first steering group as a consumer representative. Bastian has been called "Australia's consumer champion," and her way of life includes delivering uncomfortable messages to health professionals (Richards 1999). She earned a reputation as a remarkable consumer advocate when she turned a critical eye on consumer health activities that she had helped to establish. As coordinator of Homebirth Australia, she had initiated a study to document the safety of home births. The results showed that the mortality rate was higher than among hospital births (Bastian et al. 1998).

Bastian is the author of *The Power of Sharing Knowledge: Consumer Participation in the Cochrane Collaboration* (1994), which sets out the arguments for involving consumers in the Cochrane Collaboration. In her view, a shift to consideration of people's needs and a new relationship with consumers "may well be as radical and far-reaching as the shift to more evidence-based decision making in health care." Professionals are seen as having "a variety of interests which may or may not be consistent with public interests." This constitutes a bias that can only be redressed through public participation, including "the direct involvement of people's voices and influence." Importantly, consumer representatives must be "a bridge to the community" rather than a road to power or prestige. She sees "the best community proxies realistically possible" as being consumer advocates from consumer and community groups. She rejects social scientists from the role of presenting evidence of consumer views on the basis of their research: "The appropriateness of researchers speaking outside the confines of their research on behalf of the people they study is highly questionable, unless the community has designated them as their advocates."[1] She presents no argument for or substantiation of these views.

In specified topic areas, reviews prepared for the Cochrane Collaboration are required to have consumer input. In addition to its professional reviewing processes, the Cochrane Pregnancy and Childbirth Group has a consumer panel that also assesses all draft protocols for reviews, as well the completed reviews. Before a review is submitted to the *Cochrane Database of Systematic Reviews,* both professional and consumer feedback is addressed. The involvement of consumers in this way has strengthened collaboration within the Pregnancy and Childbirth Group. Carol Sakala and colleagues (2001) describe the processes of involvement. While there has been no evaluation of effect, they argue that consumer participation has strengthened the quality, relevance, and influence of their reviews and helped "to reduce bias through broader input that contributes to 'checks and balances'" (2001, p. 137).

Bastian's outline emphasizes familiar canons of community participation set out in Arnstein 1969 and tested in Willis 1995. It is possible that the rather demanding conditions set out are met within committees, and that consumers have added to the democratic nature of debate within the Cochrane Collaboration. On the other hand, there is little consideration of the potential for consumers to introduce their own form of bias. To return to the Lomas model, retailers have a role in selecting only those products for which there is a demand in their specific communities. In open democratic debate with other groups holding different views, in which no one group dominates another, these biases can be resolved. It is far from clear that these stringent conditions are being met in the Cochrane Collaboration. The exclusion of social scientists in their role of representing the views of their research participants represents one contradiction.

It is worth noting here that the emphasis is on the inclusion of consumers, rather than patients, in decision making, an emphasis not unique to the Cochrane Collaboration. Consumers represent groups of patients, and this eases the task of consulting with large numbers of individual patients in order to find out what they want from their health care providers. While this is an eminently practical approach to consultation, it is difficult to assess the ability of consumer organizations, or representatives from those organizations, to represent the range of patient views.

There is an extensive literature that analyzes the issue of the role of consumer groups representing claims on behalf of patients in health institutions. In 1976 Klein and Lewis analyzed community health councils in the National Health Service and concluded that they were a political necessity: "No Government, whether Labour or Conservative, could get rid of them without appearing to be cocking a snook at democracy, participation and consumerism — vague but vogue terms all in the rhetoric of political argument and powerfully resonant" (1976, p. 151). If political processes required consumer representation, it is also true that health activists have been influential in setting in place health policies based on good evidence. In the cases of birthing and breastfeeding, they have helped revolutionize how women give birth and care for their babies. The picture is more complicated in the case of breast cancer, where activists have been described as presenting views biased toward articulate middle-class women (Anglin 1997). Breast cancer advocacy groups are well-organized, and breast cancer carries emotive overtones. The uncertainties surrounding evidence of the effectiveness of breast cancer screening are based on studies that are difficult to understand from a lay perspective but that are well reported (see Gøzsche and Olsen 2000). This evidence is particularly controversial in light of persistent support for the program from health departments (Holland 2001–2002). In Australia, argues Karen Willis (2001), policy makers committed themselves to a national mammography screening program, but this decision owed little to research evidence and more to the heartfelt wish of activists (some of them by then in policy making positions) to "do something for women's health."

If we turn to the social science literature analyzing health consumerism, some wider implications emerge. The shift from "patient" to "consumer" has been seen as an aspect of neoliberal politics in health care, one in which consumer choice is elevated to a right that has to be defended in a new global society (Frank 2002). This is achieved through active citizenship, with consumers exercising the capacity for independent decision making based on information:

However, behind the rhetoric of "freedom of choice," "right to know," and "entitlement to participate" that has recently come to dominate discussions in health care, lie compulsions surrounding the exercise of choice and an array of predefined and limited options for action. The "good consumer" of health care is compelled to make choices, to exhibit appropriate "information seeking" behaviour, and to behave in certain prescribed ways (consulting "relevant" expertise, taking the "right" medicine, engaging in personal risk management, and so on). . . . However, one can question the extent to which this ideal of rational consumer behaviour accords with the reality of people's everyday lives. (Henderson and Petersen 2002, p. 3)

This cultural vision of the consumer is intimately linked to issues of power. Rob Irvine argues, "The idea of the consumer is used to subvert and modify relationships of power and authority in health care politics" (2002, p. 32). Irvine locates the rise in the idea of consumerism in the 1960s and 1970s, a time of declining social trust in both the professions and the state: "The consumer metaphor was mobilized as a central organizing principle and figure of speech by a range of more or less organized patient advocacy and user groups which sought greater social equality and democratic control of health care institutions" (2002, p. 33). One target was the power exercised by the medical profession, whose decision making processes were now to be mediated by the well-informed, self-actualizing consumer.

According to this analysis, consumer discourse was appropriated and reinterpreted by health administrators, who were introducing market mechanisms into health care, and, by the early 1990s, consumers were heavily featured in state health policies. Irvine argues that the rhetoric of consumer rights has provided a useful tool for government bent on managerial change in health care: "The language of the health consumer is a vehicle which transports unpopular managerial reforms into health care institutions" (2002, p. 38). In this schema, state institutions that endorse consumer representations are motivated by more than just gaining benefits for patients, and the implementation of evidence-based practice is not necessarily a central consideration.

If this analysis is correct, then the format of the Cochrane Collaboration's consumer representation articulates with the approach of the health bureaucracies that fund its centers. The inclusion of consumers is seen as one aspect of the democratic procedures in the Collaboration. Paradoxically, the inclusion of consumers could actually increase disaffection between the purveyors of evidence-based medicine and clinicians.

The Concerns of Clinicians

Conflict is inherent in the use of evidence-based medicine to diffuse responsibility for rationing. On the other hand, others see this use of evidence as a bulwark against control when the evidence lies in the hands of the profession. When decision making is assessed according to evidence produced by the medical profession, this can free the profession from state regulation: clinicians can point to the scientific basis of rational clinical decision making, and this serves to legitimate their autonomy in the face of criticism from policy makers, patients, and consumers, and even managed care. The problem, argues Stephen Harrison, is that this use of evidence is associated with a shift of power away from clinicians to academics, epidemiologists, and health services researchers (1998, p. 21).

David Armstrong (2002) supports this analysis. Evidence-based medicine, he believes, is the province of an administrative elite who are indeed using it for the purpose of sustaining the independence of the profession, but this has been achieved by undermining individual practitioners, making them subject to external control by this elite. Says Armstrong, "So instead of clinical autonomy being claimed by the professional collective and exercised by the undifferentiated practitioner, the new model involved the 'freedom' of the profession being justified politically by an elite and effected through intra-professional controls over the content of everyday clinical practice" (2002, p. 1772). If the profession is to have an unequivocal commitment to evidence-based care, this can be achieved only by denying the clinical discretion exercised by individual clinicians.

From the perspective of evidence-based medicine, there is a rational solution to the problem: individual clinicians should discard outmoded subjective clinical authority and incorporate evidence-based decision making into clinical practice. Until that time, from their perspective, the shift in power is defensible. The problem is that pressure on clinicians invoking the specter of state intervention and rationing appears to call into existence strong resistance from clinicians.

If we take account of the analyses of Harrison (1998) and Armstrong (2002), evidence-based medicine could result in the individual clinician being caught in an ever tighter web of regulation. In this scenario, evidence-based medicine is not valued for the information it delivers as much as for its rhetorical value in defending incursions into elite professional territory. This is the crucial issue raised in many of the vehement criticisms of evidence-based medicine to be found in almost every clinical field. There has been particular emphasis on the perception that a close relationship exists between evidence-based medicine and the state. B. G. Charlton and A. Miles call for the evaluation of evidence-based medicine, although "the EBM barnacle may prove difficult to dislodge now it has a grip on the minds of politicians and managers" (1998, p. 371). Black supports Klein (1996) by identifying the danger that "a vulgarized form of the new scientism will be taken up by payers, purchasers and managers, which will result in eventual disillusionment" (1999, p. 792). The problem, however, goes deeper.

The Cochrane Collaboration is built around the systematic review, preferably the review of randomized controlled trials rather than single trials. This aim is still controversial. There remains uncertainty about the methods used in meta-analysis, and an ongoing debate about whether meta-analyses provide a more trustworthy answer than further large trials, particularly in those cases where the results of a meta-analysis and a large trial are contradictory. Feinstein has no doubt about where the problem lies. He terms meta-analysis "statistical alchemy for the 21st century" (1995).

Clinicians had difficulty reconciling the results of randomized trials with the treatment decisions for individual patients. Systematic reviews have not addressed the central problem, described by Robert Fletcher as follows:

> Good clinicians think of their patients as individuals, each a unique combination of genetic endowment, social and physical environment, past experiences, and current preferences. In contrast, randomized controlled trials are about average results in groups of patients. It is a bad match.
>
> There is no perfect solution to this dilemma. (2002, p. 1188)

Together these problems have inspired provocative articles that portray evidence-based medicine as claiming more than it can achieve. Charlton, for example, echoes Feinstein by arguing that the problem of applying epidemiological data to individual patients is intractable: "And no amount of jiggery-pokery with huge data sets can make any difference" (1997). The focus on evidence is accused of denigrating clinical skills (Benech et al. 1996), but few clinicians were engaging in the debate. While evidence was undeniably an important component of clinical decision making, personal relationships with patients could be put at risk in practices restricted by guidelines based on population studies, leading to the "death of the personal doctor" (McCormick 1996).

One way of addressing these concerns would be to further integrate research with clinical practice so that the application of evidence can be properly tested in clinical settings. But clinical settings are difficult to isolate from the social and political context of life in the community. The achievements of evidence-based medicine owe much to claims that trial designs strip away context and produce objective scientific evidence of the effectiveness of interventions. The inclusion of the influence of context on clinical decision making introduces "soft" research procedures that could call into question the objectivity of research.

Such strong responses are likely to reflect more than simple ignorance of the benefits of evidence-based medicine. Armstrong (2002) presents an analysis that casts light on the problem. He reports a qualitative study involving semistructured interviews with eighty general practitioners in four South Thames health authorities in the United Kingdom. At issue was how they managed depressed patients and how they incorporated new drugs into clinical practice. Selective serotonin reuptake inhibitors were introduced as an alternative to older tricyclic drugs that were cheaper and no less effective, but were less toxic when taken as an overdose. Armstrong shows that the new drugs were gradually integrated into a repertoire of care, with doctors conducting small personal experiments to see if the drug worked as it should and to determine on which patients it had a more positive effect: "The overall result of this accumulated experience was sufficient familiarity with the range of a drug's therapeutic value and side-effects such that the GP felt confident in its use" (2002, p. 1774). Decision making rested on ways in which this understanding was adjusted to meet the physical and psychosocial needs of specific patients, and the capacity to do this rested on the quality of the communication between doctor and patient. Armstrong concludes that there was not one specific moment when evidence of the effectiveness of the drugs was considered, accepted, and incorporated into practice. Rather there was a practical process of change over time. Repertoires of care were developed to incorporate new evidence, but only after filtering it through local and specific observations of the effect on patients. Armstrong notes that this individualized way of proceeding "seems inimical to the logic of evidence-based medicine" (2002, p. 1771). The understanding of rationality in at least the general-practice clinical setting studied by Armstrong is complex and changeable. It is unlikely that clinical care can be revolutionized in a one-off, simple, and lasting way by the provision of evidence of an intervention's effectiveness; bringing about change in clinical practice will be a slow, complex process.

A similar Australian study by Justine Mayer and Leon Piterman provides supporting evidence. The Australian general practitioners in this study were sympathetic to evidence-based medicine but preferred guidelines to critical appraisal of the literature as a route to acquiring evidence. They articulated concerns about the broader implications of evidence for their practices. According to Mayer and Piterman, "The GPs were concerned with hidden political and economic motives behind evidence presented to them. They were frequently unable to tell if recommendations were based on effectiveness or cost-effectiveness. . . . Most felt that cost containment should be made explicit in guidelines. . . . Furthermore, they also felt that guidelines had the potential to reduce clinical autonomy. Many feared punitive measures (legal, financial) against those who deviated from guidelines" (1999, p. 629).

The complexity of the problem of implementation is understood within evidence-based medicine. Andy Oxman and Signe Flottorp (2001) acknowledge that knowledge is insufficient for behavior change, but they identify specific, relatively simple barriers to change as aspects of the practice environment, prevailing medical opinion, and the knowledge and attitudes of clinicians. Despite systematic reviews that call into question many tried and tested implementation strategies, there remains an implicit belief that interventions addressing these barriers will produce beneficial change. Since expected changes are likely to be small, randomized controlled trials are recommended as the best means of assessment. These positive views appear in an edited collection, *Getting Research Findings into Practice* (Haines and Donald 2002), which also carries a chapter by Theresa Marteau and colleagues pointing out that selected studies from the Cochrane Collaboration's Effective Practice and Organisation of Care Group show persistent adherence to an information deficit model in attempts to improve implementation, with much of the work being atheoretical. The introduction to the volume calls for improved understanding of the problem and recognizes that this requires "insight from a number of fields including education, psychology, sociology, anthropology, information technology, economics, and management studies" (Haines and Donald 2002, p. 3). How this is to be achieved is not discussed.

The problem of evidence being subverted by apparently irrational behavior is nothing new. The original problem, however, was that patients did not comply with evidence-based medical advice. It is worth noting here that Brian Haynes turned to the task of changing physician behavior when he found that strategies for changing patient behavior were unproductive.

The Problem of Patient Noncompliance

In the 1970s, McMaster University researchers played a major role in highlighting the importance of research into patient noncompliance with health advice. Haynes was drawn to clinical epidemiology to study the problem. There is now a large and growing literature addressing the problem. Substantial costs are said to accrue to the medical system when patients fail to follow careful medical prescription. In the United States, the cost of noncompliance to the health care system was estimated to be U.S.$100 billion dollars per annum (Gerbino 1993), accounting for 10 percent of all hospital admissions (Smith 1985). Patient noncompliance affected the conduct of trials as well when patients subverted research designs by ignoring prescriptions, by gaining irregular access to trial interventions, or by leaving a study. Such activities were recognized as introducing compliance bias into trials, creating what Feinstein refers to as "major biostatistical delusions" leading to underestimation of the effectiveness of interventions with consequent risk of overmedication of future patients (1976, p. 165).

These problems breathed new life into an old problem (Sackett and Haynes 1976; Haynes et al. 1979). Strategies were developed for controlling the actions of study participants, and these were also applicable to defaulting patients. Surprisingly, considering the size of the research effort involved, reviews of a large number of randomized trials of interventions to improve compliance with medication prescriptions showed methodological weakness in the studies and little effect on patient health outcome (Haynes et al. 1987; Haynes et al. 1996). Many of the interventions were described as so complex and labor-intensive that they would have little application in routine practice. When the review was updated in 2002, there were many more trials; only seventeen were associated with statistically significant change and nine reported improvements in long-term treatment outcomes. The trials were so disparate that it was impossible to synthesize the evidence.

Despite the argument that "effective ways to help people follow medical treatments would have far larger effects on health than any treatment itself" (Haynes et al. 1996, p. 384), close on forty years of scientific study showed little evidence of change, and one is led to wonder why this area of research continues to proliferate unchanged. In 1987 the lack of progress in dealing with noncompliance was described as a "tragedy," and, as a result of this lack of progress, "the wind seems to have gone out of the sails of the compliance research enterprise" (1996, p. 165). As in the case of interventions to increase implementation of evidence in clinical care, most of the interventions assumed that a knowledge deficit was responsible for noncompliance. When these interventions did not succeed, the idea grew that noncompliant patients were ignorant, recalcitrant, and certainly irrational (Lerner 1997). It was during the early stages of this research that Sackett lost interest, citing this as his first example of redemption from the sins of expertness: he claims to have left this field when he became too much of an expert in it (2000).

The persistence of this field of research — and the continued, large commitment of research resources to an area with little positive outcome — is remarkable. The assumption that drives it appears to be that it is irrational to act against the evidence, whether one is a clinician or a patient, and sooner or later researchers will find an intervention that gets this message across. What is substantially missing from this analysis is an account of the experience of patients as they go about the task of following advice. Like practitioner-consumers of evidence, patient-consumers have competing influences on their actions, and many of these too are social, political, and economic. Within the constraints of their lives, after weighing the courses of action open to them, they may well, rationally, conclude that compliance is not worth it for them, at that time. When circumstances change, they may decide to comply.

If we are to analyze the constraints against change in clinical care, whether that of patient or clinician, we may need to start by acknowledging that these constraints may be ephemeral or persistent, individual or systematic. The benefits to the individual may well be ephemeral in light of the burden of compliance, and the importance of this decision will vary in relation to the effect this noncompliance has on the community. If we are to carefully analyze how these decisions are made, we may need to ask patients and clinicians for their views and then derive an overarching analysis. This introduces the difficult problem that what is required is a kind of evidence different from that produced and used in evidence-based medicine.

Different Evidences

Evidence-based medicine is a finely developed enterprise, but its achievements relate only to evidence of the effectiveness of interventions. Evidence-based medicine has analyzed the application of biomedicine in clinical care, although the methods have been extended to cover other interventions in clinical care, whether devised by policy makers or educationalists. The careful way in which the task has been conducted has earned academic credibility for evidence-based medicine. In the process its adherents have almost succeeded in colonizing the meaning of the word *evidence,* so that it becomes synonymous with that evidence produced by a randomized controlled trial or other method high in its hierarchy of evidence.

Evidence-based medicine has honed its methods under intense debate, for many decades. The very success of its research has highlighted the twin problems of a lack of implementation in clinical care and a lack of compliance among patients. But if rationality is limited to that circumscribed by the evidence of randomized controlled trials, we get little new understanding of the barriers to change in relation to either patients or practitioners, and the interventions devised for overcoming these barriers continue to be hit or miss. This is a case where we need diversification of research methods, and other evidence.

Black (1996) argues that the evaluation of health care involves a quest for rigor that should not depend on adherence to one preferred method. He emphasizes the role of observational studies for the evaluation of effectiveness, and he argues for mutual recognition of complementary roles of trials and observational studies. The same argument can be extended to a range of other research methods, including those that have the social and political context of decision making as primary object. There is need here, too, for a note of caution: These studies of context are unlikely to produce evidence of the effectiveness of interventions; nor will they necessarily help to overcome constraints to change and improve compliance. There might even be questions about how ideas like noncompliance are conceptualized and whether the search for compliance is artifactual. This is evidence of a different kind.

Researchers who support a hierarchy of evidence will experience a loss of solid ground when they have to shift to other, different methods of research. Qualitative research methods have the lowest ranking in the hierarchy of evidence and, therefore, are the most destabilizing. These researchers may prefer to remained focused on the evaluation of interventions and, as far as possible, on the methods they see as tried and tested. An example here is the attempt to incorporate evidence from other methods, including qualitative designs, into systematic reviews by transposing to these methods the criteria set out for systematic reviews of randomized controlled trials: Is the question clearly focused? Is the search for relevant articles thorough? Are the inclusion criteria appropriate? Is the validity of included studies adequately assessed? And so forth. Jennie Popay and colleagues (1998) have carefully set out the rather demanding conditions for a hierarchy of qualitative research evidence for the synthesis of qualitative research. The results for such syntheses remain at best tentative (see Dixon-Woods et al. 2001) or offer little more than a traditional social science literature review (see Campbell et al. 2003). Clearly, considerable methodological development is needed here. This direction may also be a distraction from the real contribution of qualitative research. Selecting from the literature only those studies that fit specific criteria for excellence is appropriate for a systematic review of evidence for the effectiveness of interventions. But if we want to explain what is going on in a social and political context, we may need to step back from intervention research, and systematic reviews, and ask the people most concerned to tell us what is going on in their lives. Analyzing such studies requires a fundamentally different research approach, and evidence-based-medicine researchers are unlikely to possess the research skills to conduct these studies in a way comparable with the high standard that they set for intervention research. The alternative is to collaborate with researchers in other disciplines who do have these research skills.

Preferably, the researchers who conduct these complementary studies would work in collaboration with those who conduct the trials, so that one type of evidence can complement and reinforce the other. This is where the Centre for Health Economics and Policy Analysis at McMaster University provides a good starting point. There has clearly been some friction between the activities of the center and the activities of the clinical epidemiologists in the Department of Clinical Epidemiology and Biostatistics, but the relationship has stood the test of time. Another note of caution: the difficulty of setting up a series of collaborative relationships with researchers from other disciplines requires careful negotiation concerning issues of power and control. It may seem preferable to excise research methods from their disciplinary context and appoint a few relatively junior researchers from, say, the qualitative social sciences to play a handmaiden role in generating new studies under medical guidance. Separating researchers from their parent disciplines can involve the loss of the theoretical formulations that act as the basis for scientific claims. In addition, if we are going to produce highly polished and rigorous evidence to complement the evidence from evidence-based medicine, then the task requires expert involvement.

Conclusion

The products of evidence-based medicine are new, well-crafted, and subjected to international processes of quality control. If these products are not finding ready purchasers, this may reflect either a lack of appropriate marketing or a system resistant to rapid change.

The benefits of evidence-based medicine have been disseminated through standard academic channels like the academic literature and textbooks. Persuasive peer education programs have amplified the message. In the Cochrane Collaboration, the users of evidence have been directly involved in a network devoted to generating secondary analysis of evidence. Additional strategies for marketing evidence-based medicine have been identified as the involvement of policy makers and consumers or patient organizations.

Clinicians appear to have been reluctant to change clinical practices despite these efforts at marketing evidence-based medicine. It is possible that the assumptions of evidence-based medicine do not articulate with what clinicians do in clinical practice, and that this makes change difficult. The use of health administrators and consumers as additional avenues for promoting the virtues of evidence may be counterproductive when it raises the specter of an attack on the autonomy of clinicians. If the problem is a system of clinical care that is resistant to change, then we know little at present about how and why this resistance is manifest. The invocation of the assumption that clinical practice is, or should be, "rational" seems inadequate.

At the center of the evidence-based-medicine enterprise is the randomized controlled trial and systematic review. When faced with topics not readily analyzed by trial methods, one option is to force the problem into a format accessible to study by these methods. This option involves little compromise with the narrow definition of science applied in evidence-based medicine. The risk is that it will deliver evidence that lacks credibility when viewed by clinicians, because it does not readily translate into practice. The other option is to take account of other kinds of evidence produced by other methods or even generated by clinical experience in clinic settings. The risk in the latter is that these "softer" forms of evidence may undermine some of evidence-based medicine's hard-won gains in credibility in medical academic settings. A safer option may be to develop a collaborative research structure in which evidence-based research works in a strategic alliance with other disciplines.

Notes

1. H. Bastian, 1994, *The power of sharing knowledge: Consumer participation in the Cochrane Collaboration.* Available at www.informedhealthonline.org.item .aspx?tabid=37, accessed on July 26, 2004.

CHAPTER 10

The Continuing Search
for a Science of Clinical Care

> *Science is a radical movement. That is, just like religious or political*
> *radical movements, science seeks a unified and internally consistent*
> *interpretation of the world. Such a quest is always difficult, for the*
> *ideal is constantly threatened by the fuzzy, ad hoc and heterogeneous*
> *nature of the outside world as perceived in daily experience. Thus,*
> *like other radical movements, science must segregate itself from that*
> *world in order to survive.*
>
> P. M. Strong and K. McPherson, "Natural Science
> and Medicine; Social Science and Medicine:
> Some Methodological Controversies," 1982

This book recounts the development of a science of clinical care. There
was the need, argued Alvan Feinstein in 1983, for an additional basic science for clinicians, to supplement the science of biomedicine and to focus
on how biomedicine is applied at the bedside, with live patients. Many
concerns of the founders of the new science that emerged are aptly sum-
marized in the quote above. They focused on clinical care, but, instead of
employing the broad focus suggested by some, they concentrated on clinical interventions, perfecting scientific methods for showing what works
and what may cause more harm than benefit. In systematizing this area
of practice, they carved out an academic and political space that they could
defend by scientific means. The most articulate exponents promoted this
new science with a zeal that sometimes resembled a religious conviction.
But it was science they served.

Neither clinical epidemiology nor evidence-based medicine is a monolith. In different situations, different emphases were employed, but there is a close overlap in the research activities as well as in the evidence produced. There has been a cross-fertilization of ideas, and leading researchers have moved with considerable ease between countries. A strong theme in statements by the founders of the movement was that they turned to this area not for opportunistic reasons but because of concern about patient care. There was uncertainty about the effectiveness of particular clinical choices in improving the health outcomes of patients. As a result, they challenged the traditional practice of transferring knowledge directly from clinical authority to clinical trainee. They proposed instead a new science and promoted the role of the randomized controlled trial in the production of primary evidence and the use of secondary analysis to produce overview evidence from the aggregated results of trials. Review by an international collaboration of experts provided an additional source of authority. Here was additional evidence that could place the practice of clinical care on a more certain, scientific footing.

When medicine entered a troubled time in the 1960s, with health care costs rising without a corresponding increase in population health, governments called for greater accountability from medicine. The founders of evidence-based medicine were not primarily motivated by this economic crisis, but it created a knowledge vacuum that they could fill. The questions were, what tools should be used and who should the beneficiaries be?

In the United Kingdom, Archie Cochrane had no doubts. The tool was the randomized controlled trial and the beneficiary was the National Health Service and its patients. For Cochrane and the British epidemiologists who supported the National Health Service, the concern was that the health system was not doing the best it could for the population. This is an interesting phenomenon, given that scientific medicine was producing a startling range of new interventions, the very interventions being linked to burgeoning health care costs. Henrik Wulff argues that it was the uninhibited proliferation of these new medical technologies that elicited the critical response from clinicians (1986, p. 129). The same proliferation was clearly also of concern to health administrators and policy makers. From the perspectives of all these individuals, it seemed eminently rational to ask for empirical evidence that treatment A is better than treatment B in addressing the health problem of a particular set of patients.

It was in the United Kingdom that the methods for making these comparisons were first explicitly seen as research into health services. Here the methods were substantially tied to their epidemiological roots. These methods provided an opportunity to focus attention not only on the individual patient in the clinic but also on the effect of medical interventions on the health of populations. If good medical care was to be funded in light of the competing needs for these funds, then it had to be delivered in a way that was effective and efficient.

At McMaster University in Canada, the tools were the same but the intended beneficiary was primarily the clinician. In the early years it was believed that the tools could be handed over to individual clinicians to conduct their own critical appraisal of the literature, assess the effect on their own practices, and perhaps do their own research. Later the Evidence-Based Medicine Working Group recognized that the tools of evidence-based medicine were too complex for all clinicians to take into their own hands. They continue to persuade clinicians to become evidence-based practitioners and directly apply the principles of critical appraisal to their own practices, but the group now recognizes that some, or even most, clinicians will always be no more than users of evidence produced by more experienced researchers. This places a greater emphasis on systematically extracted and synthesized evidence.

In both countries the emphasis is primarily on technical aspects of care and the difficulties that concerned clinicians encounter in busy clinical practices when faced with a burgeoning literature of varying quality. Had the pioneers been unable to popularize the methods and products of evidence-based medicine, clinicians may never have found their way to its benefits. Nor would these benefits have been readily accessible without the proliferation of computer technology. Brian Haynes turned to computer technology to disseminate systematic and relevant extracts from the medical literature, and the Cochrane Collaboration built a whole international research network on this technology. Without this technology, evidence-based medicine might not have survived beyond its early years.

At McMaster University it was recognized at the inception of the department that the new ideas had to be promoted with evangelical zeal. David Sackett and those who followed after him adopted an impressive and convincing style in promoting the skills of critical appraisal and its application to the bedside. Iain Chalmers provided charismatic leadership in promoting the study of perinatal care and in setting up the international Cochrane Collaboration. But sometimes zeal and charisma are not enough. In difficult political situations, such as in South Africa, leaders must, like Jimmy Volmink, be seen as being "of the people." These qualities are required in addition to a high level of academic achievement in more than one area of medical care. Truly, this is not a task for the humble or fainthearted!

The Great People who developed evidence-based medicine were mainly men, with Suzanne Fletcher representing the exception in this book. The dearth of women in this account deserves comment. It is not clear that evidence-based medicine is unusual in its gender distribution in the upper echelons of power, in comparison with other specialist areas where similar distributions are to be found. In the early years, a successful career in evidence-based medicine for women was complicated not only by their gender but also by the fact that it is doubly difficult for women to campaign against the status quo. As the need to challenge existing power structures diminishes, a new generation of women researchers is making its way into the upper echelons of the movement. They may bring a new vision to the discipline.

The educational activities of these pioneers may seem to be just a usual aspect of academic life, but the conversions that occur in these settings count as the hidden achievements of the field. McMaster University has people constantly on the international academic circuits, spreading the word. An international audience comes to its workshops in Hamilton. The people trained in the techniques of evidence-based medicine, including those trained under the INCLEN program, provide local nodes of enthusiasm from which further initiatives grow. The various journals committed to evidence-based medicine provide a source of material to support these initiatives. The Cochrane Collaboration provides access to synthesized evidence, but it also gives researchers the opportunity to collaborate in producing these syntheses. The problem is to adapt knowledge to local conditions in a range of countries, and here again the Cochrane Collaboration provides on-the-ground support in setting up new national centers. How effectively this is being done is still not clear, but together with the charismatic leadership, these educational materials have provided a sound basis for changed clinical practice.

As a movement, evidence-based medicine has been remarkably successful. The science is respected, and the language invented has penetrated to the far reaches of health care. The unresolved question is the extent to which clinical care has been changed for the better by those who challenged the certainty of clinical authority and put in its place collective certainty about what works and what does not work. How successfully this evidence is integrated into clinical decision making is not yet clear. If there are concerns that the movement has had limited success in bringing about change at the level of clinical practice, this is often the fate of even the most successful radical movement. The task is to present a vision of a different future and move some people toward it in the hope that a groundswell of support following it will be sustained in the longer term.

The success of evidence-based medicine now poses a risk. The concepts it promotes have had growing acceptance. Within the Cochrane Collaboration, the proliferation of evidence on the effectiveness of clinical care has consistently been monitored for quality (see, for example, Olsen et al. 2001). When the concepts proliferate into other fields, they are not necessarily accompanied by the methodological backing that ensures scientific credibility. Thus we have seen evidence-based health care and evidence-based policy, and we may even read of evidence-based prisons or evidence-based libraries. There is "evidence-based purchasing of health promotion" with hardly a trial under consideration (Rada et al. 1999). In these uses of the term *evidence,* the hierarchy of evidence can be invoked but without the disclaimer that it applies only to the task of assessing the effectiveness of interventions. The risk now is that the notion of evidence from evidence-based medicine may disseminate far beyond its roots, to the extent that it loses scientific credibility.

The Criticisms

The most persistent criticism of evidence-based medicine is that its focus is too narrow. In Canada and the United States, the exclusion of the broad concepts of public health was a source of criticism, as was the lack of attention to the interpersonal, social, and political aspects of patient care. In the Cochrane Collaboration, the relationship with the state and managed care sparked resistance from critics and perhaps also from clinicians. The criticisms have been cogent and fierce.

Although external criticism of evidence-based medicine seems to have cooled in more recent years, it is worth commenting again on the reason for a narrow agenda. If we return to Zwarenstein's description of medicine as a village that does not like outsiders ("It's like village life. You can't be too far away from the mainstream if you are in a small village"; see chapter 8), some of the difficulties involved in changing medical culture become evident. In the world of academic medicine, different disciplines are segregated into relatively tight-knit groups with their own languages, cultures, and traditions. Tony Becher writes of academic tribes and territories that are fiercely defended. The disciplines devoted to "hard" science (associated with steady accumulation in the knowledge base) stand in direct contrast with disciplines devoted to "soft," applied knowledge with its "frequently reformulated interpretations" (1989, pp. 15–16). Included in the latter is humanistic medicine. The narrowness of the agenda of evidence-based medicine may be directly attributable to strategies for survival in academic medicine, requiring a rejection of the activities using "soft" forms of knowledge. Similarly, there is a distancing from specialties that are medically unpopular (public health), and which use methods that are unfamiliar and open to question (the social sciences).

While much of the criticism recounted in this book comes from outside, there has been a lack of public criticism of the movement by its founders. Even Alvan Feinstein, hovering over the field with his pen dipped in acid, primarily exhorted everyone in the field to greater, more clinical, more scientific rigor and was not prepared to reflect on those aspects of the political and economic environment that could not be addressed with a narrow technical definition of evidence. David Sackett provides the most cogent example of the lack of interest in critical deconstruction of the field. He is certainly well placed to point to productive new directions for development by reflecting publicly on the limitations of an approach that he helped set in place. This he has not done. Here is his account of his activities in the area of patient noncompliance:

Two decades ago I was an expert on the subject of compliance with therapeutic regimens. I enjoyed the topic enormously, lectured internationally on it, had my opinions sought by other researchers and research institutes, and my colleagues and I ran international compliance symposiums and wrote two books, chapters for several others, and dozens of papers about it. Whether at a meeting or in print, I was always given the last word on the matter. . . . Then it dawned on me that experts like me commit two sins that retard the advance of science and harm the young. . . . Progress towards truth is impaired in the presence of an expert especially when new evidence is rejected because it challenges the views of experts. (Sackett 2000, p. 1283)

He had come to the same conclusion with respect to evidence-based medicine: "Once again my conclusions came to be given too much credence and my opinion too much weight." He decided that he would "never again lecture, write, or referee anything to do with evidence-based clinical practice" (2000, p. 1283).

Arguably it is now time to set aside a one-sided commitment to the field and to reconsider the narrow agenda of evidence-based medicine. There may have been an overestimation of the capacity of trials alone to resolve the fundamental problems of clinical medicine, and the enthusi-astic pronouncements of the charismatic leadership may have obscured this problem. If clinicians are to be won over, this may be the time to con-sider a broader agenda. Researchers at McMaster University who are not identified with the evidence-based-medicine hierarchy argue persuasively that there has been a shift in the department to broader goals. Health out-comes are recognized as being multifactorial and long term; trials are not seen as the only way of addressing some of these problems. Murray Enkin and Alex Jadad (1998) argue for the importance of anecdotal evidence in evidence-based health care, and when they first presented their paper on this to the department, Enkin recalls, there was strong interest. No doubt McMaster University and the Cochrane Collaboration recognize the need to study the fragmented, changeable world of the patient. There is less acceptance of the argument that such studies will need to be conducted using methods that establish differences in experience rather than aggregate measures.

A Shift in Direction?

Evidence-based medicine has warily trod a path through the complexities of academic medicine. Whether this is a true path depends on the extent to which clinicians find the work acceptable. Here evidence-based med-icine faces a problem of its own making: if acceptance exists, it should be measurable, and interventions to improve implementation should be suc-cessful. Instead of embarking on this exercise, the alternative is to focus on alternative strategies that might enhance the attraction for clinicians.

As evidence-based medicine developed its recent manifestations, some initiatives dropped from the agenda, and they may be worth resuscitat-ing. Feinstein had greater interest in the complexities of clinical practice. Wulff was concerned that trials should not be seen as the sole solution for the fundamental problems of clinical medicine, and he emphasized a melding of technical evidence with a more philosophical approach to interpretive communication and ethics. Cochrane thought that the costs arising from the use of ineffective interventions should be diverted to neg-lected areas of patient care. These and other issues could still be addressed, broadening the narrower focus that has dominated.

There are persistent calls for a broadening of the agenda, and this may well hold an attraction for clinicians faced with the complexities of patient care. Walter Holland (2001–2002, p. 3) points to the problem of the narrow definition of evidence: "It is unfortunate that the term EBM has become so evocative that we forget that most medical decisions have always been based on some form of evidence. Much more and better evidence is of course now available, but . . . its interpretation is still subject to personal or political idiosyncrasies, as in the past!" In a more comprehensive science of clinical care, these additional issues would also be proper topics for rigorous research.

It will be a considerable and difficult task to integrate the understanding achieved from the various disciplines relevant to the research task in clinical care, a point emphasized by Wulff. He argued that clinicians need theoretical knowledge of the biomedical sciences as well as empirical knowledge of outcomes in patients, preferably in the form of randomized controlled trials. These must be integrated, but they also must be integrated with interpretive understanding of the patient, with attention paid to the moral norms of society. What evidence-based medicine has aimed to do is develop the second, neglected component: empirical study of the outcomes of interventions with live patients. The challenge has been to integrate the first two components, and a considerable challenge it has been. The third and fourth components have been seen as separate from the science, to be addressed after the scientific questions have been resolved, with ethics being reduced to issues of individual choice. This is where further integration is now needed.

There have been two models that move us in the direction of research that supports this expanded knowledge base for clinical care. The first is suggested by Fraser Mustard of the Canadian Institute of Advanced Research, designed to provide a network of talented individuals still located in their institutional settings to work together on the kind of problems that might be considered too challenging as a central commitment of an academic department. The other model is, of course, the Cochrane Collaboration. It has succeeded in producing a large international network of researchers working on a common set of problems in their home institutions. At this stage, however, the task it has set itself is narrow but so vast in scope that it is difficult to see any successful diversification in the short term. It also faces a pitfall in the role of consumers in the network.

The role of consumers in the Collaboration is not clear. They are involved in the generation of evidence, but they may also serve as potential retailers of the knowledge produced. Subtly, however, they may come to represent a shortcut to the study of patients and consumers of medical care. In a sense, the hard choices involved in patient decision making are relegated to those who actually make these choices. Here there is a risk that consumer biases may be incorporated into the evidence base taking the place of scientific study of consumer actions. The issue is not to see consumer participation as a substitute for the disciplines that study patient experience.

Despite these quibbles and suggestions for future directions, what evidence-based medicine has achieved is remarkable. There has been a long and ardent search for a science of clinical care that will reduce its uncertainties. But there is work still to be done.

Bibliography

Acheson, R. M. 1991. The British diploma in public health: Heyday and decline. In E. Fee and R. M. Acheson, eds., *A history of education in public health: Health that mocks the doctors' rules,* 272–313. Oxford: Oxford University Press.

All the president's scientists: Diary of a round-earther. 2000. *Mail and Guardian* (South Africa), September 8.

Andersen, B. 1990. *Methodological errors in medical research.* Oxford: Basil Blackwell.

Anderson, O. W. 1966. Influence of social and economic research on public policy in the health field: A review. *Milbank Memorial Fund Quarterly* 44, 3: 11–48.

Anglin, M. K. 1997. Working from the inside out: Implications of breast cancer activism for biomedical policies and practices. *Social Science and Medicine* 44, 9: 1403–15.

Antiplatelet Trialists' Collaboration. 1994. Collaborative overview of randomised trials of antiplatelet therapy — I. Prevention of death and myocardial infarction, and stroke by prolonged antiplatelet therapy in various categories of patients. *British Medical Journal* 308, 6923: 81–106.

Antman, E. M., J. Lau, B. Kupelnick, F. Mosteller, and T. C. Chalmers. 1992. A comparison of results of meta-analyses of randomized control trials and recommendations of clinical experts: Treatments for myocardial infarction. *Journal of the American Medical Association* 268, 2: 240–48.

Armitage, P. 1972. History of the randomised controlled trial. *Lancet* 1, 7765: 1388.

———. 1992. Bradford Hill and the randomised controlled trial. *Pharmaceutical Medicine* 6: 23–27.

Armstrong, D. 1977. Clinical science and clinical sense. *Social Science and Medicine* 11, 11–13: 599–601.

———. 1983. *Political anatomy of the body: Medical knowledge in Britain in the twentieth century.* Cambridge: Cambridge University Press.

———. 1987. Theoretical tensions in biopsychosocial medicine. *Social Science and Medicine* 25, 11: 1213–18.

———. 2002. Clinical autonomy, individual and collective: The problem of changing doctors' behaviour. *Social Science and Medicine* 55, 10: 1771–77.

Arnstein, A. R. 1969. A ladder of citizen participation. *American Institute of Planners Journal* (July): 216–24.

Atiyah, E. 1955. *The Arabs.* Harmondsworth: Penguin Books.

Atuhaire, L. K., M. J. Campbell, A. L. Cochrane, M. Jones, and F. Moore. 1986. Specific causes of death in miners and ex-miners in the Rhondda Fach, 1959–1980. *British Journal of Industrial Medicine* 43, 7: 497–99.

Balint, M. 1961. The other part of medicine. *Lancet* 1 (January 7): 40–42.

Bastian, H., M. J. N. C. Keirse, and P. A. Lancaster. 1998. Perinatal death associated with planned home birth in Australia: Population based study. *British Medical Journal* 317, 7155: 384–88.

Becher, T. 1989. *Academic tribes and territories: Intellectual enquiry and the culture of disciplines.* Milton Keynes: Open University Press and Society for Research into Higher Education.

Benech, I., A. E. Wilson, and A. C. Dowell. 1996. Evidence-based practice in primary care: Past, present, and future. *Journal of Evaluation in Clinical Practice* 2, 4: 249–63.

Bennett, K., G. Torrance, and P. Tugwell. 1991. Methodologic challenges in the development of utility measures of health-related quality of life in rheumatoid arthritis. *Controlled Clinical Trials* 12, 4 Supplement: 118S–28S.

Bensing, J. 2000. Bridging the gap: The separate worlds of evidence-based medicine and patient-centered medicine. *Patient Education and Counseling* 39, 1: 17–25.

Bernoulli, J. 1713. *Ars Conjectandi.* Basel: Thurnisiorum.

Birkelo, C. C., W. E. Chamberlain, P. S. Phelps, P. E. Schools, and D. Zacks. 1947. Tuberculosis case findings: A comparison of the effectiveness of various roentgenographic and photofluorographic methods. *Journal of the American Medical Association* 133: 359–65.

Black, D., J. Morris, C. Smith, and P. Townsend. 1980. Inequalities in health: A report of a research working group. London: Department of Health and Social Security.

Black, N. 1996. Why we need observational studies to evaluate the effectiveness of health care. *British Medical Journal* 312, 7040 (May 11): 1215–18.

———. 1999. Evidence-based surgery: A passing fad? *World Journal of Surgery* 23, 8: 789–93.

———. 2001. Evidence-based policy: Proceed with care. *British Medical Journal* 323, 7307 (August 4): 275–78.

Bloom, B. S. 1986. Controlled studies in measuring the efficacy of medical care: A historical perspective. *International Journal of Technology Assessment in Health Care* 2: 299–310.

Boston Women's Health Book Collective. 1998. *Our bodies, ourselves: For the new century.* New York: Touchstone.

Bowker, G. C., and S. L. Star. 1999. *Sorting things out: Classification and its consequences,* chap. 5. Cambridge: MIT Press.

Boyle, M. H., G. W. Torrance, J. C. Sinclair, and S. P. Horwood. 1983. Economic evaluation of neonatal intensive care of very-low-birth-weight infants. *New England Journal of Medicine* 308, 22: 1330–37.

Bradford Hill, A. 1937. *Principles of medical statistics.* London: Lancet.

———. 1951. The clinical trial. *British Medical Bulletin* 7: 278–82.

———. 1952. The clinical trial. *New England Journal of Medicine* 247: 113–19.

———. 1962. *Statistical methods in clinical and preventive medicine.* Edinburgh: E. and S. Livingstone.

———. 1963. Medical ethics and controlled trials. *British Medical Journal* 1: 1043–49.

Brickman, J. P. 1994. Science and the education of physicians: Sigerist's contribution to American medical reform. *Journal of Public Health Policy* (summer): 133–64.

Brook, R. H. 1990. Clinical scholars' leadership in health services research. In *Clinical Scholars Program Report.* Princeton: Robert Wood Johnson Foundation, June.

Browman, G. P., M. N. Levine, E. A. Mohide, R. S. A. Hayward, K. I. Pritchard, A. Gafni, and A. Laupacis. 1995. The practice guideline development cycle: A conceptual tool for practice guideline development and implementation. *Journal of Clinical Oncology* 13, 2: 502–12.

Browman, G. P., T. Newman, A. Mohide, I. Graham, M. Levine, K. Pritchard, W. Evans, D. Maroun, I. Hodson, M. Carey, and D. H. Cowan. 1998. Progress of clinical oncology guidelines development using the practice guidelines development cycle: The role of practitioner feedback. *Journal of Clinical Oncology* 16, 3: 1226–31.

Buck, C., A. Lopis, E. M. Najera, and M. Terris, eds. 1988. *The Challenge of epidemiology: Issues and selected readings.* Washington, D.C.: Pan American Health Organization.

Burke, K. 2002. NICE needs sweeping changes to maintain credibility, say MPs. *British Medical Journal* 325, 7354: 5.

Bush, J., S. Fanshel, and M. Chen. 1972. Analysis of a tuberculin testing program using a health status index. *Socio-Economic Planning Sciences* 6: 49–68.

Campbell, R., P. Pound, C. Pope, N. Britten, R. Pill, M. Morgan, and J. Donovan. 2003. Evaluating meta-ethnography: A synthesis of qualitative research on lay experiences of diabetes care. *Social Science and Medicine* 56, 4: 671–84.

Chalmers, I. 1979. Randomised controlled trials of fetal monitoring, 1973–1977. In O. Thalhammer, K. Baumgarten and A. Pollak, eds., *Perinatal Medicine,* 260–65. Stuttgart: Thieme.

———, ed. 1988. *The Oxford database of perinatal trials.* Oxford: Oxford University Press.

———. 1991. The perinatal research agenda: Whose priorities? *Birth* 18, 3: 137–45.

———. 2001. Comparing like with like: Some historical milestones in the evolution of methods to create unbiased comparison groups in therapeutic experiments. *International Journal of Epidemiology* 30: 1156–64.

Chalmers, I., and D. G. Altman, eds. 1995. *Systematic Reviews*. London: BMJ Publishing Group.

Chalmers, I., H. Campbell, and A. C. Turnbull. 1976a. Evaluation of different approaches to obstetric care. Pt. 1. *British Journal of Obstetrics and Gynaecology* 83, 12: 921–29.

———. 1976b. Evaluation of different approaches to obstetric care. Pt. 2. *British Journal of Obstetrics and Gynaecology* 83, 12: 930–34.

Chalmers, I., M. Enkin, and M. J. N. C. Keirse, eds. 1989. *Effective care in pregnancy and childbirth*. Oxford: Oxford University Press.

———. 1993. Preparing and updating systematic reviews of randomized controlled trials of health care. *Milbank Quarterly* 71, 3: 411–37.

Chalmers, I., J. Hetherington, M. Newdick, L. Mutch, A. Grant, M. Enkin, E. Enkin, and K. Dickerson. 1986. *The Oxford Database of Perinatal Trials*: Developing a register of published reports of controlled trials. *Controlled Clinical Trials* 7, 4: 306–25.

Chalmers, T. C. 1981. The clinical trial. *Milbank Memorial Fund Quarterly — Health and Society* 59, 3: 324–39.

Chalmers, T. C., J. Berrier, P. Hewitt, J. Berlin, D. Reitman, R. Nagalingam, and H. Sacks. 1988. Meta-analysis of randomized controlled trials as a method of estimating rare complications of non-steroidal anti-inflammatory drug therapy. *Alimentary Pharmacology and Therapeutics* 2, Supplement 1: 9–26.

Chalmers, T. C., R. D. Eckhardt, W. E. Reynolds, R. W. Feifenstein, N. Deane, C. W. Smith, J. G. Cigarroa, and C. S. Davidson. 1955. The treatment of acute infectious hepatitis: Controlled studies of the effects of diet, rest, and physical reconditioning on the acute course of disease and on the incidence of relapses and residual abnormalities. *Journal of Clinical Investigation* 34: 1163–234.

Chalmers, T. C., H. Levin, H. S. Sacks, D. Reitman, J. Berrier, and R. Nagalingam. 1987. Meta-analysis of clinical trials as a scientific discipline: I. Control of bias and comparison with large co-operative trials. *Statistics in Medicine* 6, 3: 315–28.

Chalmers, T. C., R. J. Matta, H. Smith, and A. M. Kunzler. 1977. Evidence favoring the use of anticoagulants in the hospital phase of acute myocardial infarction. *New England Journal of Medicine* 297, 20: 1091–96.

Chalmers, I., J. E. Zlosnik, K. A. Johns, and H. Campbell. 1976. Obstetric practice and outcome of pregnancy in Cardiff residents, 1965–73. *British Medical Journal* 1, 6012: 735–38.

Chard, T., and M. Richards, eds. 1977. *Benefits and hazards of the new obstetrics*. London: Heinemann Medical Spastics International Medical Publications.

Charlton, B. G. 1997. Restoring the balance: Evidence-based medicine put in its place. *Journal of Evaluation in Clinical Practice* 3, 2: 87–98.

Charlton, B. G., and A. Miles. 1998. The rise and fall of EBM. *Quarterly Journal of Medicine* 91, 5: 371–74.

Clarke, M., and P. Langhorne. 2001. Revisiting the Cochrane Collaboration: Meeting the challenge of Archie Cochrane — and facing up to some new ones. *British Medical Journal* 323, 7317: 821.

Cleary, P. D., and D. M. Fox. 1993. In this issue. *Milbank Quarterly* 71, 3: 45–48.

Cochrane, A. L. 1945a. Tuberculosis among prisoners of war in Germany. *British Medical Journal* 2 (November 10): 656.

———. 1945b. The medical officer as prisoner in Germany. *Lancet* 2 (September 29): 411–19.

———. 1972. *Effectiveness and efficiency: Random reflections on health services.* London: Nuffield Provincial Hospitals Trust.

———. 1979. Forty years back: A retrospective survey. *British Medical Journal* 2, 6205: 1662–63.

———. 1984. Sickness in Salonica: My first, worst, and most successful clinical trial. *British Medical Journal* 289, 6460: 1726–27.

Cochrane, A. L., with M. Blythe. 1989. *One man's medicine: An autobiography of Professor Archie Cochrane.* London: British Medical Journal.

Cochrane, A. L., H. W. Campbell, and S. C. Steen. 1949. The value of roentgenology in the prognosis of minimal tuberculosis. *American Journal of Roentgenology and Radium Therapy* 61: 153–65.

Cochrane, A. L., J. G. Cox, and T. F. Jarman. 1952. Pulmonary tuberculosis in the Rhondda Fach: An interim report of a survey of a mining community, *British Medical Journal* (October 18): 843–53.

Cochrane, A. L., A. S. St. Leger, and F. Moore. 1978. Health services "input" and mortality "output" in developed countries. *Journal of Epidemiology and Community Health* 32, 3: 200–205.

Cohen, D. 1997. Archie Cochrane: An appreciation. In A. Maynard and I. Chalmers, eds., *Non-random reflections on health services research: On the twenty-fifth anniversary of Archie Cochrane's* Effectiveness and Efficiency, 11–13. London: BMJ Publishing Group.

Coker, R. E., K. W. Back, T. G. Donnelly, N. Miller, and B. S. Phillips. 1959. Public health as viewed by the medical student. *American Journal of Public Health* 49, 5: 601–9.

Cook, D., and M. Giacomini. 1999. The trials and tribulations of clinical practice guidelines. *Journal of the American Medical Association* 281, 20: 1950–51.

Corea, G. 1985. *The mother machine: Reproductive technologies from artificial insemination to artificial wombs.* New York: Harper and Row.

Corrigan, D. J. 1828–29. Aneurism of the aorta. *Lancet* 1: 586–90.

Crowther, C. A. 1991. Hospitalisation for bed rest in twin pregnancy. In I. Chalmers, ed., *The Oxford Database of Perinatal Trials* 3376, Version 1.2, disk issue 6 (autumn).

Daly, J., A. Kellehear, and M. Gliksman. 1997. *The public health researcher: A methodological guide.* Melbourne: Oxford University Press.

Daly, M. 1979. *Gyn\ecology.* London: Women's Press.

Daniel, A. 1995. The politics of health: Medicine vs the state. In G. M. Lupton and J. M. Najman, eds., *Sociology of health and illness: Australian readings.* 2nd ed. Melbourne: Macmillan Education.

Davey Smith, G. 2001. The uses of "Uses of Epidemiology." *International Journal of Epidemiology* 30, 5: 1146–55.

Devereaux, P. J., D. R. Anderson, M. J. Gardner, W. Putnam, G. J. Flowerdew, B. F. Brownell, S. Nagpal, and J. L. Cox. 2001. Differences between perspectives of physicians and patients on anticoagulation in patients with atrial fibrillation: Observational study. *British Medical Journal* 323, 7323: 1218–22.

Devereaux, P. J., P. T-L. Choi, C. Lacchetti, B. Weaver, H. J. Schünemann, T. Haines, J. N. Lavis, B. J. B. Grant, D. R. S. Haslam, M. Bhandari, T. Sullivan, D. J. Cook, S. D. Walter, M. Meade, H. Khan, N. Bhatnagar, and G. H. Guyatt. 2002. A systematic review and meta-analysis of studies comparing mortality between private for-profit and private not-for-profit hospitals. *Canadian Medical Association Journal* 166, 11: 1399–406.

Devereaux, P. J., B. J. Manns, W. A. Ghali, H. Quan, C. Lacchetti, V. M. Montori, M. Bhandair, and G. Guyatt. 2001. Physician interpretations and textbook definitions of blinding terminology in randomized controlled trials. *Journal of American Medical Association* 285, 15: 2000–2003.

Dixon-Woods, M., R. Fitzpatrick, and K. Roberts. 2001. Including qualitative research in systematic reviews: Opportunities and problems. *Journal of Evaluation in Clinical Practice* 7, 2: 125–33.

Doll, R. 1991. Development of controlled trials in preventive and therapeutic medicine. *Journal of Biosocial Science* 23, 3: 365–78.

———. 1994. The use of meta-analysis in epidemiology: Diet and cancers of the breast and colon. *Nutrition Reviews* 52, 7: 233–37.

———. 1997. A reminiscence of Archie Cochrane. In A. Maynard and I. Chalmers, eds., *Non-random reflections on health services research: On the twenty-fifth anniversary of Archie Cochrane's* Effectiveness and Efficiency, 7–10. London: BMJ Publishing Group.

Doll, R., and A. Bradford Hill. 1950. Smoking and carcinoma of the lung: Preliminary report. *British Medical Journal* (September 30): 739–48.

———. 1964. Mortality in relation to smoking: Ten years' observation of British doctors. *British Medical Journal* 1: 1399–1410 and 1460–67.

Dowling, D. 2000. Privacy does have its limits. *Weekly Mail and Guardian*. November 10.

Drummond, M. F., G. L. Stoddart, and G. W. Torrance. 1987. *Methods for the economic evaluation of health care programmes*. Oxford: Oxford University Press.

Eisenberg, J. M. 1990. Academic general internal medicine profoundly influenced by work of scholars. In *The Clinical Scholars Program Report*, 15–18. Princeton: Robert Wood Johnson Foundation, June.

Eisenstadt, S. N. 1995. Charisma and institution building: Max Weber and modern sociology. In *Power, Trust, and Meaning: Essays in sociological theory and analysis*, 167–201. Chicago: Chicago University Press.

Elwood, P. C. 1983. British studies of aspirin and myocardial infarction. *American Journal of Medicine* 74, 6A: 50–54.

———. 1997. Cochrane and the benefits of aspirin. In A. Maynard and I. Chalmers, eds., *Non-random reflections on health services research: On the twenty-fifth anniversary of Archie Cochrane's* Effectiveness and Efficiency, 107–21. London: BMJ Publishing Group.

———. 2001. Aspirin: Past, present, and future. *Clinical Medicine* 1, 2: 132–37.

Elwood, P. C., A. L. Cochrane, M. L. Burr, P. M. Sweetnam, G. Williams, E. Welsby, S. J. Hughes, and R. Renton. 1974. A randomised controlled trial of acetyl salicylic acid in the secondary prevention of mortality from myocardial infarction. *British Medical Journal* 1, 905: 436–40.

Elwood, P. C., A. M. Fehily, H. Ising, D. J. Poor, J. Pickering, and F. Kamel. 1996. Dietary magnesium does not predict ischaemic heart disease in the Caerphilly cohort. *European Journal of Clinical Nutrition* 50, 10: 694–97.

Elwood, P. C., H. F. Thomas, P. M. Sweetnam, and J. H. Elwood. 1982. Mortality of flax workers. *British Journal of Industrial Medicine* 39, 1: 18–22.

Elwood, P. C., W. E. Waters, and P. Sweetnam. 1971. The haematinic effect of iron in flour. *Clinical Science* 40: 31–37.

Engel, G. L. 1977. The need for a new medical model: A challenge for biomedicine. *Science* 196, 4286: 129–36.

Enkin, M., and I. Chalmers, eds. 1982. *Effectiveness and satisfaction in antenatal care.* London: Spastics International Medical Publications and William Heinemann.

Enkin, M. W., and A. R. Jadad. 1998. Using anecdotal information in evidence-based health care: Heresy or necessity? *Annals of Oncology* 9, 9: 963–66.

Enkin, M., M. J. N. C. Keirse, and I. Chalmers. 1989. *A guide to effective care in pregnancy and childbirth.* Oxford: Oxford University Press.

Evans, C. E., R. B. Haynes, N. J. Birkett, J. R. Gilbert, D. W. Taylor, D. L. Sackett, M. E. Johnston, and S. A. Hewson. 1986. Does a mailed continuing education program improve clinician performance? Results of a randomized trial in antihypertensive care. *Journal of the American Medical Association* 255, 4: 501–4.

Evans, J. R. 1981. *Measurement and management in medicine and health services: Training needs and opportunities.* New York: Rockefeller Foundation.

Evans, R. G., and G. L. Stoddart. 1990. Producing health, consuming health care. *Social Science and Medicine* 31, 12: 1347–63.

Evidence-Based Medicine Working Group. 1992. Evidence-based medicine: A new approach to teaching the practice of medicine. *Journal of the American Medical Association* 268, 17: 2420–25.

Feinstein, A. R. 1963a. Boolean algebra and clinical taxonomy: I. Analytic synthesis of the general spectrum of a human disease. *New England Journal of Medicine* 269, 18: 929–38.

———. 1963b. The basic elements of clinical science. *Journal of Chronic Diseases* 16: 1125–33.

———. 1964a. Symptomatic patterns, biologic behavior, and prognosis in cancer of the lung: Practical application of Boolean algebra and clinical taxonomy. *Annals of Internal Medicine* 61, 1: 27–43.

———. 1964b. Scientific methodology in clinical medicine: I. Introduction, principles and concepts. *Annals of Internal Medicine* 61, 3: 564–79.

——. 1964c. Scientific methodology in clinical medicine: II. Classification of human disease by clinical behavior. *Annals of Internal Medicine* 61, 4: 757–81.

——. 1964d. Scientific methodology in clinical medicine: III. The evaluation of therapeutic response. *Annals of Internal Medicine* 61, 5: 944–65.

——. 1964e. Scientific methodology in clinical medicine: IV. Acquisition of clinical data. *Annals of Internal Medicine* 61, 6: 1162–93.

——. 1967. *Clinical judgment.* Malabar: Robert E Krieger Publishing.

——. 1968a. Clinical epidemiology: I. The populational experiments of nature and man in human illness. *Annals of Internal Medicine* 69, 4: 807–20.

——. 1968b. Clinical epidemiology: II. The identification rates of disease. *Annals of Internal Medicine* 69, 5: 1037–61.

——. 1968c. Clinical epidemiology: III. The clinical design of statistics in therapy. *Annals of Internal Medicine* 69, 6: 1287–311.

——. 1976. "Compliance bias" and the interpretation of therapeutic trials. In D. L. Sackett and R. B. Haynes, eds., *Compliance with therapeutic regimens,* 152–56. Baltimore: Johns Hopkins University Press.

——. 1977a. *Clinical biostatistics.* Saint Louis: C. V. Mosby.

——. 1977b. Clinical biostatistics: XXXIX. The haze of Bayes, the aerial palaces of decision analysis, and the computerized ouija board. *Clinical Pharmacology Therapeutics* 21: 482–96.

——. 1983. An additional basic science for clinical medicine. Pts. I–III. *Annals of Internal Medicine* 99: 393–97; 544–50; 705–12.

——. 1985. *Clinical epidemiology: The architecture of clinical research.* Philadelphia: W. B. Saunders.

——. 1987. *Clinimetrics.* New Haven: Yale University Press.

——. 1988. Scientific standards in epidemiologic studies of the menace of daily life. *Science* 242, 4883: 1257–63.

——. 1992. Editorial: Invidious comparisons and unmet clinical challenges. *American Journal of Medicine* 92, 2: 117–20.

——. 1995. Meta-analysis: Statistical alchemy for the twenty-first century. *Journal of Clinical Epidemiology* 48, 1: 71–79.

——. 1996. Mathematical models and clinical practice. In J. Daly, ed., *Ethical intersections: Health research, methods, and researcher responsibility,* 203–10. Sydney: Allen and Unwin.

——. 1999. Basic biomedical science and the destruction of the pathophysiologic bridge from bench to bedside. *American Journal of Medicine* 107, 5: 461–67.

Feinstein, A. R., and R. Di Massa. 1959. Prognostic significance of valvular involvement in acute rheumatic fever. *New England Journal of Medicine* 260, 20: 1001–7.

Feinstein, A. R., and R. I. Horwitz. 1997. Problems in the "evidence" of "evidence-based" medicine. *American Journal of Medicine* 103, 6: 529–35.

Feinstein, A. R., N. Koss, and J. H. M. Austin. 1967. The changing emphasis in clinical research. I. Topics under investigation: An analysis of the submitted abstracts and selected programs at the annual "Atlantic City Meetings" during 1953 through 1965. *Annals of Internal Medicine* 66, 12: 396–419.

Feinstein, A. R., H. F. Wood, J. A. Epstein, A. Taranta, R. Simpson, and E. Tursky. 1959. A controlled study of three methods of prophylaxis against streptococcal infection in a population of rheumatic children: II. Results of the first three years of the study, including methods for evaluating the maintenance of oral prophylaxis. *New England Journal of Medicine* 260 (April 2): 697–702.

Fletcher, R. H. 2002. Evaluation of interventions. *Journal of Clinical Epidemiology* 55, 12: 1183–90.

Fletcher, R. H., S. W. Fletcher, and E. H. Wagner. 1982. *Clinical epidemiology: The essentials.* Baltimore: Williams and Wilkins.

Fox, R. 1979. Training for uncertainty. In *Essays in medical sociology: Journeys into the field,* 19–50. New York: John Wiley.

Frank, A. W. 2002. What's wrong with medical consumerism? In S. Henderson and A. Petersen, eds., *Consuming health: The commodification of health care,* 13–30. London: Routledge.

Frankford, D. M. 1994. Scientism and economism in the regulation of health care. *Journal of Health Politics, Policy, and Law* 19, 4: 773–99.

Gafni, A., and S. Birch. 2003. NICE methodological guidelines and decision making in the National Health Service in England and Wales. *Pharmacoeconomics* 21, 3: 149–57.

Gavarret, J. 1840. *Principes généraux de statistique médicale.* Paris: n.p.

Gazi, C. 2000. Letter to the editor. *Sowetan* (July 7).

Gerbino, P. P. 1993. Foreword to *Annals of Pharmacotherapy* 27: S3–4.

Gesensway, D. 1995. New *Annals* editor. *ACP Observer* (March).

Glover, J. A. 1992. The incidence of tonsillectomy in school children. In K. L. White et al., eds., *Health services research: An anthology,* 16–28. Washington, D.C.: Pan American Health Organization.

Goodman, N. W. 1999. Who will challenge evidence-based medicine? *Journal of the Royal College of Physicians of London* 33, 3: 249–51.

Gøtzsche, P., and O. Olsen. 2000. Is screening for breast cancer with mammography justifiable? *Lancet* 355, 9198: 129–34.

Graunt, J. 1661. *Natural and political observations, made upon the bills of mortality.* N.p.

Gray, B. H. 1992. The legislative battle over health services research. *Health Affairs* 11, 4: 39–66.

Gray, B. H., M. K. Gusmano, and S. R. Collins. 2003. AHCPR and the changing politics of health services research. *Health Affairs* supplement: W3–283–307.

Greenland, S. 1991. Science vs advocacy: The challenge of Dr. Feinstein. *Epidemiology* 2, 1: 64–72.

Grimshaw, J., and M. Eccles. 2001. Identifying and using evidence-based guidelines in general practice. In A. Haines and A. Donald, eds., *Getting research findings into practice,* 120–34. 2nd ed. London: BMJ Books.

Gulland, A. 2002. NICE proposals for citizens council condemned by patients. National Institute for Clinical Excellence. *British Medical Journal* 325, 7361: 406.

Guyatt, G. H. 1991. Evidence-based medicine. *ACP Journal Club*, p. A-16 (supplement 2 to *Annals of Internal Medicine* 114).

Guyatt, G. H., L. B. Berman, M. Townsend, S. O. Pugsley, and L. W. Chambers. 1987. A measure of quality of life for clinical trials in chronic lung disease. *Thorax* 42, 10: 773–78.

Guyatt, G. H., and Canadian Lung Oncology Group. 2001. Investigating extrathoracic metastatic disease in patients with apparently operable lung cancer. *Annals of Thoracic Surgery* 71, 2: 425–34.

Guyatt, G. H., D. H. Feeny, and D. L. Patrick. 1993. Measuring health-related quality of life. *Annals of Internal Medicine* 118, 8: 622–29.

Guyatt, G. H., M. Meade, R. Z. Jaeschke, D. Cook, and B. Haynes. 2000. Editorial: Practitioners of evidence-based care. *British Medical Journal* 320, 7240: 954–55.

Guyatt, G. H., and D. Rennie, eds. 2002. *Users' guides to the medical literature: A manual for evidence-based clinical practice.* Chicago: AMA Press.

Guyatt, G. H., D. Sackett, D. W. Taylor, J. Chong, R. Roberts, and S. Pugsley. 1986. Determining optimal therapy: Randomized trials in individual patients. *New England Journal of Medicine* 314, 14: 889–92.

Guyatt, G., A. Yalnizyan, and P. J. Devereaux. 2002. Solving the public health care sustainability puzzle. *Canadian Medical Association Journal* 167, 1: 36–38.

Habermas, J. 1971. *Knowledge and human interests.* Boston: Beacon Press.

Hacking, I. 1990. *The taming of chance.* Cambridge: Cambridge University Press.

Haines, A., and A. Donald. 2002. Introduction to A. Haines, A. Donald, eds., *Getting research findings into practice,* 1–10. 2nd ed. London: BMJ Books.

——, eds. 2002. *Getting research findings into practice.* 2nd ed. London: BMJ Books.

Harrison, D., and M. Zwarenstein. 1993. Utilisation of public health services by caregivers of children from Khayelitsha presenting with acute diarrhoea. *South African Medical Journal* 83, 8: 573–75.

Harrison, S. 1998. The politics of evidence-based medicine in the United Kingdom. *Policy and Politics* 26, 1: 15–31.

Haynes, R. B. 1990. Loose connections between peer-reviewed clinical journals and clinical practice. *Annals of Internal Medicine* 113, 9: 724–27.

Haynes, R. B., K. A. McKibbon, and R. Kanani. 1996. Systematic review of randomised trials of interventions to assist patients to follow prescriptions for medications. *Lancet* 348, 9024: 383–86.

Haynes, R. B., P. Montague, T. Oliver, K. A. McKibbon, M. C. Brouwers, and R. Kanani. 2002. Interventions for helping patients to follow prescriptions for medication *(Cochrane Review).* In *The Cochrane Library,* issue 1. Oxford: Update Software.

Haynes, R. B., D. L. Sackett, D. W. Taylor, E. S. Gibson, and A. L. Johnson. 1978. Increased absenteeism from work after detection and labeling of hypertensive patients. *New England Journal of Medicine* 299, 14: 741–44.

Haynes, R. B., D. W. Taylor, and D. L. Sackett, eds. 1979. *Compliance in health care.* Baltimore: Johns Hopkins University Press.

Haynes, R. B., E. Wang, and M. Da Mota Gomes. 1987. A critical review of interventions to improve compliance with prescribed medications. *Patient Education and Counseling* 10: 155–66.

Henderson, S., and A. Petersen. 2002. Introduction: Consumerism in health care. In S. Henderson and A. Petersen, eds., *Consuming health: The commodification of health care*, 1–10. London: Routledge.

Hetherington, J., K. Dickersin, I. Chalmers, and C. L. Meinert. 1989. Retrospective and prospective identification of unpublished controlled trials: Lessons from a survey of obstetricians and pediatricians. *Pediatrics* 84, 2: 374–78.

Holland, W. 1983. Inappropriate terminology. *International Journal of Epidemiology* 12, 1: 5–7.

———. 2001–2002. Evidence-based medicine: A commentary. *Euro Observer: Newsletter of the European Observatory on Health Care Systems* 3, 3: 1–3.

Holmes, L., A. Lusher, and I. Chalmers. 2001. Citation of Cochrane reviews in national and international guidelines and policies, reports of the NHS Health Technology Assessment Programme, *Effective Health Care,* Finnish evidence-based medicine guidelines, and *Clinical Evidence.* Manuscript.

Hunt, M. 1997. *How science takes stock: The story of meta-analysis.* New York: Russell Sage Foundation.

Hunter, D. J. 1996. Rationing and evidence-based medicine. *Journal of Evaluation in Clinical Practice* 2, 1: 5–8.

Illich, I. 1976. *Medical nemesis: The expropriation of health.* Middlesex: Penguin.

Ingelfinger, F. J., A. S. Relman, and M. Finland. 1966. *Controversy in internal medicine.* Philadelphia: W. B. Saunders.

Irvine, R. 2002. Fabricating "health consumers" in health care politics. In S. Henderson and A. Petersen, eds., *Consuming Health: The commodification of health care,* 31–47. London: Routledge.

JAMA. 2001. Media release. August 23.

Joughin, C., and M. Zwi. 1999. *Focus on the use of stimulants in children with attention deficit hyperactivity disorder.* Primary Evidence-Based Briefing No. 1. London: Royal College of Psychiatrists.

Kassirer, J. P. 1995. Incorporating patients' preferences in medical decisions. *New England Journal of Medicine* 333, 26: 1895–96.

Klainer, L. M., T. C. Gibson, and K. L. White. 1965. The epidemiology of cardiac failure. *Journal of Chronic Diseases* 5, 18: 797–814.

Klein, R. 1983. *The politics of the National Health Service.* London: Longman.

———. 1996. The NHS and the new scientism: Solution or delusion? *Quarterly Journal of Medicine* 89: 85–87.

Klein, R., P. Day, and S. Redmayne. 1996. *Managing scarcity: Priority setting and rationing in the National Health Service.* Buckingham: Open University Press.

Klein, R., and J. Lewis. 1976. *The politics of consumer representation: A study of community health councils.* London: Centre for Studies in Social Policy.

Kuhn, L., and M. Zwarenstein. 1990. Evaluation of a village health worker programme: The use of village health worker retained records. *International Journal of Epidemiology* 19, 3: 685–92.

Kuhn, T. 1970. *The structure of scientific revolutions.* 2nd ed. Chicago: University of Chicago.

Lancet. 1826. Review from the West. 9: 471–75.

Lancet. 1995. Editorial: Evidence-based medicine, in its place. 346, 8978: 785.

Last, J. M. 1963. The iceberg: "Completing the clinical picture" in general practice. *Lancet* 2 (6 July): 28–31.

———. 1988. What is "clinical epidemiology"? *Journal of Public Health Policy* 9, 2: 159–63.

———. 1994. Professor John Last. In J. Ashton, ed., *The epidemiological imagination: A reader.* Buckingham: Open University Press.

———, ed. 1995. *Dictionary of epidemiology.* 3rd ed. New York: Oxford University Press.

Lau, J., E. M. Antman, J. Jimenez-Silva, B. Kupelnick, F. Mosteller, and T. C. Chalmers. 1992. Cumulative meta-analysis of therapeutic trials for myocardial infarction. *New England Journal of Medicine* 327, 4: 248–54.

Lau, J., and T. C. Chalmers. 1995. The rational use of therapeutic drugs in the twenty-first century: Important lessons from cumulative meta-analysis of randomized control trials. *International Journal of Technology Assessment in Health Care* 11, 3: 509–22.

Lerner, B. H. 1997. From careless consumptives to recalcitrant patients: The historical construction of noncompliance. *Social Science and Medicine* 45, 9: 1423–31.

Lessing, D. 1998. *Walking in the shade: Volume two of my autobiography, 1949–1962.* London: Flamingo.

Lewis, J. 1991. The origins and development of public health in the UK. In W. W. Holland, R. Detels, and G. Knox, eds., *Oxford textbook of public health.* Vol. 1: *Influences of public health,* 23–34. 2nd ed. Oxford: Oxford Medical Publications.

Light, D. W. 1991. Effectiveness and efficiency under competition: The Cochrane test. *British Medical Journal* 303, 6812: 1253–54.

Light, R. J., and D. B. Pillemer. 1984. *Summing up: The science of reviewing research.* Cambridge: Harvard University Press.

Lipman, T. 2001. The failings of NICE: NICE and evidence-based medicine are not really compatible. *British Medial Journal* 322, 7284: 489–90.

Lohr, K. N., K. Eleazer, and J. Mauskopf. 1998. Health policy issues and applications for evidence-based medicine and clinical practice guidelines. *Health Policy* 46, 1: 1–19.

Lomas, J. 1993a. Making clinical policy explicit: Legislative policy making and lessons for developing practice guidelines. *International Journal of Technology Assessment in Health Care* 9, 1: 11–25.

———. 1993b. Retailing research: Increasing the role of evidence in clinical services for childbirth. *Milbank Quarterly* 71, 3: 439–75.

———. 1997. Reluctant rationers: Public input to health care priorities. *Journal of Health Services and Research Policy* 2, 2: 103–11.

Lomas, J., J. E. Sisk, and B. Stocking. 1993. From evidence to practice in the

United States, the United Kingdom, and Canada. *Milbank Quarterly* 71, 3: 405–9.

Lomas, J., and G. L. Stoddart. 1985. Estimates of the potential impact of nurse practitioners on future requirements for physicians in office-based general practice. *Canadian Journal of Public Health* 76, 2: 119–23.

Loughlin, K. 2001. Epidemiology, social medicine, and public health: A celebration of the ninetieth birthday of Professor J. N. Morris. *International Journal of Epidemiology* 30, 5: 1198–99.

Louis, P.-C.-A. 1835. *Recherche sur les effets de la saignée dans quelques maladies inflammatoires.* Paris: Bailliere.

Ludmerer, K. M. 1999. *Time to heal: American medical education from the turn of the century to the era of managed care.* New York: Oxford University Press.

Magraw, R. M. 1966. *Ferment in medicine: A study of the essence of medical practice and of its new dilemmas.* Philadelphia: W. B. Saunders.

Makgoba, M. W. 2000. HIV/AIDS: The peril of pseudoscience. *Science* 2888, 5469: 1171.

Marteau, T. M., A. J. Sowden, and D. Armstrong. 2002. Changing clinical practice in the light of the evidence: Beyond the information deficit model. In A. Haines, A. Donald, eds., *Getting research findings into practice,* 68–76. 2nd ed. London: BMJ Books.

Martin, D. A., K. L. White, and C. R. Vernon. 1959. Influence of emotional and physical stimuli on pressure in the isolated vein segment. *Circulation Research* 7: 580–87.

Mather, H. G., D. C. Morgan, N. G. Pearson, K. L. Read, D. B. Shaw, G. R. Steed, M. G. Thorne, C. J. Lawrence, and I. S. Riley. 1976. Acute myocardial infarction: A comparison between home or hospital care for patients. *British Medical Journal* 1, 6015: 925–29.

Matthews, J. R. 1995. *Quantification and the quest for medical certainty.* Princeton: Princeton University Press.

Mayer, J., and L. Piterman. 1999. The attitudes of Australian GPs to evidence-based medicine: A focus group study. *Family Practice* 16, 6: 627–32.

Maynard, A., and I. Chalmers, eds. 1997. *Non-random reflections on health services research: On the twenty-fifth anniversary of Archie Cochrane's* Effectiveness and Efficiency. London: BMJ Publishing Group.

McCormick, J. 1996. Death of the personal doctor. *Lancet* 348, 9028: 667–68.

McKeown, T. 1976. *The role of medicine: Dream, mirage, or nemesis?* London: Nuffield Hospitals Trust.

McKeown, T., and C. R. Lowe. 1974. *An introduction to social medicine.* 2nd ed. Oxford: Blackwell.

McLachlan, G. 1997. Archie and the Nuffield Hospitals Trust. In A. Maynard and I. Chalmers, eds., *Non-random reflections on health services research: On the twenty-fifth anniversary of Archie Cochrane's* Effectiveness and Efficiency, 14–16. London: BMJ Publishing Group.

Medical Research Council. 1948. Streptomycin treatment of pulmonary tuberculosis. *British Medical Journal* 2: 769–82.

Molloy, D. W., G. H. Guyatt, R. Russo, R. Goeree, B. O'Brien, M. Bédard, A. Willan, J. Watson, C. Patterson, C. Harrison, T. Standish, D. Strang, P. J. Datzins, S. Smith, and S. Dubois. 2000. Systematic implementation of an advanced directive program in nursing homes: A randomized controlled trial. *Journal of the American Medical Association* 283, 11: 1437–44.

Morabia, A. 2002. The controversial controversy of a passionate controversialist. *Journal of Clinical Epidemiology* 55, 12: 1207–13.

Morris, J. N. 1955. Uses of epidemiology. *British Medical Journal* (August 13): 305–401.

———. 1957. *Uses of Epidemiology.* Baltimore: Williams and Wilkins.

———. 1969. Tomorrow's community physician. *Lancet* 2, 7625: 812–16.

———. 1992. Exercise versus heart attack: History of a hypothesis. In M. Marmot and P. Elliott, eds., *Coronary Heart Disease Epidemiology: From aetiology to public health*, 242–55. Oxford: Oxford University Press.

Morris, J. N., J. A. Heady, P. A. B. Raffle, C. G. Roberts, and J. W. Parks. 1953. Coronary heart disease and physical activity at work. *Lancet* 2: 1053–57, 1111–20.

Morris, J. N., A. Kagan, D. C. Pattison, M. J. Gardner, and P. A. B. Raffle. 1966. Incidence and prediction of ischaemic heart disease in London busmen. *Lancet* 2, 7463: 553–59.

Morris, J. N., and R. M. Titmuss. 1942. Epidemiology of juvenile rheumatism. *Lancet* 2: 59–63.

———. 1944a. Health and social change: The recent history of rheumatic heart disease. *Medical Officer* 72: 65–57, 69–71, 77–79.

———. 1944b. Epidemiology of peptic ulcer: Vital statistics. *Lancet* 2: 841–45.

Murphy, E. 1976. *The logic of medicine.* Baltimore: Johns Hopkins University Press.

Naylor, C. D. 1995. Grey zones of clinical practice. *Lancet* 345, 8953: 840–42.

Nuffield Provincial Hospitals Trust. 1968. *Screening in medical care: Revising the evidence.* Oxford: Oxford University Press.

Oakley, A. 1980. *Women confined: Towards a sociology of childbirth.* Oxford: Martin Robertson.

———. 2000. *Experiments in knowing: Gender and methods in the social sciences.* Cambridge, U.K.: Polity Press.

Oliver, S. 2001. Consumer participation in health care, planning, policy, and research. *Cochrane Consumers and Communication Review Group* 6, (September): 6–7.

Olsen, O., P. Middleton, J. Ezzo, P. C. Gøtzsche, V. Hadhazy, A. Herxheimer, J. Kleijnen, and H. McIntosh. 2001. Quality of Cochrane reviews: Assessment of sample from 1998. *British Medical Journal* 323: 829–32.

Oxman, A. D. 1995. Checklists for reviewing articles. In I. Chalmers and D. G. Altman, eds., *Systematic reviews*, 75–85. London: BMJ Publishing Group.

———. 2001. The Cochrane Collaboration in the twenty-first century: Ten challenges and one reason why they must be met. In M. Egger, G. D. Smith, and D. G. Altman, eds., *Systematic reviews in health care: Meta-analysis in context*, 459–73. London: BMJ Books.

Oxman, A. D., D. J. Cook, and G. H. Guyatt. 1994. Users' guide to the medical literature: How to use an overview. *Journal of the American Medical Association* 272: 1367–71.

Oxman, A. D., and S. Flottorp. 2001. An overview of strategies to promote implementation of evidence based health care. In C. Silagy and A. Haines, eds., *Evidence based practice in primary care,* 101–19. 2nd ed. London: BMJ Books.

Oxman, A. D., and G. H. Guyatt. 1988. Guidelines for reading literature reviews. *Canadian Medical Association Journal* 138: 697–703.

Paul, J. R. 1938. Clinical epidemiology. *Journal of Clinical Investigation* 17: 539–41.

———. 1966. *Clinical epidemiology.* Rev. ed. Chicago: University of Chicago Press.

Peckham, M. 1991. Research and development for the National Health Service. *Lancet* 338, 8763: 367–71.

Popay, J., A. Rogers, and G. Williams. 1998. Rationale and standards for the systematic review of the qualitative literature in health services research. *Qualitative Health Research* 8, 3: 341–51.

Porter, T. M. 1995. *Trust in numbers: The pursuit of objectivity in science and public life.* Princeton: Princeton University Press.

Rada, J., M. Ratima, and P. Howden Chapman. 1999. Evidence-based purchasing of health promotion: Methodology for reviewing evidence. *Health Promotion International* 14, 2: 177–87.

Rangachari, P. K. 1997. Evidence-based medicine: Old French wine with a new Canadian label? *Journal of the Royal Society of Medicine* 90, 5: 280–84.

Ravnskov, U. 1992. Cholesterol lowering trials in coronary heart disease: Frequency of citation and outcomes. *British Medical Journal* 305, 6844: 15–19.

Richards, T. 1999. Australia's consumer champion. *British Medical Journal* 319, 7212: 730.

Riska, E., and J. A. Taylor. 1979. Consumer and provider views on health policy and health legislation. In E. G. Jaco, ed., *Patients, physicians, and illness: A sourcebook in behavioural science and health,* 356–70. 3rd ed. New York: Free Press.

Rothman, K. J. 1986. *Medical epidemiology.* Boston: Little, Brown.

Ryle, J. 1948. *Changing disciplines.* London: Oxford University Press.

Sackett, D. L. 1969. Clinical epidemiology. *American Journal of Epidemiology* 89, 2: 125–28.

———. 2000. The sins of expertness and a proposal for redemption. *British Medical Journal* 320, 7244: 1283.

———. 2002. Clinical epidemiology: What, who, and whither. *Journal of Clinical Epidemiology* 52, 12: 1161–66.

Sackett, D. L., and R. B. Haynes, eds. 1976. *Compliance with therapeutic regimens.* Baltimore: Johns Hopkins University Press.

Sackett, D. L., R. B. Haynes, G. H. Guyatt, and P. Tugwell. 1991. *Clinical epidemiology: A basic science for clinical medicine.* 2nd ed. Boston: Little, Brown.

Sackett, D. L., R. B. Haynes, and P. Tugwell. 1985. *Clinical epidemiology: A basic science for clinical medicine.* Boston: Little, Brown.

Sackett, D. L., W. S. Richardson, W. Rosenberg, and R. B. Haynes. 1997. *Evidence-based medicine: How to practice and teach EBM.* Edinburgh: Churchill Livingstone.

Sackett, D. L., W. O. Spitzer, M. Gent, and R. S. Roberts. 1974. The Burlington randomized trial of the nurse practitioner: Health outcomes for patients. *Annals of Internal Medicine* 80, 2: 137–42.

Sackett, D. L., and S. E. Straus. 1998. Finding and applying evidence during clinical rounds: The "evidence cart." *Journal of the American Medical Association* 280, 15: 1336–38.

Sackett, D. L., S. E. Straus, W. S. Richardson, W. Rosenberg, and R. B. Haynes. 2000. *Evidence-based medicine. How to practice and teach EBM.* 2nd ed. Edinburgh: Churchill Livingstone.

Sakala, C., G. Gyte, S. Henderson, J. P. Neilson, and D. Horey. 2001. Consumer-professional partnership to improve research: The experience of the Cochrane Collaboration's Pregnancy and Childbirth Group. *Birth* 28, 2: 133–37.

Savits, D. A., S. Greenland, P. D. Stolley, and H. Kelsey. 1990. Scientific standards of criticism: A reaction to "Scientific standards in epidemiologic studies of the menace of daily life" by A. R. Feinstein. *Epidemiology* 1, 1: 78–83.

Schwartz, M. A., and O. P. Wiggins. 1988. Scientific and humanistic medicine: A theory of clinical methods. In K. L. White, ed., *The task of medicine: Dialogue at Wickenburg,* 137–71. Menlo Park: Henry J. Kaiser Family Foundation.

Scott, A., M. Shaw, and C. Joughin, eds. 2001. *Finding the evidence: A gateway to the literature in child and adolescent mental health.* 2nd ed. London: Royal College of Psychiatrists.

Shaneyfelt, T. M., M. F. Mayo-Smith, and J. Rothwangl. 1999. Are clinical guidelines following guidelines? The methodological quality of clinical practice guidelines in the peer-reviewed medical literature. *Journal of the American Medical Association* 281, 20: 1900–1905.

Shapiro, D. W., R. D. Lasker, A. B. Bindman, and P. R. Lee. 1993. Containing costs while improving quality of care: The role of profiling and practice guideline. *Annual Review of Public Health* 14: 219–41.

Shuster, A. L. 1990. Foreword to *The Clinical Scholars Program Report,* 1. Princeton: Robert Wood Johnson Foundation, June.

Shyrock, R. H. 1947. The American physician in 1846 and in 1946: A study in professional contrasts. *Journal of the American Medical Association* 134: 417–24.

———. 1961. The history of quantification in medical science. In H. Woolf, ed., *Quantification: A history of the meaning of measurement in the natural and social sciences.* Indianapolis: Bobbs-Merrill.

Sigerist, H. 1941. *Medicine and Human Welfare.* Oxford: Oxford University Press.

Silagy, C. A., F. Stead, and T. Lancaster. 2001. Use of systematic reviews in clinical practice guidelines: Case of smoking cessation. *British Medical Journal* 323, 7317: 833–36.

Silverman, D. 1985. *Qualitative methodology and sociology.* Aldershot: Gower.

———. 1989. Telling convincing stories: A plea for cautious positivism in case-studies. In B. Glasner and J. D. Moreno, eds., *The qualitative-quantitative distinction in the social sciences*, 57–77. Kluwer Academic Publishers.

Smith, M. 1985. The cost of noncompliance and the capacity of improved compliance to reduce health care expenditures. In *Improving medication compliance: Proceedings of a symposium in Washington, D.C., November 1, 1984*, 35–44. Washington, D.C.: National Pharmaceutical Council.

Smith, M. L., and G. V. Glass. 1977. Meta-analysis of psychotherapy outcome studies. *American Psychologist* 32, 9: 752–60.

Smith R. 2000. The failings of NICE. *British Medical Journal* 321, 7273: 1363–64.

Smith, R., and I. Chalmers. 2001. Britain's gift: A "medline" of synthesized evidence. *British Medical Journal* 323, 7327: 1437–38.

Spitzer, W. O., D. Sackett, J. Sibley, R. Roberts, M. Gent, D. J. Kergin, B. Hackett, and A. Olynich. 1974. The Burlington randomized trial of the nurse practitioners. *New England Journal of Medicine* 290, 5: 251–56.

Starr, P. 1982. *The Social Transformation of American Medicine*. New York: Basic Books.

St. Leger, A. S., A. L. Cochrane, and F. Moore. 1979. Factors associated with cardiac mortality in developed countries, with particular reference to the consumption of wine. *Lancet* 1, 8124: 1017–20.

Stoeckle, J. D., and L. M. Candib. 1969. The neighbourhood health center: Reform ideas of yesterday and today. *New England Journal of Medicine* 280, 25: 1385–90.

Strong, P. M., and K. McPherson. 1982. Natural science and medicine; social science and medicine: Some methodological controversies. *Social Science and Medicine* 16, 6: 643–57.

Stuart, G. W., A. J. Rush, and J. A. Morris. 2002. Practice guidelines in mental health and addiction services: Contributions from the American College of Mental Health Administration. *Administration and Policy in Mental Health* 30, 1: 21–33.

Susser, M., and E. Susser. 1996. Choosing a future for epidemiology: I. Eras and paradigms. *American Journal of Public Health* 86, 5: 668–73.

Taranta, A., E. Kleinberg, A. R. Feinstein, H. F. Wood, E. Tursky, and R. Simpson. 1964. Rheumatic fever in children and adolescents: A long-term epidemiologic study of subsequent prophylaxis, streptococcal infection, and clinical sequalae. V. Relation of rheumatic fever recurrence rate per streptococcal infection to pre-existing clinical features of the patients. *Annals of Internal Medicine*, Supplement 5, 60: 68–86.

Titmuss, R. 1943. *Birth, poverty, and wealth*. London: Hamish Hamilton.

Torrance, G. W. 1976. Social preferences for health states: An empirical evaluation of three measurement techniques. *Socio-Economic Planning Sciences* 10: 129–36.

Torrance, G. W., M. H. Boyle, and S. P. Horwood. 1982. Applications of multi-attribute utility theory to measure social preference for health state. *Operations Research* 30, 6: 1043–69.

Torrance, G., W. Thomas, and D. Sackett. 1972. A utility maximization model for evaluation of health care programs. *Health Services Research* 7, 2: 118–33.

Trengove-Jones, T. 2000. Democracy and the pandemic. *Weekly Mail and Guardian* (June 30).

Trostle, J. A. 1988. Medical compliance as an ideology. *Social Science and Medicine* 27, 12: 1299–1308.

Tudor Hart, J. 1997. Response rates in Wales, 1950–96: Changing requirements for mass participation in human research. In A. Maynard and I. Chalmers, eds., *Non-random reflections on health services research: On the twenty-fifth anniversary of Archie Cochrane's Effectiveness and Efficiency*, 7–10. London: BMJ Publishing Group.

———. 2001. The failings of NICE: Rationing is a respectable word for a disgraceful retreat. *British Medical Journal* 322, 7284: 490.

Tugwell, P., L. Chambers, G. Torrance, D. Reynolds, M. Wolfson, K. Bennett, E. Jamieson, and S. Stock. 1993. The population health impact of arthritis: POHEM Workshop Group. *Journal of Rheumatology* 20, 6: 1048–51.

Viseltear, A. J. 1982a. C.-E. A. Winslow and the early years of public health at Yale, 1915–1925. *Yale Journal of Biology and Medicine* 55, 2: 137–51.

———. 1982b. John R. Paul and the definition of preventive medicine. *Yale Journal of Biology and Medicine* 55, 3–4: 167–72.

Volmink, J., and P. Garner. 1997. Systematic review of randomized controlled trials of strategies to promote adherence to tuberculosis treatment. *British Medical Journal* 315, 7120: 1403–6.

Volmink, J., P. Matchaba, and P. Garner. 2000. Directly observed therapy and treatment adherence. *Lancet* 355, 9212: 1345–50.

Volmink, J., P. Matchaba, and M. Zwarenstein. 2001. Reducing mother-to-child transmission of HIV infection in South Africa. In *Informing judgment: Case studies of health policy and research in six countries*, pp. 173–92. N.p., Cochrane Collaboration and Milbank Memorial Fund.

Waitzkin, H. 1979a. A Marxian interpretation of the growth and development of coronary care technology. *American Journal of Public Health* 69, 12: 1260–68.

———. 1979b. Medicine, superstructure, and micropolitics. *Social Science and Medicine* 13A, 6: 601–9.

———. 1991. *The politics of medical encounters: How patients and doctors deal with social problems.* New Haven: Yale University Press.

———. 2000. *The second sickness: Contradictions of capitalist health care.* Rev. ed. Lanham, Md.: Rowman and Littlefield.

Wale, J. 2001. The role of the Cochrane Collaboration for consumers and research. *Cochrane Consumers and Communication Review Group* 6 (September): 10–11.

Weber, M. 1947. *Theory of social and economic organization.* Trans. Talcott Parsons. New York: Oxford University Press.

Wells, P. S., J. Hirsh, D. R. Anderson, A. W. A. Lensing, G. Foster, C. Kearon, J. Weitz, R. Dovidio, A. Cogo, P. Prandoni, A. Girolami, and J. S. Ginsberg. 1995. Accuracy of clinical assessment of deep-vein thrombosis. *Lancet* 345, 8961: 1326–30.

Wennberg, J. E., B. A. Barnes, and M. Zubkoff. 1982. Professional uncertainty and the problem of supplier-induced-demand. *Social Science and Medicine* 16, 7: 811–24.

Wennberg, J. E., and A. M. Gittelsohn. 1973. Small area variations in health care delivery. *Science* 182, 117: 1102–8.

White, K. L. 1988. *The task of medicine: Dialogue at Wickenburg*. Menlo Park: Henry J. Kaiser Family Foundation.

———. 1991. *Healing the schism: Epidemiology, medicine, and the public's health*. New York: Springer-Verlag.

———. 1997. Archie Cochrane's legacy: An American perspective. In A. Maynard and I. Chalmers, eds., *Non-random reflections on health services research: On the twenty-fifth anniversary of Archie Cochrane's* Effectiveness and Efficiency, 3–6. London: BMJ Publishing Group.

White, K. L. (editor in chief), J. Frenk, C. Ordóñez, J. M. Paganini, and B. Starfield, eds. 1992. *Health services research: An anthology*. Washington, D.C.: Pan American Health Organization.

White, K. L., and M. M. Henderson, eds. 1976. *Epidemiology as a fundamental science: Its uses in health services planning, administration, and evaluation*. New York: Oxford University Press.

White, K. L., D. A. Martin, and C. R. Vernon. 1959. Venous pressure, emotions, and congestive heart failure. *Journal of Chronic Diseases* 10: 163–85.

White, K. L., T. F. Williams, and B. G. Greenberg. 1961. The ecology of medical care. *New England Journal of Medicine* 265, 18: 885–91.

Wilcox, A. J. 2003. A conversation with Zena Stein. *Epidemiology* 14, 4: 498–501.

Willis, K. 1995. Imposed structures and contested meanings: Policies and politics of public participation. *Australian Journal of Social Issues* 30, 2: 211–27.

———. 2001. Who will benefit? The case of screening for breast cancer using mammography. In J. Daly, M. Guillemin, and S. Hill, eds., *Technologies and Health: Critical compromises*, 219–33. Melbourne: Oxford University Press.

Winslow, C-E. A. 1926. Public health at the crossroads. *American Journal of Public Health* 16 (November): 1075–85.

Wright, P., and A. Treacher, eds. 1982. *The problem of medical knowledge: Examining the social construction of medicine*. Edinburgh: Edinburgh University Press.

Wulff, H. R. 1976. *Rational diagnosis and treatment*. Oxford: Blackwell Scientific Publications.

———. 1986. Rational diagnosis and treatment. *Journal of Medicine and Philosophy* 11, 2: 123–34.

Wulff, H. R., and P. C. Gøtzsche. 2000. *Rational diagnosis and treatment: Evidence-based clinical decision-making*. 3rd ed. Oxford: Blackwell Science Publications.

Wulff, H. R., S. A. Pedersen, and R. Rosenberg. 1986. *Philosophy of medicine: An introduction*. Oxford: Blackwell Scientific Publications.

Zwarenstein, M., P. Barron, S. Tollman, N. Crisp, J. Frankish, I. Toms, D. Harrison, and G. Solarsh. 1993. Primary health care depends on the district health system. *South African Medical Journal* 83, 8: 558.

Zwarenstein, M., J. H. Schoeman, C. Vundule, C. J. Lombard, and M. Tatley. 1998. Randomised controlled trial of self-supervised and directly observed treatment of tuberculosis. *Lancet* 352, 9137: 1340–53.

———. 2000. Randomised controlled trial of lay health workers as direct observers for treatment of tuberculosis. *International Journal of Tuberculosis and Lung Disease* 4, 6: 550–54.

Zwarenstein, M., J. Volmink, I. Irwig, and I. Chalmers. 1995. Systematic review: "State of the science" health care decision-making. *South African Medical Journal* 85, 12: 1266–1267.

Index

Page references to biographical material on individuals are in italic typeface.

Text:	10/13 Galliard
Display:	Galliard
Compositor:	BookMatters, Berkeley
Printer and binder:	IBT Global
Indexer:	Marcia Carlson